Innovative Hypnotherapy

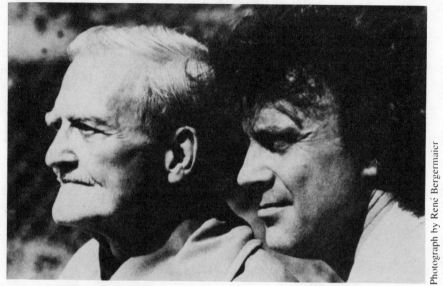

Photograph by René Bergermaier

Milton H. Erickson, MD
(1901–1980)

Ernest L. Rossi, PhD

Innovative Hypnotherapy

by MILTON H. ERICKSON

The Collected Papers of
Milton H. Erickson on Hypnosis
Volume IV

Edited by Ernest L. Rossi

IRVINGTON PUBLISHERS, INC.
NEW YORK

Library of Congress Cataloging-in-Publication Data is available.

ISBN 0-8290-1209-5

10 9 8 7 6 5 4 3 2 1

Printed in the United States of America

Foreword

This series of Milton Erickson's papers contains a fascinating array of original contributions related to every phase of hypnotic theory and practice. The papers contain stores of invaluable data that can be productively mined by researchers and clinicians for treasures useful in hypothetical structuring and experiment, as well as catalyzing psychotherapy. Dr. Erickson is perhaps the most creative and imaginative contemporary worker in the area of hypnosis and his inspired writings in this series rank among the enduring classics in the field.

Lewis R. Wolberg, M.D.
Clinical Professor of Psychiatry,
New York University School of Medicine

Emeritus Dean, Postgraduate Center
for Mental Health

Acknowledgments

The Editor wishes to acknowledge the assistance and suggestions of many colleagues and members of the American Society of Clinical Hypnosis in the preparation of these volumes. In particular: Marian Moore, Robert Pearson, Florence Sharp, and Andre Weitzenhoffer. Significant editorial and secretarial skills have been contributed by Margaret Ryan.

The following journals and publishers have generously permitted the replication of papers in these volumes:

American Journal of Clinical Hypnosis, American Journal of Psychiatry, American Medical Association, American Psychiatric Association, American Psychological Association, Appleton-Century-Crofts, *Archives of Neurology and Psychiatry, British Journal of Medical Psychology, Bulletin of the Georgetown University Medical Center, Diseases of the Nervous System, Encyclopaedia Britannica,* Family Process, Harper and Row, Paul B. Hoeber, Inc., *Journal of Abnormal and Social Psychology, Journal of Clinical and Experimental Hypnosis, Journal of Experimental Psychology, Journal of General Psychology, Journal of Genetic Psychology, Journal of Nervous and Mental Disease, Journal of the American Society of Psychosomatic Dentistry and Medicine,* Journal Press, Julian Press, Macmillan Company, Medical Clinics of North America, Merck, Sharp and Dohme, *Perceptual and Motor Skills,* Physicians Postgraduate Press, *Psychiatry, Psychoanalytic Quarterly, Psychosomatic Medicine,* W. B. Saunders Company, Springer Verlag, William Alanson White Psychiatric Foundation, Williams and Wilkins, and Woodrow Press.

Contents

Editor's Preface

These four volumes of Milton H. Erickson's selected papers have been collected for clinicians and researchers who wish to explore in depth the work of one of the most seminal minds in the history of hypnosis and psychotherapy. When Erickson began publishing his studies in the early 1930s, hypnosis was in a curious position: most investigators agreed that hypnosis had played a central role in the early studies of psychopathology and our first efforts at psychotherapy, but the authoritative approaches associated with its use were supplanted on the one hand by the seemingly more sophisticated approaches of the psychoanalytic schools, and on the other hand by experimental psychology.

The situation might have continued in just this manner, with hypnosis regarded as nothing more significant than a colorful curiosity in our therapeutic past. Into this situation, however, came the accident that was Milton H. Erickson. He was an accident of nature born with a number of congenital sensory-perceptual problems that led him to experience the world in ways so different that his acute mind could survive only by realizing at a very early age the relativity of our human frames of reference. To these early problems was added the rare medical tragedy of being stricken by two different strains of polio at the ages of 17 and 51. His efforts to rehabilitate himself led to a personal rediscovery of many classical hypnotic phenomena and how they could be utilized therapeutically.

Erickson's experimental and therapeutic explorations with the hypnotic modality span more than 50 years. His successful rejuvenation of the entire field may be attributed to his development of the nonauthoritarian, indirect approaches to suggestion wherein subjects learn how to experience hypnotic phenomena and how to utilize their own potentials to solve problems in their own way. The contents of these four volumes can be best understood as working papers on a journey of discovery. There is little that is fixed, final, or permanently validated about them. Most of these papers are heuristics that can stimulate the mind of the reader and evoke the awe of discovery, the potentials for which are unlimited in the dimension of human consciousness.

The problem of how to present these papers in the best order could have been solved in many ways. A simple chronological order seemed unsatisfactory because the record of much of Erickson's earliest work was published only at a later date. Many papers dealing with the same theme which should obviously be grouped together were published in different phases of his career. Because of this the editor decided to make a balanced presentation wherein each volume identifies a major area of exploration with appropriate sections wherein the papers are presented in an approximation of chronological order.

Each of the first four volumes of this series contains a number of unpublished papers selected by the editor from several boxes of manuscripts entrusted to him by Erickson for this purpose. A companion volume, in preparation, will contain only previously unpublished lectures and hypnotic demonstrations by Erickson throughout his career. Many of these exist in various forms of neglect and deterioration all over the world wherever he gave his numerous presentations. The editor is currently assembling as many of these as can be accurately transcribed and reviewing them with Erickson for his elucidating commentaries. So subtle are his approaches that even a detailed study of his demonstrations often leaves the investigator without a full understanding of what Erickson is doing. Because of this the editor would like to take the occasion of the publication of these four volumes to make an appeal to whomever is in possession of previously unpublished records of Erickson's work to make them available to us for possible inclusion in this companion volume. It is only through such cooperation that we can all grow together.

Ernest L. Rossi

Preface

Considerable progress has been made in the evolution of Erickson's approaches to hypnosis and psychotherapy based, in large part, on the original publication of these volumes in 1980. These volumes remain the foundation for all who seek to understand and draw fresh inspiration from Erickson's most original writings. The papers herein contain rich seeds that can sprout within the imaginations of young investigators, as well as seasoned clinicians of all schools of therapeutic thought. Indeed, it is a testament to the depth and breadth of Erickson's genius that I have received as many letters about these volumes from people in the fields of literature and the arts as I have from professionals in psychology and psychiatry.

My call for help in collecting tape recordings of Erickson's many seminars and teaching workshops throughout the world has been heard! Since 1980, Irvington has been able to publish an additional four volumes of Erickson's tape-recorded seminars, workshops, lectures, and demonstrations that were generously sent to us by professionals of many nations. The titles of these volumes are:

Healing in Hypnosis (Vol. I)
Life Reframing in Hypnosis (Vol. II)
Mind-Body Communication in Hypnosis (Vol. III)
Choices in Hypnosis (Vol. IV) (Forthcoming, January 1990)

Yet more material remains! If all goes well, we will have a few more volumes to add to this series. The extensive appreciation that has been expressed by readers from all fields of science and the humanities that has made the continuing publication of these volumes possible could have developed only if they were meeting an important public and professional need. What is that need? Perhaps each reader will have to answer that question for him/herself. For me it has been an opening and vast expansion of my world view and psychological understanding. Even now, after 15 years of continuing work with this material, I experience daily insights and a sense of serendipitous discovery as I reread and reflect on its evolving meaning for understanding consciousness, character, and the creative choices of our time.

Ernest L. Rossi
Malibu, California
January 1989

General Introduction

Ernest L. Rossi

In these papers, written over a period of more than four decades, we see a renaissance of new approaches to hypnotherapy and a remarkable creativity in facilitating symptom relief, depth psychotherapy, and the actualization of personal potentials. One senses in Erickson's innovative approaches an unusual respect and appreciation for the complexity of the human psyche. We see him as an explorer who is constantly mindful of his own limitations while fully aware of the patient's own potentials for self-cure and development. We see in these papers his efforts to break out of the limiting assumptions that underlay many "schools" of psychotherapy. From the fragments of three or four incomplete manuscripts initiated by Erickson during the 1950s and 1960s and stitched together by the editor for this general introduction we can gain an appreciation of his views in the following areas:

1. The Limiting Preconceptions of Most "Schools" of Psychotherapy
2. The Importance of Current Realities in Psychotherapy
3. Limitations of Hypnotherapy

(1)THE LIMITING PRECONCEPTIONS OF MOST "SCHOOLS" OF PSYCHOTHERAPY

In the development of psychotherapy as a field of medical endeavor there has been an extensive elaboration of theory and an astonishing rigidity of procedure. This is particularly the case in the many divergent psychoanalytically oriented schools of thought. This undue emphasis upon an extensive theoretical superstructure as a requisite for all psychotherapy, together with a rigidity of therapeutic approach toward all patients, arises from three general assumptions. The first of these is that a psychotherapy based upon observable behavior and related primarily to the demands of the immediate and future life situations of the patient must necessarily be inadequate, superficial, and lacking in validity—as compared with a therapy that restructures the patient's understanding of the remote past.

The second assumption is that the same rigid and stereotyped approach to therapy (the routines of "classical analysis," "nondirective" therapy, etc.) is applicable to all patients at all times in all situations. This assumption neglects the immediate significance of (a) the individuality of life experiences, reactions, and learnings; (b) the context of the problem in relation to the actual life situation; and (c) the character of the symptomatology manifested, whether basically psychological, physiological, somatic, or varying combinations of all three.

The third assumption is that effective psychotherapy occurs through an interpretation and explanation to patients, either directly or indirectly, concerning the inner meaning of their experiential life formulated in terms of the speculations postulated by a particular school of psychotherapy. To illustrate this assumption, consider the following: A hungry infant nursing avidly at its mother's breast is not to be regarded as merely an infant satisfying a physiological hunger. Instead, its nursing is to be interpreted as an aggressive reaction in a state of resentment to the experience of physiological hunger and an endeavor to incorporate its mother as a defense against a threatening world. Thus, a physical life process, universal to all mammals, is accorded a highly specific interpretation implying complicated mentation in a newborn infant.

That the many schools of psychotherapy are based upon vastly divergent, often opposing and contradictory formulations of human behavior—and yet achieve essentially the same general therapeutic results—has not lessened reliance upon these general assumptions. Neither has it led the proponents of the various schools to critically and comparatively reappraise the tenets of their teachings. The elaborateness of these theoretical interpretations of human behavior, together with the routinized character of the therapeutic procedures, has made psychotherapy a prolonged, involved, and expensive undertaking that is largely unavailable to the vast majority of patients. Thus, the ideal of a readily available and easily applicable psychotherapy has been defeated. Instead, the various schools of psychotherapy, particularly those that are analytically oriented, have elaborated their own separate and different philosophies to which patients must adapt even when it may not be in their best interests to do so.

(2) THE IMPORTANCE OF CURRENT REALITIES IN PSYCHOTHERAPY

The assumption that psychotherapy must necessarily be so complex and so prolonged a procedure contradicts the general experience of daily living. Simple daily events of brief and fleeting character can, and frequently do, exert profound and lasting influences upon the human personality. Such events can derive wholly out of the immediate present and can evoke important responses that bear upon the individual's present and future. Such significant responses to daily events, despite the earnest beliefs held by so many adherents of interpretative schools of psychotherapy, are not necessarily reflections and new editions of traumatic infantile experiences. This is not to disparage in any way the importance of psychic trauma in infancy and childhood. Rather, it is to emphasize the fact that traumatic experiences can occur at any age level and may reflect only the actual life situation involved. The traumas need not require antecedent infantile prototypes in order to be understood.

The current and anticipated life situations are of vast importance to patients undergoing psychotherapy, since the task confronting them is primarily an effective adjustment to the demands and forces of the present and the future, regardless of what may have been their historical past. Preoccupation with only the past and a disregard of the needs, opportunities, and capabilities of the current situation may easily, and often does, unduly prolong psychotherapy.

In accord with the importance of current daily life experiences more recognition should be given to interpersonal relationships as special and remarkably potent influences in psychopathology and in psychotherapy. The efficacy of the relationship, whether destructive or constructive, can be more a function of its intensity, duration, and character than of the various "psychodynamic interpretations" proffered by many established schools of thought. Human experience is far more replete with examples of psychotherapeutically effective interpersonal relationships that have corrected maladaptive behavior than all the combined efforts of organized psychotherapy. There are as yet no scientific measurements of the kindly word, the challenging note, the whispered doubt, the anguished gasp, the threatening tone, the mocking noise, the contented murmur, the encouraging sound, the expectant silence. Upon such forces as these can rest the success or failure of psychotherapy. The potency of the therapy derives from the therapist's capacity for sympathetic and empathetic response rather than from years of familiarization with the tenets and precepts upon which many of our current schools of analysis and psychotherapy are founded. Overemphasizing indoctrination and neglecting the importance of interpersonal relationships in all their subtle aspects have made the *practice* of medicine an assembly line of routines and procedures, while the *art* of medicine and living are subjugated to the products of the laboratory and intellectual theorizing.

This may be illustrated by citing two different types of clearly recognizable problems requiring profound psychological and somatic readjustments. The first instance is that of the adult quadruple amputee, who is suddenly confronted with the appalling task of extensively readjusting and reordering his pattern of living. This is not a psycho-therapeutic problem to be dealt with by years of painstaking exploration of his past and a laborious "psychodynamic analytical reorientation." Instead, the problem of psychotherapy is one of meeting the imperative needs, psychological and somatic, of the immediate present and impend-ing future, with only a secondary and limited utilization of his historical past.

The second case is that of a 15-year-old boy, rejected by both parents since the age of eight and boarded the year round in schools and summer camps, with only a Christmas Eve visit at home. He had reacted to his rejection by developing mucous colitis at the age of 10, and this resulted in much pain, distress, and defecatory frequency. A colectomy had been recommended by several surgeons but had been rejected by the parents. Two years of intensive daily psychoanalysis from ages 11 to 13 served only to increase his symptomatology. This was finally discontinued at his parents' insistence. When he was 15, his parents offered him the alternative of surgery or hypnosis. The boy chose hypnotherapy. The therapy was oriented entirely around the question of defecatory needs and mechanisms as a continuing daily reality, properly one of physiological pleasure and satisfaction. No effort was directed toward the resolution of the other problems of family and personal adjustment. The therapeutic results, after four hours of hypnotherapy directed exclusively toward the boy's somatic symptomatology and functioning, were a correction of his colitis, his successful completion of high school and college, and the continuance of excellent social and personal adjustments, which remained free from the original physical symptomatology.

Although this patient's problems constituted a symptom-reaction ob-viously related to problems in the past, it resulted in a distortion of current everyday realities that rendered it a greater and more disturbing problem for him than the original unhappiness. Hence, psychotherapy for this patient was focused on his immediate life situation—which should be the case in the treatment of many psychosomatic problems. The essential therapeutic consideration was not to interpret and define his excretory behavior to him as symbolically epitomizing his emotional attitudes toward his parents. Instead, the therapeutic consideration was the reality value in daily living of adequate and pleasurable physiological functioning as a personal right to be sensed and appreciated for itself, and kept apart from other unresolved and unrelated problems. In this way the patient achieved a new balance of psychological functioning that indirectly facilitated a progressive, favorable personality adjustment without further psychotherapy.

So it is with many other psychosomatic problems. The establishment of a new and propitious balance of personality forces, sometimes even very slight, may tip the scales in favor of a spontaneous, progressive recovery similar to the natural biological healing that frequently results from the removal of a single element in an organic disease complex. All of this is in accord with the experience of everyday life, wherein a single, seemingly insignificant, stimulus or experience can shatter or establish the destiny of an individual or even a nation.

Unquestionably, the influence of past traumatic events can be found, to some degree, in all cases where psychotherapy is needed. These influences, however, are not necessarily the exclusive causative factors that must be understood by the patient in order to effect a cure. *For the processes of new learnings and new experiences do not cease with childhood; they continue throughout life, bringing with them ever new and different possibilities of favorable or unfavorable personal adjustments.*

(3)THE LIMITATIONS OF HYPNOTHERAPY *

Experience of more than 50 years in the field of experimental and therapeutic hypnosis is the basis for the following discussion of the uses and limitations of hypnotherapy. Since ancient times medicine men have known of the restorative value of normal sleep. Undoubtedly, the chants of the earliest medicine men helped many patients into such a restorative sleep, just as the crooning of a mother helps her fitful child into a peaceful state of quietness and sleep.

With the rise of mesmerism and the recognition of hypnosis as a therapeutic tool in the past two centuries, however, the erroneous view has developed that hypnosis is in itself a curative force. In some mysterious way it is supposed to transcend normal psychophysiological forces to effect miraculous cures. Serious students of hypnosis know from experience that all hypnotic phenomena can be found in the normal behavior of everyday living. There is no transcendence of normal abilities in hypnosis. *In all my experience I have never found any validity to the claims of paranormal powers, miraculous healing, or extrasensory perception arising out of hypnosis.* In all such cases that I have personally investigated I have found that the so-called paranormal powers and miraculous healing were simply activated states or normal psychophysiological processes. The so-called ESP was based on the unconscious utilization of minimal cues. We all have many more potentials than we realize. Hypnotherapy consists of the evocation and utilization of these often hidden potentials.

Patients have problems precisely because they do not know how to utilize all their abilities. In my view, then, the induction of hypnosis as a

* Editor's note: This section is a highly condensed and edited synthesis of many unpublished notes in MHE's files.

simple state of quiescent receptivity is in itself not curative (apart from the restorative value of rest and sleep mentioned above). *The value of hypnosis lies entirely in its use as a modality for facilitating healing processes by evoking psychological and physiological responses conducive to the well-being of the total person.*

For hypnosis to be identified as a therapy in itself is an error analogous to identifying intelligence with education. Well-trained *therapists* have extensive knowledge of the psychological and physiological processes relevant to their field of speciality (the various specialities in medicine, dentistry, and psychology). Well-trained *hypnotherapists* know how to purposefully evoke and utilize these psychophysiological processes in an orderly manner to facilitate therapeutic goals.

An Introduction To Unorthodox Therapy

Milton H. Erickson

The task of the physician is to heal. It is neither to censure nor to judge but simply to render services that may enable patients to live their lives in a better and more adequate fashion. The kind of therapy warranted should be that which is considered clinically to meet the patient's needs and to offer the best possible therapeutic results without regard for social niceties or questions of etiquette. There should be only one ruling principle—the patient's welfare.

This apologia is offered because of the author's discovery of how much he was bound unconsciously by conventionalities. This discovery was first made when once he presented to a sophisticated medical audience a verbatim account of a patient's interpretative account of behavior involving mayhem and homicide. Several of the physicians, including some with more than 30 years of experience, became nauseated and actually ill. Yet they knew that the purpose of the presentation was to determine the justifiability of a lobotomy for a patient who could not be classified other than as a criminal. This patient had a long history of escaping the legal consequences for serious crimes by a careful and deliberate establishment of a history of mental illness of an episodic character. The verdict, whenever this patient was tried in court, had always been "not guilty by reason of insanity," and a resulting brief confinement in a mental hospital from which an escape was made or from which there was given a discharge because the patient had "recovered" or was "in remission." All of this was known to that group of more than 50 physicians. Yet the patient's own account of the crimes and interpretation of them—not acceptable in a court of law, since no attorney was present at the time of communication and since the patient was not legally responsible—rendered more than a dozen physicians ill, and another dozen found themselves unable to endure hearing a full account of the patient's behavior upon which the surgical decision was based, behavior that violated so many of the niceties, proprieties, and conventions of society.

The author's next discovery of the hold of social conventionality upon the individual occurred when he found himself questioning the propriety of reporting scientifically an account of successful psychotherapy accom-

Editor's Note: Written by Milton H. Erickson.

plished by a simple violation of conventional behavior. Nevertheless, the account was written and was read by a highly respected colleague, who urged that the account be presented to a group of psychiatrists. This was done, and to the author's amazement and personal horror, he discovered that he unconsciously lowered his voice and increased the rapidity of his speech as he read the account. As for his audience, despite their full approval of the psychotherapy, they were tense, frozen-faced, and unwilling to discuss the report. Also, the colleague who had encouraged the author to present the account found that he, too, "tightened up unconsciously," to his own astonishment.

That ingrained conventional attitudes should have such force for sophisticated, medically trained people in matters that rightly should be considered as only medical in nature suggests how strongly others might react. Yet medical problems, whatever they are, should be faced, and patients' needs should be met without regard for irrelevant social teachings. The author is reminded of the patient whose opening remark was, "I've been kicked out of every doctor's office in——[a city of more than two million inhabitants], and I suppose you will kick me out, too." His disorder was somewhat akin to Gilles de la Tourette's Disease. Furthermore, this patient's behavior was not socially destructive, though it was repulsive. Nor has this patient been the only one to seek help from the author with a comparable opening remark. Additionally, one need only call to mind the well-known neglect of rectal examinations and the undue failure to detect rectal carcinoma caused by both public and medical obeisance to "One just doesn't do such things."

With this apologia, the case histories in this volume are reported, some in which hypnosis was employed, some in which hypnosis could not be employed. These case histories present "unorthodox therapy" (if success-ful psychotherapy can ever properly be called unorthodox), illustrating a type of direct psychotherapy that unfortunately too few therapists are competent to do. If it were not for the extensive hold that social conventions have upon both physician and patient, more therapists could venture into this highly delicate field. But in all justice, the reader should bear in mind that the hold of social conventions upon the patients also played a significant role in both their illness and their therapy.

I. General Introductions to Hypnotherapy

While most of the papers in this first section are fairly conventional introductions to the history of hypnosis and its place in medicine, there is one paper, "Hypnotic Psychotherapy" (1948), that is wildly original. This paper, published in a little-known journal and never before reprinted, is a clarion call to a new kind of hypnotherapy. When one compares this paper with all that had been previously published by other authors, one can immediately recognize Erickson as an original in the invention and application of new principles of hypnotherapy. Nothing quite like it had ever been written before. In this and other papers of this volume, the reader will find significant emphasis placed on the following four salient principles of Erickson's work:

1. *The unconscious need not be made conscious:* Unconscious processes can be facilitated so that they can function autonomously to solve each patient's problems in an individual way.
2. *Mental mechanisms and personality characteristics need not be analyzed for the patient:* They can be *utilized* as processes, dynamisms, or pathways facilitating therapeutic goals.
3. Suggestion need not be direct: *Indirect suggestions can frequently bypass a patient's learned limitations and thus better facilitate unconscious processes.* "By such an indirect suggestion the patient is enabled to go through those difficult inner processes of disorganization, reorganization, reassociating and projection of inner experience to meet the requirements of [therapeutic goals]."
4. *Therapeutic suggestion is not a process of programming the patient with the therapist's point of view:* Rather, it involves "an inner resynthesis of the patient's behavior achieved by the patient himself."

These four principles of Erickson's approach represent a paradigmatic shift (Kuhn, 1970) to an entirely new way of understanding and employing hypnotherapy. Many of the papers of this volume are a record of Erickson's exploratory application of these principles even before he had

1

a fully conscious understanding of them. As is the case with all fundamental changes in our frames of reference, it may require some time and patience for most of us to assimilate and use these new principles. As we do so, however, we may be rewarded with those same sudden bursts of change and growth that we hope to facilitate in our patients.

1. The Applications of Hypnosis To Psychiatry

Milton H. Erickson

GENERAL INTRODUCTION

For nearly 200 years there has been a slowly growing scientific interest in hypnotism. Along with this interest there has also existed much antagonism, misunderstanding and actual fear of the phenomenon because of the difficulties involved in the reaching any clear understanding of it. However, the developments in psychology, psychiatry, and psychoanalysis within the last 50 years are now serving both directly and indirectly through the elaboration of new and useful concepts to place hypnotism on a secure scientific basis free from the hampering, superstitious misconceptions that have characterized so long the general attitude toward this definite psychological phenomenon.

At the present time many of the leading psychological laboratories are subjecting hypnosis to controlled scientific study. In the last 20 years slightly more than 400 articles have been written on the subject in French, English, and German. About one-third of these articles were written in the first half of the last 20 years, and they dealt either with vague generalities or limited aspects of the subject. The articles for the last 10 years amounting to two-thirds of the total, show a markedly different approach to the subject. Not only has the volume of the work doubled, but the approach to the problems of hypnotism has been placed more and more on the scientific basis of controlled laboratory analysis and experimentation in an effort to identify the essential nature of hypnotic manifestations. The immediate outcome of this type of scientific study has been the realization of the investigative and explorative values of hypnosis as an instrument applicable to the laboratory study and analysis of the psychological aspects of human behavior, neurophysiology, and mental disease.

Reprinted with permission from the *Medical Record*, July 19, 1939, pp. 60-65, originally from an address given before the Ontario Neuropsychiatric Association, March 18, 1937, at London, Ontario.

HISTORICAL PERSPECTIVE

Before discussing these aspects of the subject, hypnotism may be considered first in a brief historical review. Although actually known for centuries, even by primitive savages, hypnotism made its semiscientific debut about 1775 in a study by Mesmer, after whom it was originally termed "mesmerism." Mesmer had no realization of its psychological nature but regarded it as a force of a cosmic type possessed of decided value in the medical treatment of certain types of patients. Mesmer's misunderstanding of his discovery, together with the general antagonism of the public to any new and incomprehensible phenomenon, led to the development of many superstitions and fearful beliefs, some of which are excellently portrayed in the story of "Trilby," especially in the characterization of Svengali. These fears and superstitions are now beginning to die, although they are frequently given new life in the cinema, the tabloid newspaper, and the comic strip.

Following Mesmer were three outstanding English physicians: Elliotson, who began his work in 1817 by employing mesmerism as a definite therapeutic aid in hospital and private practice; Esdaile, who, stimulated by Elliotson's success and writings, began to employ it medically in India in a government hospital chiefly as an anesthetic agent in surgery; and finally, James Braid, who in 1841 recognized its psychological nature and first placed mesmerism, which he renamed "hypnotism," on a scientific basis.

Since Braid, many outstanding clinicians have been interested in the subject, the foremost of whom was Charcot. Much of Charcot's work, however, served only to retard the development of definitive knowledge in this field. His misidentification of hypnosis with hysteria has led to many serious misconceptions of hypnosis, and even today the false belief is held that hypnosis and hysteria are the same. Fortunately, however, the increasing clinical literature is correcting this mistaken idea.

Perhaps the next significant, though passing, figure in the development of the clinical applications of hypnosis was Freud, who with Breuer initiated its employment as an investigative psychological instrument in the treatment of mental patients. However, he soon discarded it as a method because of certain limitations which he encountered through his use of it as a direct and immediately corrective and therapeutic agent instead of as an indirectly educative measure in therapeusis—developing, instead, certain of the discoveries he had made through his use of hypnosis.

Since this first application of hypnosis as a clinical instrument for the study of mental disorders, the development of psychology as a science has served greatly in providing concepts and methods of study and analysis permitting a more comprehensive application of hypnosis as a clinical instrument for both normal and abnormal forms of behavior. Accordingly, the problem of the study of hypnotism and its applications was taken over by both abnormal and clinical psychologists and psychiatrists.

With this recognition of hypnotism as constituting a definite problem for investigation by the relatively young sciences of psychology and psychiatry, there has come to be an increasing appreciation of the possibilities it offers in both fields, first as a laboratory instrument in the study of the nature of human behavior, and second as an explorative and perhaps therapeutic agent in dealing with mental disorders.

Naturally, the greater contribution to date has been in the field of the clinical psychologist, who has taken hypnosis out of the province of abnormal psychology and has employed it to reopen certain questions in psychology formerly considered fairly well outlined. This hypnotic experimentation by the clinical psychologist has served greatly, both directly and indirectly, to contribute new significance to such concepts as learning and forgetting, reasoning, sensation, attention, feeling and emotion, association, conditioning, and personality development, to develop new approaches to old questions, and to permit the repetition of established work under varied psychological conditions, thereby serving to make it more informative.

In consequence of the general development of clinical psychology, psychiatry has profited extensively. As pointed out by Whitehorn and Zilboorg (1933), in the ten years from 1921 to 1930, there has been a complete change in the character of psychiatric literature, with a decrease of clinical descriptive articles and a more than doubling of the psychological studies. With this influx of psychological trends, psychiatry has come to look upon hypnosis not only as a limited therapeutic approach but rather as a useful instrument for the study of mental disorders and as an actual means of approaching an understanding of causal factors in the laboratory analysis of its problems.

GENERAL CONSIDERATIONS AND TECHNIQUE

However, before taking up the question of the laboratory use of hypnosis, it may be best to mention briefly certain general considerations and then to proceed to the problem of the technique of hypnosis.

First of all are those considerations included in certain general questions always asked, foremost among which is the question of who may be hypnotized. The reply to this is that any really *cooperative* subject may be, regardless of whether he is a normal person, a hysterical neurotic, or a psychotic schizophrenic patient. Next, it has no harmful effects nor does it lend itself, as the cinema and the tabloid newspapers would have one believe, to the promotion of criminal activities (Erickson, 1932, 1934). Thirdly, despite its outward appearance, it has no actual relation to physiological sleep but is simply a psychological phenomenon (Bass, 1931). Finally, it is not supernatural but a normal though little understood psychological manifestation, readily and easily controlled by the experienced worker.

Concerning the technique of trance induction little information is available in the literature, and hence each hypnotist necessarily develops his own. The actual accounts of hypnotic procedure given in the literature are inadequate and misleading. Because of this lack of information regarding the essential refinements of technique, much of the early hypnotic work attempted by investigators leads to poor or unsatisfactory results, and this in turn accounts for much of the discredit accorded to hypnotic work.

Usually the understanding is that hypnosis may be induced by repeated suggestions of fatigue, drowsiness, and sound sleep, and that when the subjects give evidence of being asleep, they are ready for hypnotic procedure. Actually, these subjects may be in a trance, giving every evidence of this fact, but in reality it is too often a type of trance permitting only limited use of hypnotic suggestion. The employment of hypnosis as a therapeutic agent or as a laboratory method of experimentation requires, for valid results, a training process extending over several hours. In this training procedure subjects may be hypnotized, awakened, rehypnotized, and reawakened repeatedly, with each of the trance and waking states employed to teach them by slow degrees a facility of control over mental faculties and an organization of responses that increases the degree of dissociation between consciousness and subconsciousness, thus establishing in effect but not in actuality a dissociated hypnotic personality. Only by building up in each subject a capacity to function in an organized, integrated fashion while in the trance state can extensive complicated therapeutic or experimental work be done.

Because of the difficulties and labor involved in integrating various forms of hypnotic behavior, the variations in time and effort required in training individual subjects and hence the impossibility of establishing any standard of routine, and the general failure to realize the need for an integration of hypnotic responses, there are inadequate, ineffective, and often misleading results from hypnotic work.

Since the scope of this paper does not permit a detailed account of the refinements of technique, it may be best to summarize with the statement that an effective technique is one based upon repeated, long-continued hypnotic trances in which the subject reaches a stuporous state. In this trance stupor the subject is taught, by slow degrees, to obey suggestions and to react to situations in an integrated fashion. Only in this way can there be secured an extensive dissociation of the conscious from the subconscious elements of the personality which will permit a satisfactory manipulation of those parts of the personality under study.

UTILIZATION OF HYPNOTIC PHENOMENA

To proceed now to a consideration of the utilization of the various phenomena of the hypnotic state, it may be best to select those having a significant bearing upon psychiatric problems and to indicate their various investigative possibilities.

One of the important trance manifestations occurring in nearly every well-hypnotized subject is catalepsy. In the stuporous trance this catalepsy may not be distinguishable from the cerea flexibilitas of the stuporous catatonic patient. Numerous attempts have been made to understand the physiology and psychology of the waxy flexibility of the schizophrenic patient, and many studies with drugs, especially bulbocapnine on animals, have been made without clarifying the problem. The apparent identity of hypnotic catalepsy with the catalepsy occurring in mental disease suggests the advisability of approaching the neuropsychiatric problem contained in this familiar sign of mental disease by exhaustive studies of its hypnotic parallel, since the hypnotic catalepsy can be induced, directed, and controlled, and thus subjected to thorough physiological and psychological study as a phenomenon complete in itself and not as a minor part of a major constellation where many other factors may be present. Perhaps it is too optimistic to consider hypnotic catalepsy as identical with the catalepsy of mental disease, but it nevertheless offers an opportunity for a complete study of a closely parallel phenomenon that can be studied thoroughly at the convenience of the investigator. Approaches to this problem have been made at Yale (Williams, 1930) and various other universities, but further and more clinically oriented work is needed. Aside from the psychiatric aspects, the investigation of this problem should contribute much to a knowledge of muscle tonus and neurophysiology. It is conceivable that an understanding of hypnotic catalepsy would contribute materially to a better knowledge of certain of the phenomena of catatonia.

Another hypnotic phenomenon which has a direct bearing upon psychiatric problems is the amnesia which develops for all trance events following profound hypnosis. Thus, subjects in deep trance may perform any number of complicated actions and yet have no knowledge of their actions upon awakening from the trance (Erickson, 1934), and indeed, they may even be unaware of the fact that they have been in a trance.

That the whole problem of amnesia in itself constitutes a nuclear part of many psychiatric questions, particularly in considering the domination of the personality by long past and forgotten experiences, is readily realized. The same sort of amnesic phenomena found in the psychiatric patient is to be found in hypnotic amnesia, with the exception that the hypnotic amnesia can be controlled, manipulated, directed, removed, and even reestablished at the desire of the investigator. Thus, there is an opportunity to synthesize or to manufacture amnesic states, and then to analyze their effects upon the personality; then to restore the memories, studying the processes by which associations can be built up and forgotten experiences reintegrated into the conscious life of the personality. In brief, one can, by hypnosis, manufacture a state of amnesia, making it all-inclusive or limiting it to certain considerations, studying and analyzing that amnesia fully, with the entire possibility at any time of removing it in part or in full, making differential analyses at each step of the procedure.

In addition to this laboratory approach to the dynamics of amnesia, there is also a clinical application of hypnosis to the problem of amnesia as encountered in psychiatric practice. Recent literature contains a number of accounts of patients who have forgotten their identity or who have forgotten some experience of vital importance to them. In ordinary psychiatric practice the meeting of such a problem is almost entirely one of painstaking but often futile trial-and-error procedure. By means of hypnosis, as has been demonstrated particularly by Beck (1936) and by Erickson (1933, 1937a; Erickson & Kubie, 1939), psychological situations can be created in the trance state, dormant associations awakened by hypnotic suggestion, and the amnesic material reconstructed. An example of the varying techniques which may be employed may be found in Erickson's *The Investigation of a Specific Amnesia* (1933), concerning a young woman who had forgotten the identity of a Christmas gift. By means of the employment of automatic writing, crystal-gazing, and dream suggestion the amnesic data was obtained. All of these are techniques which cannot be used in the waking state, but in the peculiar psychic state of hypnotic sleep they can be most effectual. The development of clinical techniques in the hypnotic exploration of amnesias should serve materially to advance knowledge concerning the development of amnesias, the repressive forces at work, and the mental mechanisms involved in their development and in their removal.

Another type of experimental hypnotic work employing certain characteristic phenomena of the trance state has been the utilization of hypnotic suggestibility as a means of testing in a laboratory the postulated fundamental causes of mental disease. Luria in his book *The Nature of Human Conflict* (1932), Huston, et al. (1934), Erickson (1935) in various studies of hypnotically induced complexes, and Brickner and Kubie in their study, *A Miniature Psychotic Storm* (1936), have all shown the significant value of hypnosis as a means of paralleling or duplicating on a miniature scale the major phenomena of mental disorders. All of these workers were concerned with the production of psychoneurotic and emotional disturbances in normal subjects similar to the complex manifestations of actual mental disorder as a means of reaching an understanding of the processes involved.

Utilizing the marked suggestibility found in hypnotic states, Luria (1932) and Huston and his coworkers (1934) suggested disagreeable experiences, which, upon acceptance, would give rise to significant internal conflicts from which could derive severe neurotic and emotional symptoms. This procedure was followed by the administration of a word-association test accompanied by voluntary and involuntary motor responses to determine the presence in both hypnotic and waking states of evidences of internal conflict. Subsequently, hypnotic psychotherapy was employed to remove these internal conflicts, and readministration of the word-association test and its accompaniments disclosed the disappearance of the previous evidence of internal psychic distress. Briefly, these workers demonstrated the possibility of producing in normal subjects miniature artificial psychoses which would serve to govern their personality reactions, which could be removed at the will of the investigator, and which presumably might parallel in their structure actual mental disorders. Erickson's study (1935) demonstrated the possibility of developing in a subject an artificial neurosis characterized by compulsions, phobias, and obsessions, in such a fashion that an actual neurosis already present in the subject became a part of this induced neurosis, with psychotherapy of the artificial neurosis serving to remove the original difficulty.

Brickner and Kubie (1936), interested in the dynamics of compulsive behavior, undertook a study in which a hypnotic subject was given posthypnotic suggestions leading to compulsive and obsessive behavior. By this means they were able to observe the slow genesis and final working out of an abnormal type of behavior, identifying each element of the reaction pattern as it appeared and relating it to accepted theoretical concepts. Such studies as these reveal the possibilities for subjecting various types of human behavior to a complete study in a state of isolation. Before Luria's work (1932) the whole psychological and psychiatric concept of a complex was a clinical assumption, but as a result of the experimental work mentioned above, laboratory proof and methods for such proof are now available to show that a complex is an experimentally demonstrable concept signifying certain psychic phenomena and furthermore, that a complex can be induced in a subject, its effects upon the personality postulated and then corrected by direct observation, and that it can then be removed by psychotherapy and its effects upon personality reactions abolished (Huston et al., 1934). Likewise, my own study (1935) and that of Brickner and Kubie (1936) have shown some of the fundamental processes entering into the development of compulsive, obsessive, and phobic behavior, demonstrating clearly the cause-effect relationships of definite experiences and their direct manifestations in behavior patterns.

Still another type of hypnotic work which gives great promise psychiatrically lies in the neurophysiological changes which may be induced in the profoundly hypnotized subject. Sears (1932) has reported some extensive studies on hypnotic anesthesia wherein the subject has had localized anesthesias induced comparable to the anesthesias that develop particularly in such psychoneuroses as hysteria and various conversion syndromes. This work is highly suggestive of the possibilities of reducing many of the conversion symptoms found in mental disorders to laboratory problems accessible to investigation in a controlled fashion.

An even farther-reaching aspect of this possibility may be found in the work reported to the American Psychiatric Association in May, 1936 (Erickson, 1938a, 1938b), which gave an account of the production by means of hypnotic suggestion of a state of deafness which gave every evidence of being a neurological deafness and yet which could be removed and reestablished readily and easily by appropriate suggestion. Similar in character are two other investigations concerning the effect of hypnosis upon psychophysiological and neurophysiological functioning in the sensory fields as shown by the hypnotic induction of color blindness (Erickson, 1939d), and the hypnotic induction of hallucinatory color vision accompanied by pseudonegative afterimages (Erickson & Erickson, 1938). That deafness and color blindness comparable in degree and character to that found in organic conditions can be induced by hypnotic techniques suggests strongly the value of hypnotic techniques for psychophysiological and neurophysiological research.

However, one of the greatest advantages of hypnosis as applied to psychiatry seems to me to be the possibilities it affords in the development of significant psychological situations permitting definite control and study of personality reactions. Thus, by hypnotic suggestion one can create definite psychological environments permitting an adequate study of personality reactions within those situations and free from other and disturbing elements. For example, should it be desired to make a study of the effects of a state of affective depression upon behavior in general, hypnotic subjects can be placed in a state of profound depression which will serve to govern their conduct in any number of ways. At the same time this depression can be removed and direct contrasts made between depressed behavior and normal behavior. An account of such experimental work can be found in the investigations mentioned earlier (Huston et al., 1934; Luria, 1932).

Just as situations can be created permitting a study of the genetic development of behavior patterns, so can hypnosis be applied to the calling forth of even long-forgotten patterns of response. To make this clear, let us consider the psychiatric concept of regression, which may be defined as a reversion to simpler and earlier forms of behavior—a thing that we see daily in the "second childhood" of senile patients and in the "regression" of schizophrenic patients. Platonow (1933) approached this problem, and his work has been repeated (Erickson, 1939b), by suggesting to profoundly hypnotized adult subjects that they were children and had not yet reached the years of adult life. To those subjects, in that suggested state of childhood, intelligence tests were administered, and it was found that there had occurred an actual evocation of the simpler and earlier forms of response, both intellectual and muscular, with an amnesia for things learned subsequent to the suggested age level.

Control studies with normal subjects in the waking state asked to respond as children disclosed the impossibility of normal adults responding genuinely at a childhood level. Personal work on this problem has shown that normal adults may be "regressed" by hypnotic suggestion literally to a state of infancy, with this regression including not only intellectual and emotional patterns of response but even muscular reflex responses. Just how significant this laboratory regression of normal subjects will prove is still a question warranting much more investigation; how much value it will be in reaching an understanding of the regression found in psychoses is still another question. But at least it does offer the best and most promising approach to date to one of the most significant and difficult of psychiatric problems.

Along this same line hypnotic regression can be employed profitably in the elucidation of another important psychiatric problem—namely, that of the abreaction or the reliving of past experiences. In this procedure subjects are reoriented or regressed to a previous period of their lives and allowed to relive as a current experience some long-past event. An example of such investigatory work is to be found in a report published in the *Archives of Neurology and Psychiatry* (Erickson, 1937a). A patient who had been drugged and beaten to unconsciousness had recovered from his injuries but had developed an amnesia for the experience. Several years later, during hypnosis, he was reoriented to that period of his life and allowed to relive that experience as if it were actually happening at the time. By this procedure a complete account was obtained, together with a redevelopment of unconsciousness characterized by a loss of reflexes, and with a duplication of the original confused mental state. In brief, the patient was enabled to reexperience in the hypnotic state a profound traumatic experience which had long been forgotten. The application of this procedure in the securing of adequate psychiatric data on patients is at once apparent, and it is highly suggestive of the possibilities for reorienting patients to those periods of their lives wherein their original maladjustments and abnormalities first appeared. With such reorientation there is then the possibility of attacking directly the problems of psychotherapy involved.

Still another application of hypnosis to psychiatry lies in the development of an experimental approach to the study of psychic dynamisms. We all realize that personality reactions and emotional attitudes may manifest themselves directly or indirectly, consciously or at a level at which people are unaware of their conduct, or if they become aware of their conduct, may be unaware of their motivations. To date our knowledge of mental mechanisms has been based on the observance of their occurrence and the explanation of their appearance on a post hoc, propter hoc basis, relating the dynamism to those events which have preceded it, and then verifying the conclusions by noting whether or not the insight afforded by knowledge of the relationships serves to elucidate the nature of the response.

By the application of hypnosis the entire approach to the problem of psychic dynamisms can be changed. For example, the existence of unconscious mentation or subconscious thinking has long been accepted, but its proof has rested on observations made after its appearance. Recent experimental work (Erickson, 1938a) shows that it is possible to create a psychological situation and to declare that a person subjected to such a situation would be forced to react in a certain way that would lead to a demonstration of unconscious mentation. In the experimental work mentioned a normal hypnotic subject was instructed to write a simple sentence, complete and meaningful in itself and which could be read by anyone else and found to have that meaning; and yet, in an unnoticeable way, it would contain a significance apparent only to the subject's unconscious mind. The subject achieved this difficult task by writing her guess concerning the length of time required to perform a certain act. The subject as well as the entire group present read the writing as "30 seconds." Yet, upon indirect questioning and the employment of automatic writing, it was found that the writing actually read 38 seconds, written with some scrawling of the word thirty and the transformation of the letter *y* into the numeral *8*. Thus, two trains of thought, simultaneously operative, were recorded by different types of symbolic thinking, one of which was kept from the awareness of the subject's conscious mind. In this same report, with another hypnotic subject, it was possible to carry on a written conversation having a conscious import but which was developed entirely in accord with an import known only to the unconscious mind of the subject and to the investigator without the subject becoming aware consciously of the actual nature of the conversation.

One other important consideration needs to be mentioned—namely, posthypnotic behavior, since this phenomenon enters so intensively into both experimental and therapeutic use of hypnosis. Briefly defined, posthypnotic behavior is that which occurs in response to hypnotic commands and subsequent to the trance state in which it is suggested. Through its utilization therapeutic efforts are made to direct, influence, and control behavior favorably and to enable patients to meet their various problems adequately. Similarly, it is used experimentally in the laboratory as a measure of manipulating a subject psychologically to permit a study of the dynamics of behavior, and its field of usefulness there is now being realized (Erickson & Erickson, 1941).

CONCLUSION

Within the limits of this report it has been possible only to sketch briefly a few of the applications of hypnosis to psychiatry. Many important considerations have been omitted. It has been my purpose only to indicate certain possibilities for definitive research in psychiatry by the use of hypnosis. That the eventual results of such research will be good or bad cannot yet be stated, but at least it can be said that hypnotic techniques applied to psychiatric problems give every promise of leading to better understandings of troublesome questions. In addition to this is the fact that hypnosis itself constitutes a form of psychic behavior worthy of understanding. And it is only reasonable that a thorough understanding of one type of mental behavior should contribute materially to an understanding of many problems of mental disorder.

2. Hypnosis in Medicine

Milton H. Erickson

Hypnosis or hypnotism is a psychological phenomenon of exceeding interest to both layman and scientist. Its history is as old as that of the human race, and it has been utilized by the most primitive of peoples, ancient and modern, in the practice of religious and medical rites to intensify belief in mysticism and magic. The striking character of this psychological manifestation, its inexplicable and bewildering phenomenology, and the seemingly miraculous results it produces—together with its long use for the bewilderment of the observer—have served to surround it with an aura of the supernatural and the unreal. As a consequence, the attitude of the general public toward this phenomenon, now scientifically established, has been, and too often still is, one of superstitious awe, misunderstanding, incredulity, antagonism, and actual hostility and fear. This attitude is perpetuated by the exploitation of hypnosis by the charlatan and the stage performer and the well-intentioned but mistaken and inadequate utilization by inexperienced experimenters and medical men.

The scientific history of hypnosis began about 1775 with Anton Mesmer, whose name is still attached to it, but unfortunately, even this scientific beginning was founded on a mystical belief that it was constituted of a peculiar cosmic fluid with healing properties.

Mesmer's use of hypnosis began with his discovery that suggestion in various forms could be used to induce a condition resembling sleep in certain types of patients, and that, in this state, therapeutic suggestions could be given them to alleviate and even remedy their complaints and symptoms. Unfortunately, Mesmer failed to recognize the purely psychological character of his discovery and attributed it to a cosmic force he termed "animal magnetism." Although Mesmer successfully treated large numbers of patients on whom orthodox medical procedures had failed, he fell into disrepute because of the mysticism with which he surrounded his therapy. Nevertheless, his discovery and utilization of it served to lay a foundation for the therapeutic use of hypnosis and for a recognition of the validity of psychotherapy as a medical procedure.

Since Mesmer's time there has been a succession of scientific men,

Reprinted with permission from *The Medical Clinics of North America*, May, 1944, New York Number.

chiefly medical, who have contributed greatly to its scientific growth. Elliotson, the first British physician to use a stethoscope, used hypnosis effectively about 1817 in his medical practice and published extensively on its suitability for certain types of patients. Esdaile, through Elliotson's writings, became so interested that he succeeded in having a government hospital built in India primarily for the use of hypnosis, where he extended its use to all types of patients, especially surgical.

In 1841 James Braid, an English physician who bitterly opposed "mesmerism," was induced to make a physical examination of a mesmerized subject. He recognized both the validity of the phenomenon and its psychological character, with the result that he coined the terms *hypnosis* and *hypnotism* and initiated the first scientific studies of hypnosis as a psychological condition of extensive medical and scientific significance.

Since then, clinicians first and psychologists later, among them many outstanding scientists, have contributed increasingly to a better understanding and utilization of hypnosis as a scientific tool and as a medical procedure of immense value for certain types of patients. Particularly has interest been developing rapidly during the last 25 years among psychiatrists and psychologists. During the last 15 years there has been an increasing wealth of publications dealing with the effective use of hypnosis in the fields of psychiatry and experimental psychology.

Regrettably, however, there is still a persistence of outmoded ideas and concepts of hypnosis which vitiate experimental studies and therapeutic efforts. For example, some psychologists are still publishing studies based upon techniques and psychological concepts belonging to the 19th century, and some medical men still employ it for direct symptom relief rather than as an educative procedure for the correction of personality disorders.

As yet the scientific study of hypnosis is still in its infancy despite the development of a healthy, intense interest in it as a scientific problem of merit. There is still lacking an adequate general appreciation of the need to integrate hypnotic studies with our present-day concepts and understandings of personality, of inter- and intrapersonal relationships, and psychosomatic interrelationships and interdependencies.

GENERAL QUESTIONS

In any discussion of hypnosis certain general questions arise concerning who may be hypnotized, the possible detrimental effects of hypnosis, its possible antisocial use, the nature of the hypnotist-subject relationship, the controllability of the hypnotic state, the relationship between hypnotic sleep and physiological sleep, and the possibility that hypnosis may crystallize or precipitate abnormal or pathological conditions in subjects that otherwise might have remained indefinitely dormant.

Because of space limitations reply to these questions must necessarily be brief and dogmatic, and the reader is referred to the following references upon which reply is based: Brickner & Kubie, 1936; Bass, 1931; Beck, 1936; Erickson, 1933, 1935, 1937a, 1938a, 1938b, 1939a, 1939c, 1943b, 1943c; Erickson & Erickson, 1941; Erickson & Brickner, 1943; Erickson & Hill, 1944; Erickson & Kubie, 1939, 1941; Farber & Fisher, 1943; Fisher, 1943; Gill & Brenman, 1943; Harriman, 1941, 1942a, 1942b; Liebman, 1941; Raeder, 1933; Sears, 1932; Vogel, 1934; White, 1941.

Briefly, there are no injurious or *detrimental effects* upon the subject other than those that can develop in any other normal interpersonal relationship; hypnosis cannot be used for *antisocial* or criminal purposes—most subjects can be induced to commit make-believe or pretended crimes, but pretenses should not be accepted as realities; the *hypnotist-subject relationship* is entirely one of voluntary cooperation, and no subject can be hypnotized against his will or without his cooperation; the hypnotist-subject relationship is analogous to that which exists between physician and patient, lawyer and client, minister and parishioner. Furthermore, a subject can be a hypnotist and a hypnotist can be a subject; they can work with each other in alternating roles, and often do in experimental work. Belief that hypnosis is a matter of a weak will dominated by a strong will is entirely a misconception. The best subjects are highly intelligent, normal people; the feebleminded and the psychotic and many psychoneurotics are either difficult or impossible to hypnotize.

Since hypnosis depends primarily upon cooperation by the subject, the control of the trance state rests largely with the subject. No subjects can be kept in a trance for an unreasonable length of time without their full cooperation, and the removal of the hypnotist from the hypnotic situation by one means or another disrupts the interpersonal cooperation necessary for the continuance of the trance. Thus, no subject can be left accidentally or intentionally in a trance for an indefinite period.

The relationship between the hypnotic trance and *physiological sleep* is one of appearance only. Hypnosis is a psychological phenomenon with secondary physiological manifestations, and sleep is physiological with secondary psychological manifestations. Blood distribution, muscle tonus, motor behavior, and reflex behavior in the trance state are not the same as in physiological sleep, and the two phenomena primarily serve entirely different purposes. Physiologically, there is much more resemblance between the hypnotic and the waking states than with physiological sleep.

As for hypnosis *crystallizing or precipitating abnormal or psycho-pathological conditions,* this is a post hoc observation. The relationship is temporal and not causal, as in the case of mental illness first noticed following a routine appendectomy.

Finally, as for *detrimental effects* of hypnosis, none have been observed in personal experience with hundreds of subjects, some of whom have been hypnotized hundreds of times. Furthermore, as every experienced hypnotist knows, the great difficulties involved in producing changes in the personality of a desired therapeutic character make evident the illogic of assuming that the time- and situation-limited hypnotic trance can bring about significant harmful effects, when earnestly desired beneficial effects are so hard to achieve.

THE TECHNIQUES OF HYPNOTIZING

The technique of inducing hypnosis, contrary to long-established and traditional superstitious ideas of eye fixation, crystal balls, and passes of the hand, is primarily a function of the interpersonal relationship existing between the subject and the hypnotist.

Hypnosis is not a mystical, magical thing that follows a definite rule-of-the-thumb or a special abracadabra. Practically all normal people can be hypnotized, though not necessarily by the same person, and practically all people can learn to be hypnotists. Hence any technique that permits the hypnotist to secure adequate and ready cooperation in this highly specialized interpersonal relationship of hypnosis constitutes a good technique. The able hypnotist is the one who is able to adapt technique to the personality needs of each subject. Thus, some subjects want to be dominated, others coaxed, still others to be persuaded. Some subjects want to dominate the situation and place the hypnotist in the role of an assistant who merely guides. Some prefer to be hypnotized by a wealth of repetitious suggestions, and there are those who like to resort to an introspective experiencing of the process of going into a trance. Sometimes the situation is one of authority-subservience, or it may be one of father-child, or again physician-patient, and often that merely of two equals intensely interested in an important problem.

Properly, hypnotists should have a good appreciation of their own personality and capabilities so that they may adapt themselves to the specific personality needs of each subject. In the majority of instances, especially in medical hypnosis, the physician-patient relationship is ideal and satisfies adequately the personality needs of the subject.

The actual procedure best employed when the problem is not controlled experimental work consists of giving the subjects a preliminary explanation of what they may expect, thereby correcting any misapprehensions they may have. At the same time this suggests indirectly to them their course of behavior and response. This is followed by a series of suggestions to the effect that they will get tired and sleepy, that they will wish to sleep, and will feel themselves going to sleep, that they will notice increasing lassitude of the body and an increasing feeling of comfort and satisfaction as they continue to sleep until they fall into a deep, sound, restful sleep. Every effort should be made to make the subjects feel comfortable, satisfied, and confident about their ability to go into a trance, and the hypnotist should maintain an attitude of unshaken and contagious confidence in the subject's ability. A simple, earnest, unpretentious, confident manner is of paramount importance, unless one wishes to be a vaudeville performer. Only then are histrionics warranted.

Once the hypnotic trance has been induced, there is need to keep a subject in the trance until the necessary work has been completed. This is best done by instructing the subjects to sleep continuously, to let nothing disturb them, to enjoy their trance state, and above all to enjoy their feeling of comfort, satisfaction, and full confidence in themselves, their situation, and their ability to meet adequately and well any problem or task that may be presented to them.

The awakening of the hypnotic subject is a simple procedure, even with those subjects who willfully insist upon remaining in the trance. Usually, simple instruction to awaken is sufficient. If the subject resists awakening, simple persuasive suggestions will suffice.

Of great importance in inducing trance states and trance behavior is the allotment of sufficient time for the subject to make those neuro- and psychophysiological changes necessary for certain types of behavior. To rush or force a subject often defeats the purpose.

HYPNOTIC PHENOMENA

While certain phenomena are characteristic of the hypnotic trance, their manifestations vary with the individual subject and with the depth of the trance—that is, whether light or deep hypnosis. Even so, phenomena usually found in deep hypnosis may, in the individual subject, occur in light hypnosis and vice versa, depending upon the subject's personality and psychological needs at the time. There is no absolute rule—hence, efforts to describe accurately various levels of trance depth are chiefly of academic interest.

Most normal people develop light hypnosis easily, and at least 70 percent of all subjects, with adequate training—by which is meant repeated hypnosis and thus continued practice in going into the hypnotic state—can develop deep trances.

For medical purposes either the light or the deep trance may be satisfactory, depending upon the nature and the character of the therapeutic goal to be achieved. Also, should the light trance be unsuitable, recourse may at once be had to the progressive induction of a more profound trance. Experience is the only able teacher of what type of trance is necessary, and failure to secure results in the light trance can always be corrected by resorting to the deep trance.

The phenomena of the trance of most interest to the medical man are several. Foremost of these is *rapport,* a condition in which the subject responds only to the hypnotist and is seemingly incapable of hearing, seeing, sensing or responding to anything else unless so instructed by the hypnotist. It is in effect a concentration of the subject's attention upon, and awareness only of, the hypnotist and those things the hypnotist wishes included in the trance situation, and it has the effect of dissociating the subject from all other things. The hypnotist may transfer this rapport by appropriate suggestions.

Catalepsy is a second phenomenom which illustrates clearly the tremendous psychosomatic significance of hypnosis. This is a peculiar state of muscle tonus which parallels *cerea flexibilitas* of the stuporous catatonic patient. The subject holds his arm up in the air, maintains any awkward position given him by the hypnotist, and shows a failure of normal fatigue reactions. Concomitant with it are a loss of the swallowing reflex, a dilatation of the pupils, a loss of facial mobility, and a definite slowing of all psychomotor activity. Yet, upon instructions by the hypnotist, the subject can perform adequately at a motor level equal to the waking capacity and often at a level that transcends it.

Sensory changes, or alterations in sensory behavior, of both a positive and a negative character are frequent and often undetected. Blindness and deafness to things not included in the hypnotic situation often develop to a degree that resists clinical tests. There also occur spontaneously anesthesia, analgesia, and other types of sensory disturbances. Additionally these sensory phenomena can be induced by appropriate suggestion. A detailed account of these types of psychosomatic manifestations has been reported (Erickson, 1943). Their presence is often of great importance in therapy, since they serve so well to make subjects appreciate their trance depth and to direct the hypnotist's attention to unexpected psychosomatic implications that need to be considered in the hypnotic procedure.

Amnesia and other memory alterations constitute another type of hypnotic phenomena of extreme interest to the medical practitioner. Usually after a deep trance subjects have a more or less complete amnesia for all trance events. This amnesia can be controlled by the hypnotist through instruction to the subjects, or the subjects themselves can deliberately set about recovering the amnestic material. In either instance the forgotten memories may be recovered in full or in part according to the instructions given or in accordance with each subject's needs. This amnesia is of profound importance in psychotherapy since it permits the therapist to deal with painful memories without arousing the subject's waking resistance and defensive reactions.

In contradistinction to hypnotic amnesia is the capacity of the hypnotic subjects to develop *hypermnesia*—that is, increased memory ability—and to recover memories of past experiences long forgotten and actually inaccessible in the waking state. Traumatic, painful, forgotten experiences and memories that often constitute a point of origin in serious personality disturbances are frequently readily accessible under hypnosis, can be easily recalled by the patient, and a foundation laid in the trance state for their integration into the waking life of the patient. The importance of the recovery of lost memories in psychotherapy is fully established, and hypnosis often proves a royal road to those memories, although it still leaves the task of integrating that memory into the waking life of the patient a painstaking task for the therapist. In addition to this recovery of past forgotten memories, hypnosis can enable subjects to recover memories of lost experiences in phenomenal and minute detail ordinarily not possible. By such hypermnesia minor clues to a personality disturbance or emotional conflict otherwise not accessible become available.

Based to some degree upon the mechanisms of amnesia and hypermnesia is another phenomenon termed *regression*. By this is meant the capacity of hypnotic subjects, upon suitable suggestions and instructions, to develop an amnesia for a definite period of life and to revivify and reestablish the memories and patterns and habits of an earlier period. Thus, a 25-year-old subject can be induced to develop a profound amnesia for all events of his life subsequent to the age of 15 years and to reassume his actual modes and habits of behavior and response belonging to his 15-year-old level of development.

The actual technique of so reorienting a subject to an earlier age level is complicated and difficult, and the process easily results in errors unless extreme care in suggestion is exercised, nor can regression behavior be accepted too readily and uncritically. However, experimental and therapeutic studies have disclosed the feasibility and usefulness of this procedure, and in addition have shown that profound psychosomatic changes accompany the process. Two such instances are given in the issue of *Psychosomatic Medicine* previously mentioned, and other studies are listed in the bibliography.

Suggestibility, necessarily a primary feature of hypnosis, is always present and constitutes the basic consideration upon which the trance and its attendant phenomena are based. Additionally, suggestibility plays another role after the trance is induced, in that any desired behavior can be suggested to the subject and an adequate performance can be secured, provided that the suggestions are not offensive to the subject. Thus, in the medical situation, the recovery of memories, the development of amnesias, identifications, and anesthesias, the causing of dreams, emotional conflicts, hallucinations, disorientation, and so forth can be produced in the patient during the course of therapy as a measure of meeting problems, developing insights, and reorganizing the psychic life.

Automatic writing and *crystal-gazing,* two somewhat comparable phenomena, both long known but superstitiously regarded, are easily elicited in the trance state and are often of great value in psychotherapy. In response to suggestion the subject writes automatically and without awareness and thus may be induced to uncover amnesic material or to disclose necessary information otherwise inaccessible or which the personality is not yet strong enough to face. Or the subject may see vividly and clearly in a crystal the enactment of long-forgotten traumatic experiences and thus achieve a realization of their actuality and reality to him as a person.

Posthypnotic suggestion is one of the most significant of all hypnotic phenomena. By this measure subjects can be given instructions in the trance to govern their future behavior, but only to a reasonable and acceptable degree. Thus, the subject may be instructed that at some future date he is to perform a certain act. At the specified time the subject executes his bidding, but believes his performance self-ordered and spontaneous. As a therapeutic measure, posthypnotic instructions are of great value, but if improperly used they are ineffectual and futile. They need to be used primarily as a measure of providing the patients with an opportunity to develop insight and to integrate their behavior.

Somnambulism is another form of hypnotic behavior always significant of a deep trance state. In this condition subjects behave and respond as if they were wide awake and may even deceive observers with their seeming wakefulness. This state is the most suitable for the deeper forms of psychotherapy and can be induced by repeated hypnosis in at least 70 percent of all subjects.

THE VALUES OF HYPNOSIS

To the medical doctor, the values of hypnosis in medical science are of first importance. That hypnosis can contribute to the scientific study of human behavior, normal and abnormal, is self-evident, since it permits experimentation and investigation not ordinarily feasible and under conditions difficult or even impossible to obtain in the waking state. Thus, it possesses values of a basic character in the development of a more adequate scientific understanding of the medical problems arising from disturbances in human behavior and adjustment. These values alone would warrant continued hypnotic work.

Additionally, hypnosis possesses other values of paramount interest to the physician as an individual. Foremost of these is the education it gives the physician in understanding, sympathizing and dealing effectually with that vast array of emotional conflicts, fears, anxieties, uncertainties, psychoneurotic complaints and psychosomatic disturbances that constitute so large a part of the problems presented to every medical practitioner. These are problems that cannot be treated with drugs or surgery nor with the simple statement that "there is nothing wrong with you physically."

Such patients are in need of therapy, therapy of the class that falls under the heading of the "art of medicine." This is essentially a physician-patient relationship that permits the physician to enable the patient to capitalize upon every positive thing he has to reach a satisfactory adjustment in life rather than become psychologically invalided.

The physician who learns hypnosis and thus learns how and when and why to give suggestions effectively to hypnotic subjects is literally taking a postgraduate course in how to suggest to patients the attitudes, insights, understandings, and methods of behavior that will enable them to adjust more adequately in life. In the general practice of medicine it is not only the drug dispensed but the physician's manner of handling the patient that constitutes the actual turning point in the patient's illness, his attitude toward himself and toward life. The entire history of medical practice emphasizes the tremendous factor of the human relationship, and physicians who have trained themselves in hypnosis have acquired special experience that stands them in good stead in building up their art of medicine, even though they may not utilize hypnosis directly.

As an actual medical therapeutic procedure, hypnosis possesses definite and demonstrated values. Certain early psychoneuroses, behavior problems, personality maladjustments, circumscribed neuroses, and psychosomatic disturbances are frequently susceptible to intelligently conceived hypnotic psychotherapy. Such therapy, however, should not be directed merely to the alleviation of a symptom or to the forcing of the patient to adopt better adjustment patterns. Therapeutic effects thus achieved are short-lived and account for the majority of failures. Successful hypnotic psychotherapy should be systematically directed to a reeducation of patients, a development of insight into the nature of their problems, and the promotion of their earnest desires to readjust themselves to the realities of life and the problems confronting them. Too often hypnosis is employed simply to relieve a symptom, and there is a failure to capitalize upon the peculiar intense, effective physician-patient relationship engendered by the hypnosis which constitutes the actual point of departure in effecting a psychotherapeutic reordering of the patient's life adjustment and a healthy integration of the personality.

Another field of application now just developing for the utilization of hypnotic therapy lies in the treatment of the acute psychiatric war disturbances occurring in front-line action. Under these conditions present findings indicate that the induction of a deep trance, the building of an intensely satisfying interpersonal relationship between the physician and each patient and then permitting the patients to verbalize in this protected situation their fears and anxieties, their horror and distress, and then to take inventory of themselves, of their self-confidence, their abilities, their ambitions and desires is effecting a high percentage of recovery—as, indeed, might logically be expected.

ILLUSTRATIVE CASE HISTORY

To illustrate the actual application of hypnosis to a specific medical problem, the following case history is presented. This account has been selected because it demonstrates clearly both the medical and the psychological aspects of a total problem reflected in a single symptom which could easily have been the point of departure for a serious, prolonged neurotic disturbance, and also because the account permits the reader to recognize readily the psychological significance and the rationale of each step in the therapy employed. The total time spent in treating the patient was slightly over three hours. Such an expenditure of time was warranted by the nature of the case and justified by the results obtained, and it illustrates the need in hypnotic therapy to allot time as freely as is done in surgery.

That so systematic and elaborate a procedure of hypnotic therapy was necessary for the patient described is open to question. Perhaps a simpler approach would have succeeded, but adequate therapy of the patient was the goal sought, and there was no thought of experimentation to determine how economical of effort the therapist might be in handling this particular problem. Failure in attempts at hypnotic therapy always increases the difficulty of further efforts at therapy. Hence, for the benefit of the individual patient, extensive care and effort is always warranted.

The patient, a woman in her middle thirties, was referred to me by her physician for hypnotic therapy because of hysterical urinary retention of fourteen days' duration, and an increasing neurotic reaction of fright, terror, and panic over her condition. The history secured contained the following significant facts.

She had been recently married after having despaired of marriage for many years because of her belief that she was not physically attractive. Following a brief honeymoon, she had developed an acute nonspecific urethritis and cystitis, which, because of her educational background in medical· science, had frightened her seriously. The infection yielded rapidly to medication, but during the course of her treatment she had been catheterized several times. This had embarrassed and distressed her greatly. Just before her discharge from the hospital as recovered, her husband received notice to report for induction, a notification arriving much sooner than had been anticipated. She reacted to this with intense grief but soon composed herself and began to rearrange her plans for the future.

Some hours thereafter she had found herself unable to void. Repeated futile efforts over a period of several hours had increased her anxiety and discomfort seriously and she had to be catheterized.

Thereafter catheterization twice daily for two weeks was necessary, since various measures of encouragement, reassurance, and sedation failed. The patient responded to this with increasing alarm and terror because of her helplessness. Nor was the general situation helped by the patient's own realization that her symptom might be hysterical, since she regarded hysteria as much worse than an organic disability.

The actual therapeutic procedure was simple. She was given an evening appointment so that ample time free from interruption would be available. The history furnished by her physician was confirmed and elaborated by a casual, comfortable questioning and discussion of the patient's problem as a means of alleviating her anxiety.

She was then sent to the lavatory with firm instruction to discover if her symptoms still persisted and to make certain that she really needed treatment. Thus, she was given the first real doubt about the continuance of her difficulty. To have sent her to the lavatory with instruction to void would have courted therapeutic failure, since inability to obey such a command would seemingly have demonstrated my incapacity to handle her problem. But to be sent to discover if she really needed treatment had the effect of convincing her of my complete confidence in my therapy and of my unwillingness to use it unless actually required. She returned to report that her symptom was still present, whereupon she was asked if she wished me to proceed with therapy. Upon her assent, the explanation was offered that before therapy would be undertaken at all, it would be necessary to discover how capable a hypnotic subject she was as a preliminary to dealing with her problem therapeutically. She expressed some disappointment at this delay in therapeutic hypnosis, but recognized the desirability of permitting me to follow my own procedure.

Accordingly, a light trance was induced and simple hypnotic phenomena elicited, and this was followed by the induction of a fairly deep trance during which the patient was called upon for a continued manifestation of hypnotic phenomena. This procedure was simply a means of teaching her effectively that she could execute hypnotic instructions readily and adequately and constituted a process of building up her confidence in her ability to obey any instructions given to her.

She was then sent to the lavatory in the trance state with firm instructions *not* to empty her bladder but instead to have a bowel movement. However, with careful emphasis, these instructions were qualified by further suggestion that she probably would *not* have a bowel movement, since she really *did not need* to have one, and this idea was stressed repeatedly. Thus, by implication she was given to understand effectively that excretory activity was not a matter of response to hypnotic suggestion, however strong, but *a function of an actual bodily need that could be aided by hypnotic suggestion.* Additionally, the failure to urinate in this situation would have a new and important meaning to the personality—namely, one of obedience to the hypnotist's instructions and not one of personal inability. Also, in relation to the bowel movement, the patient would have the perverse satisfaction, characteristic of neurotic behavior, of failing to obey the therapist's instructions in relation to an unimportant consideration and not in relation to her actual symptom.

The patient obeyed instructions as intended, whereupon the suggestion was offered that she might like to discuss in detail, while still in the trance state, her general immediate life situation. She agreed, and there followed a detailed, systematic, comprehensive, psychotherapeutic discussion and appraisal of her deprecation of her appearance, her despair about ever getting married, her sexual adjustment, her infection and the fears it engendered, her husband's impending induction, and the neurotic utilization of invalidism to escape problems. Every effort was made to give the patient insight into her situation and to organize her thinking constructively so that she would be able to face her problems adequately instead of retreating from them into neurotic illness. However, at no time was any direct psychological interpretation made of her urinary retention. In fact, it was not even mentioned specifically. Instead, reliance was placed upon the patient's own thinking and intelligence to make the proper psychological interpretation of her symptom when she became ready for that realization.

When the patient seemed to have adequate understanding of her situation and its probable significance to her personality, return was made indirectly to her symptom. In the guise of casual conversation she was reminded of the practice of little children at play to suppress the need for urination until the last possible moment and then to rush frantically to the bathroom where any unexpected delay would result in a wetting of their clothes.

As soon as the patient understood this general statement, she was asked with much urgency to tell me approximately how long it would take her to reach her home after I dismissed her, what route she would follow, an approximation of the distance from the pavement to the front door, the location and the length of the stairway leading upstairs, and how far down the upstairs hallway the bathroom was located.

When the patient had given this information as accurately as she could she was given a rapid series of urgent, strongly persuasive suggestions to the effect that:

1. She would leave for home feeling generally comfortable and at ease and not thinking about anything specific but just simply absorbed in quietly enjoying the ride home.
2. That during the last 20 minutes of the trip home there would come to her mind vague fears that she might wet herself, which she would promptly suppress, only to have them recur with increasing frequency and insistency until finally they would become an annoying and even distressing conviction that if she did not arrive home soon she would surely wet herself.
3. That the last five minutes of the trip home she would spend in a state of feverish anxiety and that she would be unable to think of anything except whether she would be able to hold out long enough to rush through the door, up the stairway, and into the bathroom where she then could relax completely and be comfortable all over.
4. That when she was relaxed and was comfortable all over, she could then have a full recollection and understanding and memory of all those things she needed to know to meet her life situation without handicaps.

These suggestions were given repetitiously, urgently and with great rapidity until it was certain the subject understood them sufficiently well to execute them. Then, after instruction to have amnesia for all trance events and suggestions, she was awakened and promptly dismissed.

Her husband, who had accompanied her, was instructed to drive home quietly, commenting only on the beauty of the night, acceding to any demands of his wife that he drive faster but to keep within the speed limits, and asking no questions of any sort.

Subsequent reports from the husband, the patient, and the referring physician disclosed the effectiveness of these suggestions and success of the therapy, both in relation to her symptom and her adjustment to her husband's military status. Inquiry a year later disclosed no recurrence of her problem.

CONCLUSION

To summarize, the age-old attitude of superstitious awe, fear, incredulity, and antagonism toward hypnosis is now being rapidly replaced by an appreciation of its scientific values. In its place is a growing, constructive recognition of hypnosis as both a therapeutic medical procedure and a means of acquiring a sympathetic understanding and appreciation of human nature and behavior requisite to the adequate practice of psychotherapy and the art of medicine.

3. Hypnotic Techniques for the Therapy of Acute Psychiatric Disturbances in War

Milton H. Erickson

Ever since the first primitive medicine man attempted to use hyponosis in some form to treat his savage patients, there has persisted a general tendency to regard hypnosis, its techniques, its methods, and its applications as something beyond the ken of common man, as mysterious, magical, and occult, based upon and derived from special powers, a ritual of mystical passes and an abracadabra of verbal commands. Only recently has the rapid growth of scientific interest in hypnotism made possible the recognition of hypnosis as a special and highly significant intrapersonal state or condition clinically important, deriving from interpersonal relationships and valuable for both intra- and interpersonal significances. Also, there has been a progressive realization that practically all normal people as well as many of those suffering from certain types of mental disturbances can be hypnotized under proper circumstances; and, similarly, that anyone reasonably interested and intelligent can learn to hypnotize even as anyone can learn to do surgery. Special talents and abilities, other than a reasonable degree of aptitude, are necessary only to achieve historical prominence. In other words, the field of hypnosis is open to any person willing to qualify by interest, study and experience, and the intelligent use of hypnosis depends essentially upon a background and foundation of personal interest and training.

The technique for the induction of hypnotic trances is primarily a function of the interpersonal relationships existing between subject and hypnotist. Hence, hypnotic techniques and procedures should vary according to the subject, circumstances, and the purposes to be served. Furthermore, since hypnosis is dependent fundamentally upon the subject's cooperativeness and his willingness to be hypnotized, any technique eliciting the necessary cooperation is adequate in this highly specialized interpersonal relationship. Indeed, competent hypnotists avoid any rigidity in technique and properly adapt it to the personality needs of their subjects in the immediate situation.

A variety of individual approaches may be employed, but they need to

Read at the Centenary Meeting of The American Psychiatric Association, Philadelphia, Pa., May 15-18, 1944 and reprinted with permission from the *American Journal of Psychiatry*, 1945, *101*, 668-672.

be directed especially to the development in the subject of full confidence and security in the hypnotist, his willingness to participate in any legitimate procedure and his readiness to yield to an experience which is understandable, though perhaps painfully, of value to him as a personality. To this end, some subjects need to feel themselves dominated by the hypnotist, others want to be coaxed or persuaded, some wish to go into the trance as a result of joint cooperative endeavor, and there are those who wish, or more properly need, to be overwhelmed by a wealth of repetitious suggestions guiding every response they make. The actual interpersonal relationship established between subject and hypnotist may be one purely of authority-subservience, of father-child, or more frequently physician-patient. In the armed forces, however, hypnotists occupy a position of special vantage. They combine the significant prestige of both an officer and a physician, and this is further enhanced by the training of the ranks in habitual, unquestioning obedience, which leads easily to the ready acceptance of hypnotic suggestions. However, in this regard, much more is to be accomplished when medical officers minimize their authoritarian status as officers and deal with their patient primarily at a medical level, thereby transforming their authority into additional prestige as a physician concerned not with authority but with professional interest and effort.

Another important consideration in inducing trances, especially among members of the armed forces, where group relationships predominate, is the utilization of the group situation itself. Even among civilians, where greater emphasis is placed upon individualism, the induction of a trance in the group situation, aside from the exceptional case, decreases the time and effort required and leads to a more rapid and better training of the individual subject. Especially is this true when a trained or unusually capable subject is used as an object lesson for the group. Even those subjects who resist hypnosis in a group situation respond privately much more readily after having observed group trance behavior.

The use of drugs to induce hypnotic trances is often feasible in excited, fearful, emotionally unstable, disturbed, or unconsciously uncooperative patients. Alcohol, paraldehyde, the barbiturates, and even morphine can be used, although alcohol is the drug of preference because of its rapid transient effects, its relief of inhibitions and anxieties, and the absence of narcotic effects. Although in certain cases narcotic drugs are decidedly useful, there is always the possibility of narcotic effects masking or excluding hypnotic responses. However, experience and clinical judgment are the means of learning how and when to use drugs as an adjunct to hypnosis.

Trance states for therapeutic purposes may be either light or deep, depending upon such factors as the patient's personality, the nature of the problem, and the stage of therapeutic progress. Sometimes light hypnosis is all that is needed even in a severe problem, and sometimes deep hypnosis is required for a relatively mild disturbance. Clinical experience and judgment are the best determinants, and there is always the possibility of recourse to the other type of trance in case of failure to achieve results.

Another highly significant general consideration in the medical use of hypnosis, often overlooked or completely disregarded, is its striking usefulness even when it is not the indicated therapeutic procedure. This usefulness lies in its effectiveness in building up patient morale and in establishing a physician-patient relationship of profound trust, confidence, and security that so often constitutes a vital factor in helping the patient to adjust adequately to the problems of invalidism. Especially is this so when the invalidism involves serious psychic distress, anxiety, and fear such as characterize the acute psychiatric disturbances of war.

An illustrative example, cited from personal experience to demonstrate the usefulness of hypnosis when not the indicated therapy, is the instance of a recovered drug addict hospitalized for major surgery. She developed an acute anxiety state, was unable to sleep, and refused sedative or narcotic medication because of her intense fear that it might lead to a recurrence of her drug addiction. Sympathetic interest, reassurance, and postponement of the operation for another day failed to lessen her panic reactions. The induction of a hypnotic trance with extensive posthypnotic suggestions governing sleep; the development of an emotional feeling of comfort, security, and trust; and the induction of subsequent trances resulted in an uneventful pre- and postoperative course of events.

The actual technique for inducing hypnotic trances varies greatly from one hypnotist to another and from one subject to the next. No set, rigid technique can be followed with good success since, in medical hypnosis, the personality needs of the individual subject must be met, and such is the purpose of hypnosis rather than the mere induction of a trance. Additionally, there is an equally important need for the hypnotist to use that technique which permits him to express himself most satisfactorily and effectively in the special interpersonal relationship which constitutes hypnosis.

The procedure most uniformly successful in initiating hypnosis consists in prefacing the actual induction of the trance by a simple, informative discussion of hypnosis as a scientific medical phenomenon, taking care to develop the patient's interest in it as a personal experience. During such discussion patients should be given opportunity to express their attitudes, fears, misconceptions of hypnosis; simple, unpersuasive explanations, corrections, and reassurances can be offered. Also, such a discussion is an effective means of giving the intended subjects a wealth of information and suggestions to govern their own hypnotic responses.

The group approach is an effective manner of accomplishing this, despite its seemingly time-taking and laborious nature. My procedure, which is also being used by several former associates now in the army and employing hypnosis therapeutically for acute psychiatric war disturbances, consists in presenting before a group of 10 to 30 interested persons, among whom are intended hypnotic patients, a comprehensive lecture and a demonstration of hypnosis, using first a trained subject and then volunteer subjects.

The results obtained are invariably profitable. A favorable and appreciative attitude toward hypnosis is engendered; new subjects useful in the future are secured; fears, doubts and misconceptions are dispelled; and the intended hypnotic patients develop a most helpful, satisfying sense of comfort and confidence in hypnosis.

How successful this approach may be is shown by the following instance. After a lecture and demonstration before a group of 15 persons, 12 of whom were intended for future intensive hypnotic work, it was possible to begin the proposed work with all 12 subjects without further individual preparation. While such success is not always to be achieved, the sense of belonging to the group, the freedom to participate or merely to observe, the visual instruction afforded, and the opportunity to identify with the subjects employed are potent factors in securing the confidence, cooperation, and rapport necessary to hypnotize the individual subject. While this approach is not always applicable, my tendency is to rely upon it as often as possible.

The procedure of the trance induction with the individual subject is relatively simple after the preliminary establishment of rapport and confidence. A series of suggestions is given to the effect that the subjects will feel themselves relaxed, tired and sleepy, that they will become increasingly tired and will wish to sleep and will feel themselves beginning to go to sleep, and that as this continues they will want, with progressive intensity, to enjoy more and more the comfort and satisfaction of a deep, sound, restful sleep in which their only desire is to sleep with no other interest than to enjoy that sleep.

A second step of technique I have found of immense value, and which I usually employ concomitantly with the sleep suggestions, is the development of the subject's own feeling of active participation in the process of going into a trance. The reason for this is that in medical hypnosis there is a great need for the patient to participate actively in any reorganization of his psychic life. Hence his behavior should not be limited to the level of passive receptiveness and responsiveness so often mistakenly assumed to be all that hypnosis permits.

To secure active participation, hand levitation suggestions are given as the first step. That is, the subject is told that, as he goes to sleep, his hand will gradually and involuntarily begin to lift up in the air. This he may not notice at first, but when he does become aware of it, he will find fimself tremendously interested and absorbed in sensing and enjoying that effortless, involuntary movement of his hand and arm. Thus, the subject is given the opportunity of observing his hypnotic response as a personal experience that is occurring within himself. There follow suggestions that soon the direction of the hand movement will change, that he is to be greatly interested in discovering what the new direction may be. This suggestion does result in an alteration of the hand movement, an alteration recognized by the subject as not determined in direction by specific hypnotic suggestions but determined by the continuing processes within himself as a hypnotic subject. This gives him a growing realization of his active participation in a progressive intrapsychic experience in which he plays an undefined but definite directive role governed by forces within him.

This can be followed by suggestions directing the subject's attention to those other possible psychosomatic manifestations characteristic of hypnotic behavior, reported upon previously (Erickson, 1943a, b, c, d) with the result that the subjects become absorbed in sensing their own psychosomatic phenomena as a personal experience in which they are active. Thus the situation is transformed from one of passive responsiveness for the patient to one of active interest, discovery, investigation, and participation in these changes produced by hypnosis. This is further enhanced by his realization that these changes in him are the result of his response to hypnosis itself and that they are occurring within him and are not forced upon him by specific suggestions. Thus, from intrapsychic evidence he has full opportunity to understand hypnosis as a significant and vital personality experience.

The crucial step of bridging the gap between light hypnosis and a deep trance can often be accomplished easily by letting the subject assume the entire responsibility for this further progress instead of resorting to the use of overwhelming, compelling suggestions by the hypnotist.

The method I usually employ is to suggest that the subject continue to sleep more and more deeply and to his own satisfaction and that, as he does so, his hand—automatically, involuntarily, and perhaps without his knowledge—will slowly move up and touch his face. However, his hand will not and must not touch his face until he is in a deep trance. Then, the touching of his face will be merely a signal for his own realization that he is in a profound trance.

Thus, suggestions are given to the subject, but the execution of them, the rapidity and time of response, and their effectiveness are made the responsibility of the subject, and they are contingent upon processes taking place within him and related to his own needs. In this way the suggestions are made to serve a more important function than that of eliciting passive obedience to the hypnotist. Consequently, hypnosis becomes a vital personality experience in which the hypnotist plays primarily the role of an instrument, merely guiding or directing processes developing within the subject.

This measure of securing the hypnotic subject's participation in the development of responses to suggestions is of value not only in inducing trances but also in eliciting hypnotic behavior of all sorts, whether simple experimental phenomena or therapeutic objectives. Indeed, in medical hypnosis the result obtained should derive primarily from the subject's activity and participation since it is his needs and problems that must be met.

Too often the unwarranted, unsound assumption is made that, because hypnosis can be induced by suggestion, whatever develops from the trance must be completely the result of suggestion and is only expressive of suggestions, that hypnosis as a special psychological state is in itself of no importance, and that what the hypnotist says, does, and understands is all-important. However, in the hypnotic situation the factor of paramount importance is hypnosis as a potent personality experience of peculiar and special importance to the subject.

This discussion of technique should demonstrate that the hypnotic subject can participate actively in his own hypnotic trance in an indefinite but nonetheless signigicant manner, and in direct relation to his own needs; and that hypnotic technique oriented to this understanding can resonably offer the hypnotic patient an opportunity to deal with his own needs and problems in accord with his own psychological structure and experiences.

The reasons for this exposition of hypnotic technique are several. Personal experience with acute personality disturbances and the experience of former associates now in the army employing hypnosis for the therapy of acute psychiatric war disturbances suggest the value of much more extensive utilization of hypnosis as a therapeutic procedure. Also, hypnosis lends itself readily to easy and repeated use and requires no equipment other than training and experience. Additionally, it gives the patient an opportunity to reassociate and reorganize the psychological complexities and disturbances of his psychic life under special conditions that permit him to deal with his problems constructively, free from overwhelming distress.

In the actual application to acute psychiatric disturbances hypnosis can reasonably be expected to offer several therapeutically significant advantages.

Experience to date with narcosis therapy, which is proving a most useful procedure, has indicated the great importance of the interpersonal relationship of physician and patient. In this connection hypnosis as a means of building up a favorable rapport between patient and physician can scarcely be equaled.

Experience also shows that narcosis therapy without verbalization by the patient of his fears and anxieties is ineffective. The hypnotic state can give the patient this same important avenue of self-expression without the handicap of narcotic effects and even make possible for him the verbalization of traumatic material otherwise repressed and unavailable to him.

Also, properly oriented, hypnotic therapy can give the patient that necessary understanding of his own role in effecting his recovery and thus enlist his own effort and participation in his own cure without giving him a sense of dependence upon drugs and medical care. Indeed, hypnosis offers the patient a sense of comfort and an attitude of interest in his own active participation in his therapy.

Probably of even greater significance is the opportunity hypnosis gives the patient to dissociate himself from his problems, to take an objective view of himself, to make an inventory of his assets and abilities, and then, one by one, to deal with his problems instead of being overwhelmed with all of them without being able to think clearly in any direction. Hypnosis offers an opportunity to control and direct thinking, to select or exclude memories and ideas, and thus to give the patient the opportunity to deal individually and adequately with any selected item of experience.

Finally, hypnosis offers both to the patient and the therapist a ready access to the patient's unconscious mind. It permits a direct dealing with those unconscious forces which underlie personality disturbances, and it allows a recognition of those items of individual life experience significant to the personality and to which full consideration must be given if psychotherapeutic results are to be achieved. Hypnosis alone can give the ready, prompt, and extensive access to the unconscious, which the history of psychotherapy has shown to be so important in the therapy of acute personality disturbances.

4. Hypnotic Psychotherapy

Milton H. Erickson

Since the most primitive times hypnosis has been employed almost universally in the practice of religious and medical rites to intensify belief in mysticism, magic, and medicine. The impressive, bewildering character of hypnotic manifestations and the profoundly inexplicable, seemingly miraculous psychological effects upon human behavior achieved by the use of hypnosis, have served to bring about two general contradictory attitudes toward it. The first of these is the unscientific attitude of superstitious awe, fear, disbelief and actual hostility, all of which have delayed and obstructed the growth of scientific knowledge of hypnosis.

The second attitude is one of scientific acceptance of hypnosis as a legitimate and valid psychological phenomenon, of profound importance and significance in the investigation and understanding of human behavior, and of the experiential life of the individual. This attitude had its first beginnings with the work of Anton Mesmer in 1775, who tempered his scientific approach to an understanding of hypnosis by mystical theories. Nevertheless, Mesmer did succeed in demonstrating the usefulness and effectiveness of hypnosis in the treatment of certain types of patients otherwise unresponsive to medical care. Thus he laid the foundation for the therapeutic use of hypnosis and for the recognition of psychotherapy as a valid psychological medical procedure.

Since then there has been a long succession of clinically trained men who demonstrated the usefulness of hypnosis as a therapeutic medical procedure and as a means of examining, understanding and reeducating human behavior. Among these was James Braid, a Scotch physician who, in 1841, first discredited the superstitious mystical ideas about the nature of hypnosis, or "mesmerism," as it was then called. Braid recognized the phenomenon as a normal psychological manifestation, coined the terms of "hypnosis" and "hypnotism," and devised a great variety of scientific experimental studies to determine its medical and psychological values.

Following Braid, many outstanding scientists, including both clinicians and later psychologists, accepted his findings and contributed increasingly to the scientific development of hypnosis despite the hampering heritage

Reprinted with permission from *The Medical Clinics of North America*, May, 1948, New York Number.

of traditional misconceptions, fears, and hostilities that have surrounded it
and still do among the uninformed.

As yet, a scientific knowledge of hypnosis is still in its infancy. Theories
of its nature are too general and too inadequate. Methods of application
constitute a problem warranting extensive investigation. A general
appreciation of the need to integrate hypnotic studies with current
knowledge is only slowly developing. The types of disorders for which it is
best suited are still undetermined. New variations in techiques need to be
developed.

As for the utilization of hypnosis in psychotherapy, this too, is still in its
infancy. Traditions and traditional ways of thinking, the rigid self-
sufficiency of various schools of psychotherapy, and the human tendency
to fear the new and untried have hampered studies in this field. Only
during the past 25 years has there been an increasing number of studies
demonstrating hypnosis to be of outstanding value in investigating the
nature and structure of the personality, in understanding normal and
abnormal behavior, in studying interpersonal and intrapersonal relationships and psychosomatic interrelationships. Also, there have been extensive developments in the utilization of hypnosis as an effective instrument
for psychotherapy. During the Second World War there was a tremendous
increase in the recognition and utilization of hypnosis as a valuable form
of psychotherapy.

Any discussion of hypnotic psychotherapy or hypnotherapy requires an
explication of certain general considerations derived directly from clinical
observation. In the following pages an effort will be made to indicate
some of the misconceptions, inadequate understandings, oversights, and
failures of differentiation which hamper or militate against the acceptance
and usefulness of hypnotherapy. Also, material will be given to illustrate
techniques, and explanations of their use will be given.

DIFFERENTIATION BETWEEN TRANCE INDUCTION
AND TRANCE STATE

One of the first considerations in undertaking hypnotic psychotherapy
centers around the differentiation of the patient's experience of having a
trance induced from the experience of being in a trance state. As an
analogy, the train trip to the city is one order of experience; being in the
city is another. To continue, the process of inducing a trance should be
regarded as a method of teaching patients a new manner of learning
something, and thereby enabling them to discover unrealized capacities to
learn, and to act in new ways which may be applied to other and different
things. The importance of trance induction as an educational procedure in

acquainting patients with their latent abilities has been greatly disregarded.

Both the therapist and the patient need to make this differentiation, the former in order to guide the patient's behavior more effectively, the latter in order to learn to distinguish between conscious and unconscious behavior patterns. During trance induction the patient's behavior is comprised of both conscious and unconscious patterns, while the behavior of the trance state should be primarily of unconscious origin.

The failure of such distinction or differentiation between the induction and the trance often results in patients attempting to perform the work of the trance state in the same fashion as they learned to develop a trance. That is, without proper differentiation, patients will utilize both conscious and unconscious behavior in the trance instead of relying primarily upon unconscious patterns of behavior. This leads to inadequate, faulty task performance.

Although patients can, and frequently do, make this distinction spontaneously, the responsibility, though often overlooked, rests properly with the therapist. To ensure such differentiation, the trance induction should be emphasized as a preparation of the patient for another type of experience in which new learnings will be utilized for other purposes and in a different way. This education of patients can be achieved best, as experience has shown, by teaching them how to become good hypnotic subjects, familiar with all types of hypnotic phenomena. This should be done before any attempt is made at therapy. Such training, while it postpones the initiation of direct therapy, actually hastens the progress of therapy since it gives the patient wider opportunities for self-expression. For example, the patient who can develop hypnotic hallucinations, both visual and auditory, manifest regressive behavior, do automatic writing, act upon posthypnotic suggestions, and dream upon command is in an advantageous position for the reception of therapy.

As for the trance state itself, this should be regarded as a special, unique, but wholly normal psychological state. It resembles sleep only superficially, and it is characterized by various physiological concomitants, and by a functioning of the personality at a level of awareness other than the ordinary or usual state of awareness. For convenience in conceptualization, this special state, or level of awareness, has been termed "unconscious" or "subconscious." The role in hypnotic psychotherapy of this special state of awareness is that of permitting and enabling patients to react, uninfluenced by their conscious mind, to their past experiential life and to a new order of experience which is about to occur as they participate in the therapeutic procedure. This participation in therapy by the patients constitutes the primary requisite for effective results.

ROLE OF SUGGESTION IN HYPNOSIS

The next consideration concerns the general role of suggestion in hypnosis. Too often the unwarranted and unsound assumption is made that, since a trance state is induced and maintained by suggestion, and since hypnotic manifestations can be elicited by suggestion, whatever develops from hypnosis must necessarily be completely a result of suggestion and primarily an expression of it.

Contrary to such misconceptions, the hypnotized person remains the same person. His or her behavior only is altered by the trance state, but even so, that altered behavior derives from the life experience of the patient and not from the therapist. At the most the therapist can influence only the manner of self-expression. The induction and maintenance of a trance serve to provide a special psychological state in which patients can reassociate and reorganize their inner psychological complexities and utilize their own capacities in a manner in accord with their own experiential life. Hypnosis does not change people nor does it alter their past experiential life. It serves to permit them to learn more about themselves and to express themselves more adequately.

Direct suggestion is based primarily, if unwittingly, upon the assumption that whatever develops in hypnosis derives from the suggestions given. It implies that the therapist has the miraculous power of effecting therapeutic changes in the patient, and disregards the fact that therapy results from an inner resynthesis of the patient's behavior achieved by the patient himself. It is true that direct suggestion can effect an alteration in the patient's behavior and result in a symptomatic cure, at least temporarily. However, such a "cure" is simply a response to the suggestion and does not entail that reassociation and reorganization of ideas, understandings, and memories so essential for an actual cure. It is this experience of reassociating and reorganizing his own experiential life that eventuates in a cure, not the manifestation of responsive behavior which can, at best, satisfy only the observer.

For example, anesthesia of the hand may be suggested directly, and a seemingly adequate response may be made. However, if the patient has not spontaneously interpreted the command to include a realization of the need for inner reorganization, that anesthesia will fail to meet clinical tests and will be a pseudo-anesthesia.

An effective anesthesia is better induced, for example, by initiating a train of mental activity within the patient himself by suggesting that he recall the feeling of numbness experienced after a local anesthetic, or after a leg or arm went to sleep, and then suggesting that he can now experience a similar feeling in his hand. By such an indirect suggestion the patient is enabled to go through those difficult inner processes of disorganizing, reorganizing, reassociating, and projecting of inner real experience to meet the requirements of the suggestion, and thus the induced anesthesia becomes a part of his experiential life instead of a simple, superficial response.

The same principles hold true in psychotherapy. The chronic alcoholic can be induced by direct suggestion to correct his habits temporarily, but not until he goes through the inner process of reassociating and reorganizing his experiential life can effective results occur.

In other words, hypnotic psychotherapy is a learning process for the patient, a procedure of reeducation. Effective results in hypnotic psychotherapy, or hypnotherapy, derive only from the patient's activities. The therapist merely stimulates the patient into activity, often not knowing what that activity may be, and then guides the patient and exercises clinical judgment in determining the amount of work to be done to achieve the desired results. How to guide and to judge constitute the therapist's problem, while the patient's task is that of learning through his own efforts to understand his experiential life in a new way. Such reeducation is, of course, necessarily in terms of the patient's life experiences, his understandings, memories, attitudes, and ideas; it cannot be in terms of the therapist's ideas and opinions. For example, in training a gravid patient to develop anesthesia for eventual delivery, use was made of the suggestions outlined above as suitable. The attempt failed completely even though she had previously experienced local dental anesthesia and also her legs "going to sleep." Accordingly, the suggestion was offered that she might develop a generalized anesthesia in terms of her own experiences when her body was without sensory meaning to her. This suggestion was intentionally vague since the patient, knowing the purpose of the hypnosis, was enabled by the vagueness of the suggestion to make her own selection of those items of personal experience that would best enable her to act upon the suggestion.

She responded by reviewing mentally the absence of any memories of physical stimuli during physiological sleep, and by reviewing her dreams of walking effortlessly and without sensation through closed doors and walls and floating pleasantly through the air as a disembodied spirit looking happily down upon her sleeping, unfeeling body. By means of this review she was able to initiate a process of reorganization of her experiential life. As a result she was able to develop a remarkably effective anesthesia which met fully the needs of the subsequent delivery. Not until sometime later did the therapist learn by what train of thought he had initiated the neuro-psycho-physiological processes by which she achieved anesthesia.

SEPARATENESS OF CONSCIOUS AND
SUBCONSCIOUS LEVELS OF AWARENESS

Another common oversight in hypnotic psychotherapy lies in the lack of appreciation of the separateness of the possible mutual exclusiveness of the conscious and the unconscious (or subconscious) levels of awareness. Yet all of us have had the experience of having a word or a name "on the tip of the tongue" but being unable to remember it so that it remained unavailable and inaccessible in the immediate situation. Nevertheless, full knowledge actually existed within the unconscious, but unavailably so to the conscious mind.

In hypnotic psychotherapy too often suitable therapy may be given to the unconscious, but with the failure by the therapist to appreciate the tremendous need of either enabling the patient to integrate the unconscious with the conscious or of making the new understandings of the unconscious fully accessible, upon need, to the conscious mind. Comparable to this failure would be an appendectomy with failure to close the incision. It is in this regard that many armchair critics naively denounce hypnotic psychotherapy as without value, since "it deals only with the unconscious." Additionally, there is even more oversight of the fact, repeatedly demonstrated by clinical experience, that in some aspects of the patient's problem direct reintegration under the guidance of the therapist is desirable; in other aspects the unconscious should merely be made available to the conscious mind, thereby permitting a spontaneous reintegration free from any immediate influence by the therapist. Properly, hypnotherapy should be oriented equally about the conscious and unconscious, since the integration of the total personality is the desired goal in psychotherapy.

However, the above does not necessarily mean that integration must constantly keep step with the progress of the therapy. One of the greatest advantages of hypnotherapy lies in the opportunity to work independently with the unconscious without being hampered by the reluctance, or sometimes actual inability, of the conscious mind to accept therapeutic gains. For example, a patient had full unconscious insight into her periodic nightmares of an incestuous character from which she suffered, but as she spontaneously declared in the trance, "I understand those horrible dreams, but I couldn't possibly tolerate such an understanding consciously." By this utterance the patient demonstrated the protectiveness of the unconscious for the conscious. Utilization of this protectiveness as a motivating force enabled the patient subsequently to accept consciously her unconscious insights.

Experimental investigation has repeatedly demonstrated that good unconscious understandings allowed to become conscious before a conscious readiness exists will result in conscious resistance, rejection, repression and even the loss, through repression, of unconscious gains. By working separately with the unconscious there is then the opportunity to temper and to control the patient's rate of progress and thus to effect a reintegration in the manner acceptable to the conscious mind.

ILLUSTRATIVE CASE HISTORY

A 28-year-old-married man sought therapy because he believed implicitly that he did not love his wife and that he had married her only because she resembled superficially his mother, to whom he was strongly attached. In the trance state he affirmed this belief. During hypnotherapy he learned, in the trance state, that his marital problem had arisen from an intense mother-hatred disguised as oversolicitude and that his wife's superficial resemblance to the mother rendered her an excellent target for his manifold aggressions. Any attempt to make his unconscious understandings conscious confronted him with consciously unendurable tasks of major revisions in all of his interpersonal relationships and a recognition of his mother-hatred, which to him seemed to be both intolerable and impossible.

In psychotherapy other than hypnotic, the handling by the patient of such a problem as this would meet with many conscious resistances, repressions, rationalizations, and efforts to reject any insight. The hypnotherapeutic procedures employed to correct this problem will be given in some detail below. No attempt will be made to analyze the underlying dynamics of the patient's problem, since the purpose of this paper is to explicate methods of procedure, new techniques, the utilization of mental mechanisms, and the methods of guiding and controlling the patient's progress so that unconscious insight becomes consciously acceptable.

Early in the course of this patient's treatment it had been learned that he did not consciously dare to look closely at his mother, that he did not know the color of his mother's eyes or the fact that she wore dentures, and that a description of his mother was limited to "she is so gentle and graceful in her movements, and her voice is so soft and gentle, and she had such a sweet, kind, gracious expression on her face that a miserable neurotic failure like me does not deserve all the things she has done for me."

When, during hypnotherapy, he had reached a stage at which his unconscious understandings and insights seemed to be reasonably sufficient to permit the laying of a foundation for the development of conscious understandings, he was placed in a profound somnambulistic trance. He was then induced to develop a profound amnesia for all aspects of his problem and a complete amnesia for everything about his mother and his wife, except the realization that he must have had a mother. This amnesia included also his newly acquired unconscious understandings.

There are special reasons for the induction of such a profound amnesia or repression. One is that obedience to such a suggestion constitutes a relinquishing of control to the therapist of the patient's repression tendencies. Also, it implies to the patient that if the therapist can repress, he also can restore. In undertaking hynotherapy it is important in the early stages to have the patient develop an amnesia for some innocuous memory, then to restore that memory along with some other unimportant but forgotten memory. Thus, an experiential background is laid for the future recovery of vital repressed material.

The other reason is that such an amnesia or induced repression clears the slate for a reassociation and reorganization of ideas, attitudes, feelings, memories, and experiences. In other words, the amnesia enables patients to be confronted with material belonging to their own experiential lives but which, because of the induced repression, is not recognized by them as such. Then it becomes possible for those patients to reach a critical objective understanding of unrecognized material from their own life experience, to reorganize and reassociate it in accord with its reality significances and their own personality needs. Even though the material has been repressed from both the working unconscious and the conscious, personality needs still exist and any effort to deal with the material presented will be in relationship to their personality needs. As an analogy, the child on a calcium-deficient diet knows nothing about calcium deficiency or calcium content but, nevertheless shows a marked preference for calcium-rich food.

After the induction of the amnesia, the next step was a seemingly casual, brief discussion of the meaning of feminine names. Then it was suggested that he see, sitting in the chair on the other side of the room, a strange woman who would converse with him and about whom he would know nothing except for a feeling of firm conviction that her first name was Nelly. Previous hypnotic training at the beginning of hypnotherapy had prepared him for this type of experience.

The patient's response to that particular name, as intended, was that of a hallucination of his mother whom he could not, because of the amnesia, recognize as such. He was induced to carry on an extensive conversation with this hallucinatory figure, making many inquiries along lines pertinent to his own problem. He described her adequately and objectively. He was asked to "speculate" upon her probable life history and the possible reasons therefor. He was asked to relate to the therapist in detail all that

Nelly "said" and to discuss this material fully. Thus, careful guidance by the therapist enabled him to review objectively, critically, and with free understanding a great wealth of both pleasant and unpleasant material, disclosing his relationships to his mother and his comprehension of what he believed to be her understandings of the total situation. Thus he was placed in a situation permitting the development of a new frame of reference at variance with the repressed material of his life experience, but which would permit a reassociation, an elaboration, a reorganization, and an integration of his experiential life.

In subsequent therapeutic sessions a similar procedure was followed, separately, with two other hallucinated figures, "spoken of" by Nelly as her son Henry and his wife Madge, neither of whom the patient could recognize because of his induced amnesia.

The hypnotic session with Henry was greatly prolonged since Henry "told" the patient a great wealth of detailed information which the patient discussed with the therapist freely and easily and with excellent understanding. The patient's interview with the hallucinatory Madge was similarly conducted.

Of tremendous importance in the eventual therapeutic result was the patient's report upon the emotional behavior he "observed" in the hallucinated figures as they related their stories, and his own objective, dispassionate appraisal of "their own emotions."

To explain this procedure it must be recognized that all of the material the patient "elicited" from the hallucinatory figures was only the projection of the repressed material of his own experience. Even though a profound repression for all aspects of his problem had been induced, that material still existed and could be projected upon others, since the projection would not necessarily lead to recognition. To illustrate from everyday experience, those personality traits disliked by the self are easily repressed from conscious awareness and are readily recognized in others or projected upon others. Thus, a common mental mechanism was employed to give the patient a view of himself which could be accepted and integrated into his total understandings.

The culminating step in this procedure consisted in having him hallucinate Nelly and Henry together, Madge and Henry, Nelly and Madge, and finally all three together. Additionally, he was induced to develop each of these various hallucinations in a great number of different life settings known from his history to be traumatic, such as a shopping trip with his wife which had resulted in a bitter quarrel over a minor matter, a dinner table scene, and a quarrel between his wife and his mother.

Thus the patient, as an observant, objective, judicious third person, through the mechanisms of repression and projection, viewed freely, but without recognition, a panorama of his own experiential life, a panorama which permitted the recognition of faults and distortions without the blinding effects of emotional bias.

In the next session, again in a profound somnambulistic trance, he was emphatically instructed to remember clearly, in full detail, everything he had seen, heard, thought, and speculated upon and appraised critically in relationship to Nelly, Henry, and Madge. To this he agreed readily and interestedly. Next he was told to single out various traumatic incidents and to wonder—at first vaguely, and then with increasing clarity—whether or not a comparable incident had ever occurred in his life. As he did this, he was to have the privilege of remembering any little thing necessary in his own history. Thus he was actually given indirect instructions to break down by slow degrees the induced amnesia or repression previously established.

The patient began this task slowly, starting with the simple declaration that a cup on the table, in a dinner scene he had hallucinated, very closely resembled one he had had since childhood. He next noted that he and Henry had the same first name, wondered briefly what Henry's last name was, then hastily observed that Madge and Henry evidently lived in the same town as he did, inasmuch as he had recognized the store in which they quarreled so foolishly. He commented on Nelly's dentures and, with some reluctance, related his fears of dentists and of losing his teeth, and being forced to put up a "false front." As he continued his remarks, he became more and more revealing. Gradually he tended to single out the more strongly emotional items, spacing them with intervening comments upon relatively innocuous associations. After more than an hour of this type of behavior, he began to have slips of the tongue, which he would immediately detect; he became tense, and then, upon reassurance by the therapist, would continue his task. For example, in comparing Nelly's light-brown eyes with Madge's dark-brown eyes, he made the additional comment, "My wife's eyes are like Madge's." As he concluded his statement, he showed a violent startle reaction and, in a tone of intense surprise, repeated questioningly. "My wife?" After a moment's hesitation he remarked to himself, "I know I'm married. I have a wife. Her name is Madge. She has brown eyes like Madge. But that is all I know. I can't remember any more—nothing—nothing!" Then, with an expression of much anxiety and fear, he turned to the therapist and asked pleadingly, "Is there something wrong with me?"

Shortly he discovered the similarity between Nelly and his mother, then continued, with excellent understanding, by appraising Nelly as an unhappy neurotic woman deserving normal consideration and affection. This led to the sudden statement: "That applies to my mother too—Good God, Nelly is my mother, only I was seeing her for the first time—her eyes are brown—like Madge's. My wife's eyes are brown—her name is Madge—Madge is my wife."

There followed then a whole series of fragmentary remarks relating to traumatic situations, of which the following are examples:

"The fight at the store—that coat she bought—we almost broke our engagement—birthday cake—shoestring broke—Good God, what can I ever say to her?" After each utterance he seemed to be absorbed in recalling some specific, emotionally charged event in detail. After about 20 minutes of this behavior he leaned forward, cupped his chin in his hands, and lost himself in silent reflection for some minutes, terminating this by asking in a questioning manner, "Nelly, who is Nelly?" but immediately absorbed himself in reflection again. For some time longer he sat tense and rigid, shifting his gaze rapidly here and there and apparently thinking with great feeling. About 15 minutes later he slowly relaxed and, in a tired voice, declared. "That was hard. Henry is me. Now I know what I've been doing, what I've been doing here, and been doing all my life. But I'm not afraid anymore. I don't need to be afraid—not anymore. It's an awful mess, but I know how to clean it up. And I'm going to make an appointment with the dentist. But it's all got to take a lot of thinking—an awful lot, but I'm ready to do it."

Turning to the therapist he stated. "I'm tired, awful tired."

A series of questions and answers now disclosed that the patient felt satisfied, that he felt comfortable with the rush of new understandings he had experienced, that he knew that he was in a trance, and that he was at a loss to know how to let his conscious mind learn what he now knew in his unconscious. When asked if he wanted some suggestions in that regard, he eagerly indicated that he did.

He was reminded of how the induced amnesia had been broken down by the slow filtering out of ideas and associations by outward projection where he could examine them without fear or prejudice and thus achieve an understanding. With each new understanding he had experienced further reorganization of his experiential life, although he could not sense it at first. This, as he could understand, was a relatively simple task, involving nothing more than himself and his thinking and feelings. To become consciously aware of his new understandings would involve himself, his thinking, his everyday activities, his own personal relationships, and the interpersonal relationships of other people. This, therefore, would be an infinitely more difficult task. Upon full understanding of this, an agreement was reached to the effect that he would continue to be neurotic in his everyday life, but as he did so, he would slowly and gradually develop a full conscious realization of the meaningfulness of his neuroticisms, first of the very minor ones and then, as he bettered his adjustments in minor ways, to progress to the more difficult problems. Thus, bit by bit, he could integrate his unconscious learnings with his conscious behavior in a corrective fashion which would lead to good adjustment.

The above paragraph is but a brief summary of the discussion offered the patient. Although he believed he understood the explanation the first time, it is always necessary, as experience has shown repeatedly, to reiterate and to elaborate from many different points of view and to cite likely incidents in which unconscious insights can break through to the conscious before patients really understand the nature of the task before them. A possible incident was cited for him by which to learn how to let unconscious learning become conscious. On some necessary trip to the store where the quarrel had occurred he would notice some clerk looking amused at something. He would then experience a strong feeling of amusement for no known reason, wonder why, discover that his amusement was tinged with a mild feeling of embarrassment, suddenly recall the quarrel with his wife in its true proportions, and thus lose his conscious resentments. A few other such incidents were also suggested and, as subsequently learned, were acted upon. He was then awakened from the trance and dismissed.

The patient's first step to effect a conscious integration, in accord with his trance declaration, was to visit, with much fear, his dentist, thereby discovering, in the dental chair, how grossly exaggerated his fears had been. Next, he found himself humming a song while putting on his shirt, instead of examining it compulsively for wrinkles, as had been his previous habit.

Examination of all the family photographs initiated a process of identification of himself, his mother, and his wife. He discovered for the first time that he resembled his father strongly and could not understand why he had previously believed so fully that he was the image of his mother. By way of the photographs he discovered the dissimilarities between his wife and his mother, and that dentures had actually altered his mother's facial appearance.

At first his adjustments were made singly and in minor matters, but after a few weeks larger and larger maladjustments were corrected. Usually, these were corrected without his conscious awareness until sometime later, a measure which had been suggested to him. For example, he had always visited his mother regularly at the hour of her favorite radio program, and he had always insisted on listening to another program which he invariably criticized unfavorably. Unexpectedly, one day, he became aware that, for several weeks, he had been making his visits at a different hour. With much amusement he realized that his mother could now listen to her favorite program, and, at the same time he experienced the development of much insight into the nature of his attitudes toward his mother.

During this period of reintegration he visited his therapist regularly, usually briefly. Sometimes his purpose was to discuss his progress consciously, sometimes to be hypnotized and given further therapy.

One of his last steps was to discover that he loved his wife and always had, but that he had not dared to know it because he was so convinced in his unconscious that any man who hated his mother so intensely without knowing it should not be allowed to love another woman. This, he now declared, was utterly unreasonable.

The final step was postponed for approximately six months and was achieved in the following manner.

Walking down the street, he saw a stranger swearing fluently at a receding car that had splashed water on him. He felt unaccountably impelled to ask the stranger why he was swearing in such a futile fashion. The reply received, as reported by the patient, was, "Oh, it don't do no good, but it makes me feel better, and besides, it wasn't the driver's fault, and my swearing won't hurt him."

The patient related that he became obsessed with this incident for several days before he realized that it constituted an answer to the numerous delays in the execution of many half-formulated plans to stage a quarrel with his mother and "have it out with her." He explained further that an actual quarrel was unnecessary, that a full recognition of his unpleasant emotional attitudes toward his mother, with no denial or repression of them, and in the manner of the man in the street, would permit a true determination of his actual feelings toward his mother. This was the course he followed successfully. By following the example set by the stranger, he successfully established good relationships with his mother.

The remarkable parallelism between this final step and the hypnotic procedure of having him project his experiential life upon hallucinatory figures is at once apparent. It illustrates again the value of the hypnotic utilization of the dynamics of everyday behavior.

COMMENTS

In presenting this case material, the purpose has not been to give an understanding of the dynamics involved in the patient's illness nor of the varied nature of his maladjustments. Rather, the purpose of the entire paper is that of demonstrating the values of hypnotic psychotherapy, methods of application, and techniques of utilization. A most important consideration in hypnotherapy lies in the intentional utilization, for corrective purposes, of the mental mechanisms or dynamics of human behavior.

Repressions need not necessarily be broken down by sustained effort. Frequently their maintenance is essential for therapeutic progress. The assumption that the unconscious must be made conscious as rapidly as possible often leads merely to the disorderly mingling of confused, unconscious understandings with conscious confusions and, therefore, a retardation of therapeutic progress.

The dissociation of intellectual content from emotional significances often facilitates an understanding of the meaningfulness of both. Hypnosis permits such dissociation when needed, as well as a correction of it.

Projection, rather than being corrected, can be utilized as a therapeutic activity, as has been illustrated above. Similarly, resistances constituting a part of the problem can be utilized by enhancing them and thereby permitting the patient to discover, under guidance, new ways of behavior favorable to recovery. The tendency to fantasy at the expense of action can be employed through hypnosis to create a need for action.

SUMMARY

In brief, there are three highly important considerations in hypnotic psychotherapy that lend themselves to effective therapeutic results. One is the case and readiness with which the dynamics and forms of the patient's maladjustments can be utilized effectively to achieve the desired therapy.

Second is the unique opportunity that hypnosis offers to work either separately and independently, or, jointly with different aspects of the personality, and thus to establish various nuclei of integration.

Equally important is the value of hypnosis in enabling the patient to re-create and to vivify past experiences free from present conscious influences, and undistorted by his maladjustment, thereby permitting the development of good understandings which lead to therapeutic results.

5. Hypnosis in General Practice

Milton H. Erickson

Hypnosis can help you in treating almost any patient. Divested of the mystery which it holds for the uninitiated, this long-known psychological phenomenon has a definite place in general medical practice.

As every doctor knows, it is not enough to prescribe and advise correctly—the patient himself must put the recommended regime into action. Whether he does or not will depend on many things, among them his understanding of himself, his illness and the required treatment, plus the degree of rapport he has with his physician. Here's where hypnosis can be a valuable therapeutic aid.

In a hypnotic state the patient gains a more acute awareness of his needs and capabilities. He is freed from mistaken beliefs, false assumptions, self-doubts and fears which might otherwise stand in the way of needed medical care. Whether he really is sick or just believes that he is (which, by the way, can be equally damaging), the new insights he gets through hypnosis improve his attitude toward his condition. Rapid development of a sound relationship with the doctor is also facilitated, since trust and confidence in others is based, to a large extent, on a real understanding of one's self.

HYPNOTIC RESPONSIVENESS STIMULATES COOPERATION

Another significant change occurs while the patient is hypnotized. He becomes much more responsive to ideas and is able to accept suggestions and to act upon them more readily than in his ordinary state of awareness. The patient's increased responsiveness under hypnosis helps the doctor to secure the kind of cooperation that is essential to successful medical treatment.

To repeat: all patients who come to you seeking the help, the inspiration, and the motivation they need to recover and maintain recovery can benefit from hypnosis. There is the obstetrical patient who is entitled to the easiest possible delivery and the allaying of her anxiety; the

Reprinted from *State of Mind*, 1957, *1*.

surgical patient who fears a needed operation; the dermatological or
allergic patient who cannot stand the itching of his skin; the rheumatoid
arthritic patient who progressively handicaps and limits himself, the
patient with minor illness who invalids himself completely; the obese
patient who "tries" but does not cooperate; the patients with unhealthy
habits ranging from thumb-sucking to alcoholism. I could go on indefinitely, but I think I can better make my point by citing two case histories
which illustrate widely different applications for hypnosis in general
practice.

HYPNOSIS AIDS DIAGNOSIS

The first case concerns a middle-aged nurse who had an extremely
domineering personality. She had been referred to me by another
physician to whom she had complained of fatigability, insomnia, weakness, and vague gastric pains. She had accepted referral somewhat
reluctantly and by the time she appeared in my office had already
diagnosed her problem herself as "globus hystericus." She demanded that
hypnosis be used as a therapeutic approach and only grudgingly consented
to give her case history. From her description of her physical complaints it
appeared to me that her self-diagnosed ailment was in reality a symptom
displacement. I offered the suggestion that she might have a peptic ulcer
and that she go to see an internist. This she flatly refused to do unless I
employed hypnosis on her. In a light trance, she was persuaded to have an
X-ray, and the report disclosed that she did, in fact, have a peptic ulcer.
She told me that she had been given a wealth of medical advice and
prescriptions, all of which, she announced, she intended to reject.

Another somewhat deeper trance was induced in which she was given a
whole series of suggestions to the effect that she could dominate the entire
situation (which was important to her) by taking control of therapy
herself. I told her she could do this by utilizing fully and cooperatively all
advice and instructions given her, by assuming a comfortable and happier
attitude toward her situation and by realizing that such an attitude would
free her of tensions. She was further advised that she had no real need for
her presenting complaint of "globus" and that she could dismiss it now
that she had radiographic confirmation of her true condition. A month
later she went to the internist for a reexamination and was delighted with
his announcement that she was symptom-free, with no X-ray evidence of
an ulcer.

She returned to me twice more for trance induction, to be continued in
her "own handling of her physical problems," as she put it.

HYPNOSIS "KILLS" PAIN

Another middle-aged woman came under my care for quite a different reason. This patient was suffering from metastatic carcinoma of the lung and was experiencing continuous, excruciating pain which required constant sedation with narcotics. She was well aware of the fact that she had only a few weeks to live and bitterly resented the comatose state induced by the narcotic medication.

Her husband sought my help in the hope that a hypnotic anesthesia could be induced which would free his wife of both the pain and the narcotic so that she could spend her remaining days with her family.

The woman willingly endured pain for some 12 hours to rid herself of the effects of the narcotics so that I might hypnotize her. Because of her tremendous motivation, it was possible to induce in her a profound trance state. A deep hypnotic anesthesia was achieved and she was given posthypnotic suggestions to the effect that each day this would be renewed and strengthened. As a result, she was released from the narcotic-induced comatose state and enjoyed five weeks of contact with her family before she expired. During this time she experienced no more than a slight dull ache and feeling of heaviness in her chest.

WHERE CAN YOU LEARN HYPNOSIS?

Assuming that what I've said has convinced you that hypnosis has a place in your practice, you will want to know where you can learn it.

A few universities, scattered around the country, teach formal courses in hypnosis. But for the most part you will have to get your training from people who are experienced in hypnosis and willing to teach it. Such training is best accomplished in situations where more than one person's knowledge and experience is presented, since every patient poses problems that need understanding from more than one point of view.

Preferably, hypnosis should be taught under multidisciplinary auspices as it is by an independent group in Chicago, which includes psychiatrists, obstetricians, general practitioners, dentists, and psychologists. I look forward, however, to the time when more professional schools will offer courses in hypnosis in a concentrated form that does not take doctors away from their practice for too long.

For as the age-old attitude of superstitious awe, fear, incredulity, and antagonism toward hypnosis is replaced by an appreciation of its scientific values, it will become an even more important therapeutic aid and a valuable tool in practicing the art of medicine.

6. Hypnosis: Its Renascence as a Treatment Modality

Milton H. Erickson

INTRODUCTION

Hypnosis Is as Old as Medicine and Almost as Old as Man

Civilizations now belonging to the ancient past reveal that the primitive use of hypnosis was incorporated into the healing arts of the earliest civilizations. These civilizations arose, flourished, and fell, only to be buried under the ruins of newer civilizations that succeeded one another in man's march out of the past. As man continued to think, to behave, to desire, so did he continue to use the art of hypnosis. Throughout history there has been an ever-continuing need to cast the magic spell, to bring healing sleep to the sick, and inner peace to the wounded.

Down through the ages priests and priestesses rendered their services to the ailing and troubled in Temples of Sleep, built upon the ruins of other Temples of Sleep belonging to previous civilizations. The Chinese, Hindus, Greeks, and Egyptians all had temples where suggestion and hypnosis were administered to lessen hurt and suffering. Undoubtedly, there are ancient civilizations yet-to-be-discovered that used hypnosis expressed in magical sleep, rites, and incantations. For men forever remain men with needs in common.

A rebirth of medical interest in hypnosis, although short-lived, began following World War I. The Germans in World War I exhausted their supply of chemical anesthetics and used hypnosis as an anesthetic agent. After the war, particularly in England, hypnosis was used as a calming and reeducative influence in what was then called "shell shock."

By the 1930s a new type of study of hypnosis was evolving. This was the use of hypnosis as a means of investigating psychological and physiological behavior. This was done first by the author, who was then one of Clark L.

Reprinted in *The American Journal of Clinical Hypnosis*, 1970, *13*, 71-89, with permission of the original publishers: Merck Sharp & Dohme, *Trends in Psychiatry*, 1966, 3(3), 3-43.

Hull's students. Subsequently, Hull became seriously interested in hypnosis and proceeded to demonstrate that hypnosis could be subjected to laboratory examination and study just as can other forms of human behavior. Publications originating first in his laboratory, then elsewhere, disclosed that hypnosis could be evaluated by measurable changes brought about in the physiology of the person on whom it was employed, and that by inducing changes in the person's behavior, there could be an investigation of the various forces and experiences that constitute the foundation of personality.

During World War II physicians and psychologists who had learned something about hypnosis found that it could be used not only as an anesthetic, as the Germans had shown in World War I, but to investigate the particular experiences that resulted in "combat fatigue." Further, it could be employed to reeducate the patient to a better understanding of his actual capabilities and potentialities in meeting the stresses of war. Thus, many battle casualties were salvaged. When World War II ended, many of the men from the psychological, medical, and dental fields, returning to civilian life, realized that there should be much more extensive teaching of hypnosis.

Enterprising men from the professions of medicine, dentistry, and psychology organized teaching teams and traveled throughout the country conducting seminars on hypnosis. These teams included people well-founded in psychosomatic medicine, general medicine, psychiatry, obstetrics, surgery, psychology, and dentistry. They lectured before medical societies, psychological groups, or other organizations. Properly, the qualifications for admission to these seminars was the possession of a proper academic degree. Very slowly, scientific interest continued to grow. The result was that here and there a psychology department, a physiological department, or a dental school permitted investigative work by means of hypnosis.

In 1949 the Society of Clinical and Experimental Hypnosis was organized by a small group of scientifically trained men in New York City. The organization promoted the development of hypnosis and founded a journal in that field. . . . In 1957 came the founding of the American Society of Clinical Hypnosis. . . . , which affiliated with, and stimulated the growth of numerous comparable societies throughout the world. It also aroused the interest of qualified individuals interested in hypnosis. Thus, there arose a progressive and compelling interest in hypnosis as a valuable modality in the healing arts and in the field of psychological investigation of human behavior. Iatrogenic well-being rather than iatrogenic illness became a new center of interest.

Little is really known of the actual potentials of human functioning. Hypnosis offered for scientific exploration a different field of conscious awareness, an unexplored approach to puzzling medical problems, a new awareness that scientific studies could be approached in a different way. In brief, a new field of scientific investigation had been opened.

Hypnosis, as an adjunct to the practice of medicine, has opened new fields of exploration in the study of human behavior and is changing the concepts of psychological and physiological potentialities. That it will be productive is unquestionable. But how productive, and in what way, no one can yet say.

HYPNOSIS BY DEFINITION

A Special State of Conscious Awareness

Today there are still those who think of hypnosis as a healing sleep, a magical force, a kind of demoniacal power, as has been thought for thousands of years.

But what is hypnosis as we understand it scientifically today? It is certainly not physiological sleep, even though it may seem to resemble it and may even be used to produce physiological sleep. It is not some special power or magic, nor is it some barbaric force arising from evil sources. It is, in simple terms, nothing more than a special state of conscious awareness in which certain chosen behavior of everyday life is manifested in a direct manner, usually with the aid of another person. But it is possible to be self-induced. Hypnosis is a special but normal type of behavior, encountered when attention and the thinking processes are directed to the body of experiential learnings acquired from, or achieved in, the experiences of living.

In the special state of awareness called hypnosis the various forms of behavior of everyday life may be found—differing in relationships and degrees, but always within normal limits. There can be achieved no transcendence of abilities, no implantations of new abilities, but only the potentiation of the expression of abilities which may have gone unrecognized or not fully recognized.

Hypnosis cannot create new abilities within a person, but it can assist in a greater and better utilization of abilities already possessed, even if these abilities were not previously recognized.

Using Hypnosis in Medical Practice

The rationale for the use of hypnosis in the healing arts is the beneficial effect of restriction of the patient's attention to those items of behavior and function pertinent to his well-being.

To clarify by an example, lay a wooden plank 25 feet long and 20 inches across on the level ground. Anybody in a state of ordinary, conscious awareness can walk that 25 feet easily. But place that same plank at an elevation of 200 feet in the air and the problem of walking its length becomes greatly changed for the person, even though the actual task is unchanged. In the ordinary state of conscious awareness performance is too often limited by considerations which may actually be unrelated to the task. Walking that wooden plank with transparent flooring on both sides, but the ground plainly visible 200 feet below, would still remain a nerve-racking task for many persons who could do it easily on the ground. Ideas, understandings, beliefs, wishes, hopes, and fears can all impinge easily upon a performance in the state of ordinary, conscious awareness—disrupting and distorting even those goals which may have been singly desired. But in a state of hypnosis the field of conscious awareness is limited and tends to be restricted to exactly pertinent matters, other considerations being irrelevant. To cite another illustration, a badly burned patient is in desperation for pain relief. He does not want to be presented with ideas and suggestions about his pain. He is not interested in taking fluids and food. He has no appetite as a result of his suffering. He cannot sleep because of pain, fear, and anxiety about the outcome of his condition.

Under hypnosis, by contrast, the badly burned patient is open to suggestion. He is as ready to accept suggestions of hypnotic anesthesia and analgesia as he would be to accept morphine. He is also ready to accept suggestions of thirst and hunger and to respond readily to them, something that would be impeded by drug administration, as would likewise the elimination of toxins be retarded by medication for pain. Further, he enjoys natural, physiological sleep rather than a narcotic sleep.

Even if hypnosis fails to bring full relief, the symptomatology can be greatly reduced, thus lessening the amount of medication that can interfere with toxin elimination.

In the writer's own experience the shock response of a seven-year-old child to severe scalding of one arm, her shoulder, chest, and side, was utilized in inducing a hypnotic trance. Local dressing of the burned areas, but no general medication, resulted in full recovery within three weeks. Further hypnosis after the initial session was not required, since the original posthypnotic suggestions continued to remain effective throughout the hospitalization.

In another instance, which took place some years ago, a male patient in his early twenties, who had been committed to the mental hospital three years previously, was diagnosed as suffering from catatonic schizophrenia. His clinical course in the hospital came to be almost completely predictable. There would be a week during which he would show rising tension and anxiety, and always within eight days he would reach a peak of highly disturbed violent behavior, requiring either physical restraint or seclusion, and during which time no interpersonal contact could be made. This period would last four to six weeks. There could then be a six- to eight-day period during which his disturbed behavior would subside, and always within eight days he reached a state of passive, inaccessible behavior, but was unable to give any clear account of the reasons for, or the nature of, his disturbed behavior. This state of behavior would then continue for seven to nine weeks, whereupon the disturbed cycle would begin again.

During one period of remission approximately 25 hours were spent in training this patient to be a somnambulistic hypnotic subject, the purpose being purely experimental and investigative. He was given special posthypnotic suggestions to which he was "always to respond."

At the beginning of the third week of the next disturbed period following his hypnotic training, the patient was still in full physical restraint and, so far as could be determined, was still completely inaccessible by ordinary methods, requiring tube feeding and being completely incontinent. The patient was approached, his wrist was grasped gently, and he was addressed by the name of "John," an agreed-upon name assigned to him during previous hypnotic trances and to be used only in the trance condition. After he had been called by the name "John" three times at five-second intervals, each time his wrist being gently squeezed, he appeared to recognize the writer and asked what was wanted. Then he almost immediately seemed to become aware of his restraints and asked what had happened. He was told simply that it was desirable to have him talk to the medical students—a procedure of much previous experience during remission states. "John" stated that he was not feeling well, that he was full of "awful feelings" and fears and anxiety, and he expressed doubt that he could talk to the students. He also asked why he was called "John" instead of his real name Frank. This signified that he was not in a hypnotic trance, a development not anticipated, since it was hoped and expected that he would "come out" of his disturbed state into a trance state. Nevertheless, with much urging he was persuaded to take a shower, to dress, and to talk to the students. He was told that he was free to ask to be put back into restraint if he found his emotional distress becoming too much for him. Hesitantly, he agreed.

After two hours with the students, Frank stated that he was "getting sick" and asked to be put in restraint as rapidly as possible. He even assisted in an anxious, hurried manner in the securing of the restraints. When this was completely accomplished, he was so informed. Immediately he renewed his previous disturbed behavior of screaming, shouting, and struggling violently, again completely inaccessible.

The next week, the fourth week in his disturbed cycle, the same procedure was followed and similar contact was obtained.

By the fifth week it was recognized that he was in a state of beginning remission, which was achieved within a week's time. It was not considered desirable to intrude upon this spontaneous abatement of his symptoms.

During the succeeding eight-week period of remission he was used repeatedly to demonstrate hypnotic trances, and he was still a most competent subject. Unfortunately, the most intensive questioning could secure no information regarding his disturbed period experiences. He did not even seem to understand that he had had a disturbed period, but he knew that a period of time, for which he could not account, had elapsed.

During the next period of disturbed behavior it was learned that he could again be approached by the previously established posthypnotic cues of a gentle grasping of his wrist and calling him by the name of "John" three times. This could be done at intervals of four or more days. There were two failures when such an attempt was made on the third day after a successful approach. Hence, all approaches thereafter were never more frequent than four days apart.

None of the other psychiatrists was willing to follow the writer's example. Several medical students succeeded easily, but this was not a fair test since I was present. But in general the use of hypnosis as an easy approach to a disturbed psychotic patient, unapproachable by any other method, was frowned upon and discouraged, and only my rank on the professional staff made it possible for me to perform these "unorthodox" experiments.

Encouraged by this experience with Frank, I attempted a similar procedure in six other schizophrenic patients, both catatonics and hebephrenics. Similar results were obtained with these patients, three of them recovering sufficiently to be sent home. All returned to the hospital within three years' time, acutely disturbed in behavior. Nevertheless, each responded again to the posthypnotic cues given them in their previous hospitalization and shortly left the hospital.

Hypnosis was also employed successfully with three violently excited manic-depressive patients who showed brief remissions sufficiently long to permit hypnotic training. With them, as with the schizophrenic patients, extremely violent, excited episodes of disturbed behavior could be briefly interrupted for two to four hours before it would be necessary to restore the restraints or to return them to the seclusion rooms.

In the writer's experience this manner of dealing with disturbed psychotic behavior could be accomplished only by hypnosis. Even though the percentage of successes was much lower than the percentage of failures, the elicitation of reasonable normal behavior by hypnosis from acutely disturbed psychotic patients indicates, in a limited way, the remarkable effectiveness of this "special state of conscious awareness." It also indicates an important area warranting continuing research and investigation.

The problem yet remaining is to ensure that the members of the medical profession fully realize that the thinking, the emotions, and the past experiential learnings of each person play a significant role in his psychological and physiological functionings.

HYPNOSIS IN MEDICAL PRACTICE: THREE CASE HISTORIES

The following case histories illustrate how the potentials within a person can restore well-being. Hypnosis isolates the person from his immediate conscious surroundings—and so directs attention within one's self and to one's own actual potentialities. This is as important as the conventional scientific laboratory, because it is the laboratory that exists within the person.

Edward C.

Edward was one of two children. His sister was six years his senior. His father was employed in an industrial plant. Upon graduating from high school Edward secured employment in the same plant. He was quiet, thoughtful, had few friends and these were merely casual. He had no interest in girls, although he had taken two or three to a movie (but never the same girl twice). He was neither friendly nor unfriendly. One day while at work he suddenly became violently disturbed. He had to be subdued by his fellow workers until the police came to put him in handcuffs and leg irons and take him to the psychopathic ward of a city hospital. From there he was committed to the mental hospital. The psychiatric staff made a diagnosis of schizophrenia, catatonic type.

On the ward Edward sat quietly in a chair. He would listen attentively when spoken to, but would never reply. However, about three times every 24 hours he became violently disturbed. He would rush wildly through the dormitory, crawling under and over beds, around beds, shoving them away from the wall. The disturbances would last from 10 to 20 minutes, whereupon, covered with perspiration, he would return to his chair or, at night, to his bed. There was never a word of explanation received from Edward about these episodes. More than a dozen physicians endeavored repeatedly to interview the patient or to elicit some verbal response from him. Each interview was a failure—and this had been going on for three years.

Finally this writer decided to use hypnosis. I employed a technique of relaxation, with suggestions of tiredness, fatigue, sleep, and attentiveness to what was said. Within the course of 20 minutes Edward gave every evidence, physically, of being in a hypnotic trance. He showed catalepsy, would nod his head affirmatively or shake it negatively when asked various questions. It was soon determined that he would like to tell about his difficulties, but did not know how. This information was obtained by laborious questioning, answered by head movements. I explained that I was going to help him, and that this help would consist of having him sit quietly in a chair and have a dream. (A dream could be acceptable, since it was an inner experience, and direct communication is not.) This dream might occur during the coming night, but it was explained that I would like to have it occur within the next hour if that were agreeable. Edward nodded affirmatively. He was told that he was to dream informatively about his problem, about the reason why he was in a mental hospital. It was suggested that he relate the content of this dream after it occurred. He was asked to think this over for a half-hour while still in a hypnotic trance. I explained that I would return to him and ask him if he would dream that informative dream within the hour after I returned. Edward nodded his head to express his agreement. He was then left sitting in his chair in a trance. Half an hour later I returned and asked Edward if he were willing to have his dream within the next hour, and after the dream to relate it verbally. Edward nodded his head affirmatively. I took a comfortable seat near the patient and waited for 15 minutes to pass, the time Edward had said it would take before he would have his dream. Almost exactly 15 minutes passed when Edward suddenly became extremely tense and began to perspire freely. His muscles quivered. He clenched his jaws. These movements persisted for about 20 minutes. Then Edward relaxed and sighed deeply. I asked him, "Are you through dreaming," He replied, "Yes, it was awful, just awful."

I asked him to narrate the dream fully, if he could. He nodded his head affirmatively and also stated, "I can, but take me by the hand because I will get awful scared." Edward related his dream. He imagined himself being suddenly thrown into complete darkness and being seized by a terrible force. "It drags me, it yanks me, it pulls me, it twists me, it turns me. It hauls me through great piles of barbed wire, through heaps of stabbing knives. It jerks me first one way and then another. It pulls me up and it pulls me down, and all the time I am being stabbed. I can't see anything. I just feel awful pain. It goes on and on and on. And I am so scared."

I asked if there was anything I could do to comfort him. Edward replied that nobody could help him, that nothing could help him, that all he could do was sit and wait. I then asked him to sit quietly and comfortably, to rest for two or three hours, and to let nothing happen to him. During that period he was told to awaken and to go to lunch as usual. Later that same day Edward was approached again. He was silent, but looked attentively at me—his first real effort in three years to respond to a psychiatrist.

I asked if he were willing to let me hypnotize him again. Edward nodded and reached out his hand. I took a careful grasp of his hand and induced a trance within a few minutes. As soon as catalepsy indicated that Edward was in a hypnotic state, I asked if he were asleep. He answered, "I am sound asleep, I am resting comfortably, I am all alone except for your voice. I like it this way." Edward was then asked, "Are you willing to have another dream?"

He answered, "No." I persisted, "I would like you to have another dream because I think I can help you by your having this dream again." Edward answered, "If it will help, I'll try." Sick people do want to try— usually they don't know how. Edward was asked to listen most attentively, slowly and laboriously. He was told that he was to dream that same dream that he had dreamed previously. He shook his head and said, "No! No!" I continued, "I want a different setting, a different set of conditions. I want it to be the same dream with a totally different set of characters, because you can call those barbed wire heaps and the thorn bushes and the heaps of stabbing knives 'characters.' This time I want it to be the same dream with the same emotions, but with a different cast of characters. Will you do this for me, Edward, knowing that it really is for you?"

After some minutes of thought Edward asked how soon to start. I asked, "After five minutes will it be all right to begin the dream?" There was a slow, reluctant "Yes." The minutes were counted—one, two, three, four—and about 50 seconds later Edward tightened his fingers on my hand very forcibly and showed the previous behavior—tense, quivering muscles, diffuse perspiration, and shuddering of his body. Again, this lasted about 20 minutes. Then Edward suddenly relaxed and sank weakly in his chair. He stated in reply to a question, "It is all over now. It was the same dream. Hold my hand carefully. I will tell you, but don't make me dream it again."

Edward began to tell his dream. A sudden terrible darkness had enveloped him, and the same awful power seized him. But this time it dragged him and yanked him and pulled him and twisted him and turned him and shoved him down a never-ending canyon. All the way there were earthslides and great boulders fell on him or knocked him hither and yon. He bumped from one side of the canyon to the other, and dirt filled his eyes and mouth, and great stones fell on his legs. Sometimes he was hauled up over a landslide only to be covered by a second landslide. And so on and so on. Edward concluded his description, "It was just the same as the other dream except it was a canyon. That is all there is to it. Now let me rest." I thanked him and waked him. Again he sat there—silent and attentive, but unresponsive. He would neither nod nor shake his head. I saw Edward on the next day. He responded only by averting his face. The following day he was again approached. Again he turned away. This continued for a week. It was also noted that the nurses' records disclosed that Edward had not been having his periodic disturbed episodes. Then, 12 days later, Edward had his usual disturbed episode. When I approached him that afternoon, Edward did not turn his face away, but made no response to questions until he was asked if he were willing to go into a hypnotic trance. To this he nodded yes. The hypnotic state was induced in a couple of minutes. I asked, "Did those dreams help you?"

Edward said, "Yes. Those dreams are what happened on the ward, in the dormitory. They are just the same." I asked, "Would you like to have another such dream?" He replied, "No," reluctantly. I told him that his negative answer was not emphatic. It almost seemed as if he wanted to say yes. He was asked to explain. He said, "Those dreams are awful, just awful. What happens on the ward is just awful. But after those first two dreams, nothing happened again. I know it will, but I don't want it." I asked, "Since those first two dreams were helpful, maybe another dream would give you a few days' relief. Are you willing to try?" Fearfully, hesitantly, he finally said yes.

Again I explained to him, "I want you to have the same dream again, but with a different cast of characters. Not barbed wires or stabbing knives or huge boulders such as you had before. I want it to be the same dream with a different cast of characters. Will it be all right to start the dream in five minutes? I will hold your hand carefully." Edward said weakly, "Yes." This time I was very careful in taking hold of Edward's fingers because I had experienced the forcefulness of his grip. About five minutes later he showed the behavior previously manifested. Again it lasted about 20 minutes. As he finally relaxed, breathing heavily, I asked him, "Can you tell me about the dream?" He said, "Yes." "All right, tell me now." Edward related a dream of being in "a jalopy" that was filled with broken glass. It was a big jalopy, and there were four people in it. He was one of the four. The others didn't get hurt as the jalopy went down a mountain road with hairpin turns. It was falling down the mountainside, always landing on the road below. It was going at frightful speeds. He couldn't see the people. He just knew they were awful people, and all that glass around him. It filled up that whole jalopy. He was in the glass on the seat. None of the glass touched the others, but each time the jalopy jumped, the glass hit him. It went on and on and on until, all of a sudden, the darkness stopped and the dream ended. I thanked Edward quietly, told him to awaken and feel as rested as he could. He awakened, but as usual he did not speak. When spoken to, he merely looked attentive. He was obviously fatigued, and his shirt was soaked with perspiration.

There were no disturbed episodes for the next six days. On the seventh day Edward moved his chair up to the door which I customarily used to enter the ward. As I opened the door, Edward reached up with his hand, took my hand, and pulled me down into the chair beside him. I asked, "Do you want something, Edward?" Slowly he nodded yes. I asked, "Do you want to go into a trance?" After some moments he said softly, "Yes." Thus, for the first time in over three years, he had voluntarily asked for help—thanks to hypnosis.

Excitedly, I hypnotized him again. The trance state developed very rapidly, and I asked Edward to "explain." In essence his explanation was, "Those dreams are all the same. Just something different, but they mean the same. They scare me. They hurt me. They are awful. But when you make me have the dreams, I don't have to have the dreams on the ward. But today I am going to—and I don't want to. So maybe you had better have me dream." (Development of first real insight.) Again, the laborious explanation was given. "Dream the same dream with the same meaning, the same emotional significance, but with a different cast of characters. This time maybe it won't be so dark. Maybe you can see a bit more clearly. It won't be pleasant, but maybe it won't hurt so much. So go ahead as soon as you can and have your dream." Within four minutes the dream developed; 20 minutes later, streaming with perspiration, Edward said, "It was the same dream. It was bad. It was awful bad. But it didn't hurt so much. I was walking through a forest. The sky got blacker and blacker until I couldn't see anything. Then the wind began blowing. I could hear the crashing of the lightning, but I couldn't see it. There was thunder. The wind would pick me up and throw me against the trees. I went crashing against the forest, on and on for miles. Just as the dream ended, I thought I saw a house. But I am not sure." (Beginning of identification.)

Edward was asked when he thought he would have the next dream. He replied, "Not this week. Maybe next week." I asked if he would let me know. He answered, "Every day walk past me. When I want the dream, I will take your hand." (Three long years and now trust in another person!) Edward was asked to relax, to feel as comfortable as possible, and then to awaken. Upon arousing from the trance state, Edward was asked if he would like to talk. He nodded affirmatively. When I repeated the question, he shook his head no. For the next 10 days I dutifully walked past Edward. It was not until the 11th day that he reached up and took my hand as before. The nurse's note showed that Edward had had no disturbed episodes. As I sat down on the chair beside him, Edward did not wait, but developed a trance immediately. I asked if he thought he was going to have a disturbed episode. He said, "Yes, one is coming soon. I want you to help me."

Again he was asked to dream the same dream, but to dream it with less pain, less discomfort, and to dream more clearly—to see the characters more plainly. His fingers tightened on my hand, and the dream developed immediately. The observed behavior was essentially the same. The duration was again about 20 minutes. His recovery from the dream was a bit more difficult. There was much shuddering, much gasping for breath. He fended me off with his hands. He was asked to explain. He said, "I was walking along a strange street. It was very shady. The sun wasn't very bright. I came to a hideous house. I knew I didn't want to go in, but something awful hit me on the back and knocked me inside. It was an awful room. Then something that looked like a woman hit me with something that looked like a great big broom. Then something that looked like a man seemed to jump on me. Then another woman kept hitting me with a red hot iron. I tried to get away. I ran from one room to another, but they always followed me. I couldn't get away. Finally I came to the last room. I couldn't see who these people were. They were huge; they were monsters. All of a sudden the sun shone and I was out in the street. Then I was here in the chair beside you." I asked, "Is there anything more you can tell me?" His answer was no. "But I know there is something awful dreadful that is coming up in my mind. I am awfully afraid. Will you come every day and speak to me?" I told him I would. Each day Edward met me at the door to the ward and walked with me on rounds. Questions I asked him were answered only by a nod or a shake of the head. There was no verbalization. On the fourth day Edward took me by the hand and led me to a chair. For the first time he spoke, saying loudly, "I want help right away! Now!" (After three years of inaccessibility, Edward, through hypnosis, could volunteer communication.) A spontaneous trance developed immediately. I told him again to dream the same dream with the same cast of characters, but this time to make the dream "nearer," "clearer," "more understandable, but not too understandable." It was explained to him that he was not to understand the importance of the dream, but only that the characters were to be clearer.

The usual dream sequence ensued. There was much less physical agony manifested. The perspiration was markedly decreased. Edward related his dream as follows: "Out of somewhere, I don't know where, I was yanked into what seemed to be a hospital. There was a huge, awful, towering nurse, who was in charge. I was thrown into a bathtub. I was washed. They used steel brushes. They yanked me out. They dried me with towels made of ropes with knots in them. I was jerked here and there. Then another nurse, not as big as the first one, grabbed me by the hair and waved me around in the air and banged me on the floor, knocking me against the beds. Then she threw me in a great big bed right between two awful people. One of them seemed to be a woman. She was covered all over with awful sores, like cancers. She didn't seem to have any clothes on. Her teeth were awful. Her eyes were awful. Her fingers were claws. I tried to get away from her. The only way I could move was toward another person, who seemed to be a man. There were many terrible things about him. I don't know how terrible. I was afraid to look. They kept knocking me on the head to make me look. The man kept yelling at me. I couldn't get out of bed. I tried to explain it wasn't my fault. This went on and on. All of a sudden it ended. I was sitting beside you."

I asked if he wanted to remember this dream when awake. Edward said, "No, I just can't, I can't. Don't make me." I asked him when he thought he should have the next dream. In reply he asked, "Will the next dream tell me? But I am afraid to know." "If you want to," I answered. "Think it over for three or four days. Don't rush. Don't hurry. You and I can handle it. Really handle it." I asked him if he were ready to awaken. He answered, "Yes, but say something when I am awake, something nice." He aroused readily upon suggestion and said, "It seems to me that you are going to say something, but I don't know what." I replied very cautiously, "Do you know, Edward, you have come a long way. You are almost ready to be well. You are almost ready not to be afraid. You are almost ready to know something." Edward answered, "I don't know what you are talking about." He was assured that all was well.

Three days later Edward was found pacing the ward restlessly, with much tension. He seemed relieved at seeing me. As I approached, he said, "I think you had better do something for me today. I am awfully afraid, but I think you can do something for me. Something that has got to be done. I think I am ready." I led him to a quiet end of the ward and seated him. Immediately he developed a deep trance and spontaneously stated, "I think I am ready." I told him, "Well, since you think you are ready, have the same dream with the same cast of characters. But let them have a meaning that you can recognize, that you can accept, that won't scare you. I'll be here. If things get too bad, I can stop everything. I want everything to go ahead. But I'll stop things if you need them stopped." Instantly Edward stated, "All right. I am beginning a dream. I am beginning a dream. I am in the hospital. It is this hospital. There is a nurse. She is the head nurse. She looks awful mean. There is a patient. He looks like my father. He is the one in the corner bed on the west side. He looks like my father. The first time I saw him, I wanted to kill him. I wanted to kill the nurse. There is another nurse. She is nasty, too. She looks like my sister. They are taking care of a patient. That awful, great big patient. The head nurse and the other nurse are taking care of a patient. He is kicking. He is trying to get away. They are holding him tight. They put him in bed. They tell him to stay there. That patient is awful afraid. That's funny. That patient is me. I look awful scared. That big patient looks just like my father. The head nurse looks just like my sister. I know what it is all about. I can tell you now. But I wish you would wake my up and let me tell you, because I will be able to listen when I tell you. Wake me up now, right now."

He was awakened. He was tremulous. There was a rush of words. "It is this way, Doctor. My father and mother and sister came from a foreign country. Everybody respected my father there. Everybody respected my mother, my sister. They were bigshots. They came here to America. Then it all happened. Everybody made him a dumb foreigner. That is all he was—a dumb foreigner. I was born here and learned to speak English. Everybody made fun of my father. They laughed at my mother. They laughed at my sister. They even laughed when I spoke. Then my family would get mad at me and beat me up. They took it all out on me. That is why I never had any friends. They would call me 'that dumb foreign kid.' But I wasn't dumb. I couldn't have friends. I went to grade school, and they all called me the dumb foreigner. I studied hard, but I couldn't be friends. Every day my father would get drunk. He worked in a factory. Sometimes he wouldn't work. We were on welfare. Then he got a job, and I went to high school. It didn't do me any good. Every time I came home they'd drag me all around calling me a dumb immigrant. They talked about me. They made fun of me. They said I thought I was smart because I could talk English. They yelled and they screamed at me. My father would knock me down. My mother would hit me with anything. My sister was a big woman. She yelled and screamed that she couldn't get married. Every day it went on. I kept studying by myself. Then, when I got through high school, I went to get a job. When I gave my name, they said I was foreign, just like my father. Nothing I could do changed it. I got shoved around at the factory where I worked. I wanted to make friends. I wanted a girl. But everybody knew my name. I was a dumb foreigner. Things kept getting blacker and blacker. Then, all of a sudden, they got awful black. That is what my first dream was about. I was dragged through everything—every insult, every hurt, everything mean, because I was born in America. I wasn't really a foreigner. I was an American. That was what all my dreams were about. That canyon. That's the immigrant section of the city. Why weren't former nationalities forgotten? All the old folks hate it. They don't like being dumb immigrants. Those people in that awful jalopy going down the mountain road. Once we took our secondhand car and drove out in the country. All the time my father was calling me a dumb foreign kid just born in America. My mother and sister were saying it, too. I thought the ride would never come to an end. They said it was a picnic. I got my mother mixed up with the head nurse. That patient was my father. For years I wanted to commit suicide. I have been afraid because I wanted to live. I couldn't stand being alive. I can keep on telling you all these things, Doctor, because you are the first one who I have ever told anything. Some way you made it possible to talk to you. I never could tell anybody. Now I want to talk to you all about this. I am an American. I don't care about what my mother does or what my sister does. I just want to be an American. I tried to be like them and I couldn't. I tried to be the way I wanted to be, and now I know. I can be me."

Within two months, after almost daily discussions of the matter, Edward decided to change his name. He secured his father's permission to shorten his name. He discussed his emotional reaction to his parents, to his sister. He felt sorry for them. He felt helpless so far as they were concerned, but he knew he could help himself.

The years have passed. Edward never needed to return to a mental hospital. He made a good adjustment. He married an American girl of similar foreign extraction. He feels sorry for his father who drank himself to death, for his mother who died eventually of cancer, for his sister who despairingly committed suicide. Edward regrets all this. He is proud of his children. Through hypnosis Edward learned the thing so vital in human living—how to communicate.

Ann R.   Ann, 21, entered the office hesitantly, fearfully. She had been hesitant and fearful over the telephone. She expressed an absolute certainty over the telephone that I would not like to see her. Accordingly, she was urged to come. As she entered the office, she said, "I told you so. I will go now. My father is dead, my mother is dead, my sister is dead, and that is all that's left for me." She was urged to take a seat, and after some rapid thinking I realized that the only possible understanding this girl had of intercommunication was that of unkindness and brutality. Hence, brutality would be used to convince her of sincerity. Any other possible approach, any kindness, would be misinterpreted. She could not possibly believe courteous language. I realized that rapport would have to be established—and established very quickly. She would have to be convinced, beyond a doubt, that I understood and recognized her and her problem and was not afraid to speak openly, freely, unemotionally, but truthfully.

Her history was briefly taken. Then she was asked the two important questions. "How tall are you and how much do you weigh?" With a look of extreme emotional distress she answered, "I am 4 feet 10 inches. I weigh between 250 and 260 pounds. I am just a plain, fat slob. Nobody would ever look at me except with disgust."

This offered a suitable opening. She was told, "You haven't really told the truth. I am going to say this simply so that you will know about yourself and understand that I know about you. Then you will believe, really believe, what I have to say to you. You are *not* a plain, fat, disgusting slob. You are the fattest, homeliest, most disgustingly horrible bucket of lard I have ever seen, and it is appalling to have to look at you. You have gone through high school. You know some of the facts of life. Yet here you are, 4 feet 10 inches tall, weighing between 250 and 260 pounds. You have got the homeliest face I have ever seen. Your nose was just mashed onto your face. Your teeth are crooked. Your lower jaw doesn't fit your upper jaw. Your face is too damned spread out. Your forehead is too hideously low. Your hair is not even decently combed. And that dress you are wearing—polka dots, millions and billions of them. You have no taste, even in clothes. Your feet slop over the edges of your shoes. To put it simply—you are a hideous mess. But you do need help. I think you know now that I won't hesitate to tell you the truth. You need to know the truth about yourself before you can ever learn the things necessary to help yourself. But I don't think you can take it. Why did you come to see me?"

She answered, "I thought maybe you could hypnotize me so I could lose some weight." I answered her with, "Maybe you can learn to go into a hypnotic trance. You are bright enough to graduate from high school. Maybe you are bright enough to learn how to go into hypnosis. I would like to have you go into hypnosis. It's an opportunity to say a few more uncomplimentary things to you. Things I don't think you could possibly stand to hear when you are awake. But in the trance state you can listen to me. You can understand. You can do something. Not too darn much, because you are horribly handicapped. But I want you to do everything I tell you to do because the way you have gobbled up food to make yourself look like an overstuffed garbage pail indicates that you need to learn something so you won't be so offensive to the human eye. Now that you know that I can tell you the truth, just close your eyes and go deeply into a trance. Don't fool around about it, just as you don't fool around in making yourself a disgusting eyesore. Go into a completely deep, hypnotic trance. You will think nothing, see nothing, feel nothing, do nothing, hear nothing except my voice. You will understand what I say—and be glad that I am willing to talk to you. There is a lot of truth I want to tell you. You couldn't face it in the waking state. So sleep deeply in a deep hypnotic trance. Hear nothing except my voice, see nothing, think nothing except what I tell you to do. Just be a helpless automaton. Now, are you doing that? Nod your head yes and do exactly as I tell you, because you know I'll tell you the truth. The first thing I am going to do is to get you— rather order you—to tell me certain facts about yourself. You can talk even though you are in a deep trance. Answer each question simply but informatively."

"What is important about your father?" Her answer was, "He hated me. He was a drunk. We lived on welfare. He used to kick me around. That's all I ever remember about my father. Drunk, slapping me, kicking me, hating me."

"And your mother?" "She was the same, but she died first. She hated me worse than my father did. She treated me worse than he did. They only sent me to high school because they knew I hated high school. All I could do at high school was study. They made me live in the garage with my sister. She was born defective. She was short and fat. She had her bladder on the outside of her body. She was always sick. She had kidney disease. We loved each other. We only had each other to love. When she died of a kidney disease, they said, 'Good.' They wouldn't let me go to the funeral. They just buried the only thing I loved. I was a freshman in high school. The next year my mother drank herself to death. Then my father married a woman worse than my mother. She didn't let me go in the house. She would bring slop out to the garage and make me eat it. Said I could eat myself to death. I would be good riddance. She was a drunk like my mother. The social worker didn't like me, either, but she did send for some medical examinations. The doctors didn't like to touch me. Now my stepmother and my sister were all dead. Welfare told me to get a job. I got a job scrubbing floors. The men make fun of me there. They offer each other money to have sex relations with me, but nobody will. I am just not good for anything. But I would like to live. I have got a place where I live. It is an old shack. I don't earn much—eat corn meal mush and potatoes and things like that. I thought maybe you could hypnotize me and do something for me. But I guess it isn't any use."

In a most unsympathetic, peremptory fashion she was asked, "Do you know what a library is? I want you to go to the library and take out books on anthropology. I want you to look at all the hideous kinds of women men will marry. There are pictures of them in books in the library. Primitive savages will marry things that look worse than you. Look through book after book and be curious, horribly curious. Then read books that tell about how women and men disfigure themselves, tattoo themselves, mutilate themselves to look even more horrible. Spend every hour you can at the library. Do it well and come back in two weeks."

Ann was awakened from her trance with this posthypnotic suggestion and left the office in the same cringing fashion as she had entered it. Two weeks later she returned. She was told to waste no time—to go into a trance, a deep one, immediately. She was asked if she found some pictures unpleasant to her. She spoke of finding pictures of the steat-opygous women of the Hottentots, and of duckbilled women, and giraffe-necked women, of keloid scarification in some African tribes, of strange rituals of disfigurement. She was then instructed to go to the corner of the busiest section of the city (in a waking state) and there watch the peculiar shapes and faces of the things that men marry. She was to do this for one whole week, and then the next week she was to look at the peculiar faces and peculiar shapes of the things that women will marry, and to do this wonderingly.

She obediently returned, went into a trance and stated with simple wonderment that she had actually seen women almost as homely as she was who wore weddings rings. She had seen men and women who seemed to be man and wife, both of whom were hideously fat and clumsy. She was told that she was beginning to learn something.

Her next assignment was going to the library to go through all the books she could on the history of cosmetology—to discover what constituted desirable beauty to the human eye.

Ann made a thorough search and entered the office without cringing, but still clad in her polka dot dress.

Her next assignment was to go to the library and look through books dealing with human customs, dress, and appearance—to find something depicted that was at least 500 years old and still looked pretty. Ann returned, developed a trance immediately upon entering the office, sat down, and spoke eagerly, relating what she had seen in books. She was then told that her next assignment would be very hard. For two weeks she was to go first to one women's apparel store and then another, wearing her frightful polka dot dress. She was to ask what she really ought to wear—to ask so earnestly and so honestly that the clerks would answer her. She reported after this assignment that a number of elderly women had called her "dearie" and explained to her why she should not wear millions and millions of polka dots. They told her why she should not wear dresses that were unbecoming—that served to exaggerate her hideous fatness. The next assignment was to spend two weeks in obsessive thinking: Why should she, who must have been born weighing less than 20 pounds, have added such enormous poundage? Why had she wrapped herself up in blubber? From that assignment she reported she couldn't reach any conclusions.

Again, in the trance state, she was given another assignment. This time to discover if there were really any reason why she had to weigh what she did . . . to be curious about what she might look like if she weighed only 150 pounds and were dressed appropriately . . . to awaken in the middle of the night with that question in mind, only to fall asleep again restfully. After a few more trances in which she reviewed all her assignments, she was asked to recall, one by one, each of her assignments and to see whether they applied to her.

Ann was seen in two-week intervals. Within six months she came in, with great interest, to explain that she could not find any reason why she should weigh so much—or why she should dress so atrociously. She had read enough on cosmetology, on hair dressing, and makeup. She had read books on plastic surgery, on orthodontia. She asked piteously, in the waking state, if she could be permitted to see what she could do about herself. Within another year's time Ann weighed 150 pounds. Her taste in clothes was excellent. Ann had a much better job. She was enrolling in the university. By the time she graduated from the university, even though she still weighed 140 pounds, she was engaged to be married. She had had two teeth that had developed outside of the dental alignment removed and replaced. Her smile was actually attractive. Ann had a job in dress designing as a fashion artist for catalogs and newspapers. She brought her fiance to meet me. She came into the office first and said: "The darn fool is so stupid. He thinks I'm pretty. But I am never going to disillusion him. He's got stars in his eyes when he looks at me. But both you and I know the truth. I have difficulty in keeping below 150—and I am afraid I am going to reach more. But I actually know that he loves me this way. You will find Dick the handsomest man in the state."

She brought Dick into the office and winked at me. Then she left. As the door closed behind her, Dick turned to me and said, "Isn't she just a beautiful dream?" The writer agreed as he looked at "the handsomest man in the state." He was fully as homely as Ann—only more so. His features had been thrown together—but did not seem to fit together. Yet Ann truly thought he was the handsomest man in the state—even the nation.

They have been married for 15 years. They have three handsome children, two boys and a girl. This writer has looked the children over. They show every promise of growing up to be physically attractive in every way. Dick still thinks that Ann is a beautiful dream. Ann winks at me with amusement as she states, "That handsome fellow actually thinks I'm pretty." Economically they are successful. Socially they are successful. Ann talks freely of her therapy since she remembers everything that was said to her. She has stated more than once, "When you said those awful things about me, you were so truthful. I knew that you were telling me the truth, that I could trust you. I am so glad you told me the truth. But if you hadn't put me in a trance, I wouldn't have done any of the things you made me do. I just wonder—how did Dick grow up? His parents must have praised and flattered him. Yet, being handsome, it hasn't affected him in any way."

To know how to communicate with patients is all-important in medicine, in all branches of life. Semantics are important, but communication is basic. Hypnosis needs to be recognized as a science of intercommunication.

Sandra W.

Having first telephoned for an appointment, this rather beautiful 38-year-old woman entered the office and asked, "Do you use hypnosis?" She was answered, "If I find it necessary and helpful." She proceeded to take a seat and explained, "I think it is necessary in this case. Most people won't believe this, but I am sure you will. I am troubled by nude young men that float in the air just above my head. See them up there next to the ceiling? Wherever I go they follow me. No matter what street I walk on, they are always in the air just above me. They never do anything. They just float.

"Now there is a second thing I want you to do. Quite often I like to float up into the sky and travel around the world on a cloud. Some people think

I am just sitting quietly in a chair. Actually, I am up on a cloud floating around the world. Sometimes, instead of doing that, I go down to the bottom of the Pacific Ocean, where I have a beautiful castle made of glass. I spend a day or two, sometimes even a week, there. It's so lovely to look out at the fish that are swimming all around my castle. I cannot tell these things to people. They don't understand. They call me crazy. My ex-husband got a divorce because he wanted to put me in the State Hospital. I don't want to go there because I am able to work and support myself. I just don't want to have people interfering with me. Now, if you use hypnosis, can you do something about those nude young men? And can you protect me from criticism when I go down to the bottom of the Pacific . . . or when I float around the world on a cloud?

"By the way, Doctor, are you sure you are ethical? I notice that over there in that corner of the office you have a half-dozen nude dancing girls. I don't want my young men to associate with them. It wouldn't be moral. So would you keep control over your nude young women? I hope that all you do is let them dance for you."

This was the introductory meeting with a young woman who suffered from schizophrenia, catatonic type. She was working as a secretary for a real-estate firm for the summer and handling her work most satisfactorily.

"I've been married twice, but I didn't tell either of my husbands about the nude young men or of going around the world or to the bottom of the ocean. After we were married I told them about everything. George was so mad about it he beat me up something terrible. Bill just acted plain awful. He called in some psychiatrist. They said I was psychotic and they wanted to commit me to the State Hospital. They took me to court for a hearing. I figured that the fuss must be about those nude young men . . . and taking trips around the world . . . and my castle on the bottom of the ocean that disturbed Bill so often. So I just flatly denied all those things and I wasn't committed. Bill got a divorce.

"I have been teaching school regularly during the school year and always take a secretarial job during the summers. I have only been married twice so far. But neither of my husbands seemed to understand. It is awful worrisome teaching school—keeping the children's attention so that they won't notice those young men. It is so embarrassing when I take a bath, but I have gotten used to it. They won't even let me go to the bathroom alone. So I always wait until night, and then I don't turn on the light.

"One summer I told my employer about the nude young men. The next day I was fired and he gave me a check for two weeks. I never could understand that. He seemed to be such a sensible man.

"I came to you for help. What I want you to do is to hypnotize me. I don't want to be troubled by these nude young men. They are mine as those nude dancing girls are yours. I want to keep right on making my trips around the world. But lately I have been staying in my apartment for as much as week at a time—to take a trip around the world on the cloud or go down to the bottom of the Pacific and spend time in my castle. I want you to change things hypnotically. Don't take away my young men. Don't stop me from going around the world. Don't stop me from going down to the Pacific. Just see to it that I keep these things, but don't let them interfere with my everyday life. Now I am ready to go into a trance."

Indeed the patient was. In less than five minutes she gave every evidence of being in a profound somnambulistic trance. She was asked to remain in the trance and to talk freely. Her statement was rather peculiar. She said, "That poor girl that is really me is just plain psychotic, but she doesn't know it. She is hallucinating. She is going to the library and she has read up on catatonic schizophrenia. She is really afraid. She is covering up with you. She does not even know how afraid she is. Don't you ever let her find out how afraid she is because she might do something awful. Sometimes she has thought of suicide. Several times she has taken an overdose of sleeping pills. She just doesn't have anybody she can confide in. She thinks maybe you are all right, and will you be awfully kind to her? And you won't think bad about her because, even though she is psychotic, she is normal. Now and then she goes to bed with men, even if she isn't married to them. She wouldn't want you to know that. There are a lot of things she doesn't want you to know about her until she trusts you completely. You will have to do something about those nude young men. She is giving too much time to them. She is taking too much time to travel around the world . . . too much time to go down to her castle at the bottom of the ocean. She really enjoys and believes that the castle and the trip around the world exist. She enjoys looking down at Hong Kong and other cities. Do you think you can do anything for her?"

The somnambulistic patient was assured that, with her help, something could be done for "this psychotic girl. She is really me, you know." Instructions were offered. She listened carefully.

Slowly and systematically an explanation was given her of dreams. Normal dreams that everybody has, in which one dreams of falling off a mountainside. Falling and falling and falling forever, it seems. Finally, after what seems to be hours of falling, you hit bottom and wake to discover that you have only fallen out of bed. Yet, it seems as if one has been falling for days and weeks and months and years. It was suggested that she employ this same normal mechanism of behavior and, at any time, climb onto a cloud and feel herself floating gently around the world. She was to feel as if it were taking days and weeks and even months, maybe even years. Yet in actual clock time this will be accomplished in a minute or two or three. She smiled very happily and asked—couldn't she do that in her trips to the bottom of the sea, too? She was told she could even stay three months and the clock on her kitchen shelf would only show that she had been gone a minute.

Ready agreement was expressed, and the somnambulistic patient said that this arrangement could prove most satisfactory. But she asked most gently about the nude young men. The writer explained that he had a rather large closet attached to his office and that he could let the young men float in there. They could remain in the closet and that any time, night or day, she would be at liberty to come to the writer's house (the office is in the writer's home) and look in the closet to see if they were still there.

The patient continued to teach school for several years, and was a most competent teacher. At first, at least twice a week, she would drop in the writer's office and ask if she could look in the closet. She was always satisfied. The frequency of these visits decreased. Finally she was making them only once in three months. Then once in six months. Then approximately once a year. During this period of time she made many trips around the world on the cloud. She took great pride in being able to make a three-month trip in three minutes' time . . . in being able to stay months in her castle at the bottom of the Pacific in only three minutes of kitchen-clock time. After about three years the patient began having difficulties and sought further help. She explained openly that she was having "psychotic episodes." These "episodes" she "reserved" for the weekend, but they were becoming rather difficult. She wanted to know what she could do about them. She explained further that she did not see how she could put them in the closet with the nude young men. They might become disturbed. She didn't know if these episodes would disturb her in her teaching and in her summer work as a secretary. They might also disturb her employers and other people. She was asked what she thought she ought to do. Her statement was rather simple. "I think I think better and more clearly when you put me in a trance." Accordingly a trance was induced. In the state of somnambulism she said, "The poor thing, she is really having psychotic episodes. They are most distressing. She hasn't really told you the truth. She had to pretend she had a headache and get an excuse from teaching. She has missed more than the allowable number of sick leave days. She really has to do something about it. Last summer she lost two jobs as a secretary. You thought of putting her young men in the closet. Why don't you think of somewhere to put her psychotic episodes?"

The question was asked, "Could she put them in a manila envelope? Let them do whatever they want to do in the envelope and therefore not interfere with her. She could go by the office and leave the envelope for placement in the files." The patient thoughtfully considered this and asked, "Can you tell me [the next time she has a psychotic episode] to go into a hypnotic trance and put the psychotic episode in an envelope and bring it to you?" An agreement to this effect was reached.

The next week the patient appeared most unexpectedly, obviously in a somnambulistic state. "Here's the envelope. Don't open it. It is sealed carefully. The psychotic trance is in there. Put it in your filing cabinet. She will come by later and ask to see it." A few days later the patient appeared in the office and said, "I believe you have something of mine, but I don't know what it is." The sealed manila envelope was taken out of the files. She said, "So that is where my psychotic episodes went. You know, I think that is a good idea." For 15 years the writer has been receiving in the mail envelopes containing "psychotic episodes."

The patient is now living in a city 1,000 miles away. During one disturbing episode she took a sick leave and came to see the writer. She demanded to see the envelopes containing her "psychotic episodes." They were carefully taken out of the file, one by one, and shown to her. Before this task could be completed, she said, "Now I know I can trust you. Couldn't completely before. You don't have to take out the others. Now I can feel comfortable sending them to you."

At present the patient is gainfully employed and has a civil service position. She will soon be eligible for pension. She has been married eight times and has been self-supporting, but she has never been able to establish a savings account. She was last seen two years ago. She looked at least 15 years younger than her age. She felt free to tell the writer that there was a period of time when she became addicted to alcohol, joined Alcoholics Anonymous, and overcame the problem.

Hypnosis is not a cure. Neither is insulin in diabetes. This writer has used hypnosis on more than one psychotic patient to keep him a productive citizen. The above case history illustrates the value of intercommunication between people to establish good purposes. All of her marriages were brief, psychotic in character. She is not a mental hospital patient. She is a successful civil service worker—not a burden on society. How many more mentally ill patients, hopelessly sick, might be economically rehabilitated if physicians understood hypnosis as a modality of communication of ideas, understandings, and useful unrealized self-knowledge contained in what is popularly called the unconscious?

Only by hypnosis could this patient be approached and contact indefinitely prolonged.

HYPNOSIS TODAY—A TREND

Until very recently the study of hypnosis had been restricted to its external phenomena. Now it is realized that it is useless to continue to study hypnosis merely for itself alone. It is the association between the psychological aspects and the physical manifestations that now call for investigation. Today's developments are born of the realization that hypnosis opens the door to a more searching interest of how the person in his body behaves and reacts.

One need only study the mentally ill to note phonomenal changes not understandable by ordinary medical and psychological reasoning. By hypnosis one can so alter a person's consciousness of his environment that, in his reactions, he can call upon past experiences and learnings to utilize and accomplish equally phenomenal changes. How does a woman have an anesthetic childbirth by the spoken word? How does a man with hemophilia have˛bloodless dental extractions without medication? We need to understand the secrets of this sort of thing if we are to understand, psychologically, both health and illness.

The Fourth World Congress of Psychiatry held in September, 1966, in Madrid, disclosed a significant development of scientific interest in hypnosis at the complex physiological level. There was dissension about the ultimate question—why does the unwilling patient heal slowly? And the opposite question—how can this intrinsic force which delays healing be reversed in order to alter the unwilling patient psychologically so that he can heal more rapidly?

Thus today the trends in hypnosis center around a scientific understanding of the functioning of the human body, the forces that influence it, the means by which it can be influenced. Hypnosis can be used to elicit the learnings acquired by the human body, but unrealized by the person. Pain and stress are two of the greatest medicinal problems in their many aspects. These need to be dissected, analyzed, and studied. Mental disease is the breaking down of communication between people. Hypnosis permits a development of communication.

In laboratories of psychology departments, the physiological laboratories, the dental schools, and even in the everyday practice of medicine much is being learned about how to talk to people, to understand them. Any statesman can tell us that most of the world's troubles derive from a lack of intercommunication. So it is with matters of human illness and health. Hypnosis is not a simple matter. It is another important tool in exploring human behavior from a new and different approach—a tool that will lead to a definition of the still undefined "personality" and allow us to learn how the human body reacts to stimuli. Stimuli can then be given to take advantage of existing, but unrealized, body learnings.

7. Hypnotic Approaches to Therapy

Milton H. Erickson

I did bring several typewritten papers with me to read on "Approaches," but I also brought some notes that I think it might be better to talk from.

The first item that I want to mention concerns my demonstration this morning. I requested my subject's permission to say these things. I met her Wednesday—she came over and spoke to me. I've watched her and reached the conclusion that she has a tremendous number of conflicts. She has given me permission to tell you that. When she came up, the remarkable thing was her absolute honesty in telling me that she would resist. Therefore, it became a problem not of trying to force anything upon her but of trying to utilize her resistances and to adapt them in such a fashion that she could accomplish something, so that the members of the conference could obtain information on methods. After induction procedures the subject showed catalepsy of the left arm. In other words, she could yield on one point, but she'd be damned if she'd yield on the other! It was beautifully done on her part, and I think it was a most marvelous thing on her part. Another phenomenon—Dr. Pattie mentioned it to me—was that when she was asked a question, she would nod her head and keep nodding her head long after it was necessary. She didn't know that, but the rest of you knew it. She was not really aware of it. Her answer was that she wasn't really in a trance, but I think some of you realize that she was definitely out of contact with the audience on a number of occasions. She just didn't know you people were here. This was no reflection upon your impressiveness, but just an indication of her ability to forget all about you.

All this is an introduction to one important thing, and I think it is paramount in any approach to hypnotic therapy. That is that one must always protect the subject or the patient. The patient does not come to you just because you are a therapist. The patient comes to be protected or helped in some regard. But the personality is very vital to the person, and he doesn't want you to do too much, he does not want you to do it too suddenly. You've got to do it slowly, you've got to do it gradually, and you've got to do it in the order in which he can assimilate it. A certain

Reprinted with permission from *The American Journal of Clinical Hypnosis,* July, 1977, *20,* 1, 20-35 number of calories of food per day are necessary, but don't cram them all down at breakfast; if you do, you'll have a stomachache. You spread them out and you don't cram them all down in one mouthful. You take a number of mouthfuls. It's the same way with psychotherapy, as any analytically trained person will tell you. You go into some matters slowly, easily, and gently. In the matter of hypnotic psychotherapy you approach everything as slowly and as rapidly as the patient can endure the material. You don't do it by a drastic, driving technique because that can be rejected. The slow approach enables the patient to recognize there is value in this idea, there is value in that idea, and that's what you want him to do: to recognize that there *is* value in this idea and that *is* value in that idea. Furthermore, you therapists really don't know what the problems are, and it is your job to find out. The patient doesn't consciously know what the problems are, no matter how good a story he tells you, because that's a conscious story. What are the unconscious factors? You want to deal with the unconscious mind, bring about therapy at that level, and then to translate it to the conscious mind.

I think an experiment that I did in antisocial behavior illustrates the need of that approach. I took two secretaries and had them each in a deep trance, and I told them separately an utterly malicious and false story about a third secretary. The third secretary knew that I was going to do it and consented to it. I told each of the two girls that utterly malicious, false story, and a couple of days later Secretary A came to me—they both avoided the third girl—and told me she had a very bad headache. In fact, she'd had it since the last hypnotic session with me, and would I please do something about it. I took her in my office, put her in a trance, and she recalled that malicious story. She then gave me her very frank opinion of anybody that would tell such a malicious story about C. She really handed it to me, and it was necessary for me, in self-protection, to call in some of my collaborators and produce the typewritten protocols of the experiment to prove to her that it was an experiment. That was all in a trance state. Then I awakened her, and she promptly recalled a full recollection of the malicious story and she really gave me a nice bawling out—a second one, because my explanation had not yet seeped through. It was necessary again for me to call in my collaborators and bring out the protocols and explain the experiment all over to her conscious mind, so that she knew it at both levels.

Thus, one tries to do hypnotherapy at an unconscious level but to give the patient an opportunity to transfer that understanding and insight to the conscious mind as far as it is needed.

The second girl told me she had had a headache ever since the last time I had hypnotized her, and wouldn't I do something. So I gave her some aspirin and told her it would fix her up. About an hour later she came into the office and told me what sort of a liar I was. It was rather difficult to get her to consent to see the protocol of the experiment, and she cussed out my collaborators thoroughly too. After I had convinced her in the conscious state, I had to put her in a trance and go through all the whole ordeal with her a second time, because she needed to know it at both a conscious and an unconscious level. It was also necessary to call in the third girl about whom the story had been told to convince both of those girls that it was a put-up job, and she had to tell them both in the conscious state and in the unconscious state.

In therapeutic approaches, how does one protect a subject? I had one extremely bitter experience. I had a nice experimental subject that I was working with and I wanted her to do some hallucinating. I told her to see the loveliest thing she ever saw in her life. I thought that was a safe suggestion, and I gave her a mirror in which to hallucinate the loveliest thing she ever saw in her life. I learned a very drastic lesson. What was the loveliest thing she ever saw in her life. Her mother had been killed in an automobile accident, and she saw the mother's face in repose in the coffin. She burst into tears, and I lost rapport with her. It took me three weeks to regain that girl's confidence and trust. She was an excellent experimental subject. I learned that when you give suggestions, therapeutically or experimentally, you try to give them in a way that is going to permit the patient or the subject to handle them in a fashion that does not arouse too much difficulty.

In therapeutic approaches one must always take into consideration the actual personality of the individual. One must give thought as to how they express their behavior. Are they overfriendly, hostile, defiant, extroverted, introverted, so on? One must modify his own behavior—that is, the therapist actually must be fairly fluid in his behavior, because if he is rigid he is going to elicit certain types of rigid behavior in the patient. In turn, the patient's rigid behavior is unfamiliar to him, and he is not going to be able to handle him properly. Therefore, the more fluidity in the hypnotherapist, the more easily you can actually approach the patient.

I think perhaps the best way to continue is to give my thoughts as they come to me, and not try to follow a rigid outline.

Who is the important person in a therapeutic situation? Is it the therapist? I really don't think the therapist is important at all. I don't think that the hypnotist is important in the experimental situation. I think he is part of the apparatus, and nothing more. I think the apparatus should be in well-ordered condition, run properly, and so on, but I don't think that any experiment is possible where you have only apparatus. You need a subject in therapy. I don't think the therapist is *the* important person; I think the patient is *the* important person in the situation. I think, too, that the patient should be given the opportunity to dominate in any way, whether it is by complete subservience or by complete dominance of the situation. It is this that the patient comes in for, not to have the therapist take charge, but to give the therapist an opportunity of doing something, and doing something in accord with the needs of the patient, not in accord with the needs of the therapist. I disagree with a lot of therapists who think that they should sit up straight behind a couch, and take notes, and more or less direct this thought and that thought, because that is just their understanding and it is the patient's needs that should be met. Now, this is not intended as a criticism of psychoanalysis, because it is extremely valuable.

Recently I had an experience in experimental therapeutic procedure that I want to cite. It's not published; in fact, all of this material that I am going to give is unpublished. It concerns this problem of amnesia that was mentioned—the John Does. How often are these amnesia victims really amnesic? How often are they neurotics who are having their amnesia serve as a recognizable purpose?

A patient that I know was picked up by the police in Phoenix. They attempted to ascertain her identity and her age. I happened to be one of the psychiatrists called. She gave the year as 1934, and she thought the calendar on the wall was wrong. Moreover, she knew she was not in Phoenix because she knew that was not possible: she had never been in Arizona. The real truth was, of course, that she had been in Arizona for several years; and certainly it wasn't 1934, it was 1952. She was afraid of everybody, so my wife went with me as a reassuring person. The question was, how would you really handle that amnesia?

All of us have heard about age regression. Obviously, there had been a spontaneous age regression; and a few questions here indicated a definite age regression—a spontaneous one—in which the amnesia was very definite. She took a violent dislike to me because I carried a cane, and she took a violent dislike to me also because I wore a moustache. When the police officer introduced me to her as Dr. Erickson, she took a violent dislike. I asked him to repeat my name until he wondered who was the patient, because I wanted to know what the situation was. I soon found out that it was the first part of my name—not Erickson, but *Eric*kson—to which she objected. So there must have been an Eric somewhere. Where did the cane come in—the fear reactions, the trembling, the perspiration, the involuntary responses she showed to a cane?

I took her to my office and puzzled over this question. What can you do for a genuine amnesia? She was back in 1934, and then I hit upon the very happy idea: why not reverse the process? I pointed to the wall and told her "There's a calendar there, and I think if you look real hard you'll see a calendar that reads 1934." I wanted to put myself into that amnesia pattern, and it wasn't long before I had her seeing a calendar of 1934. Then we watched the leaves of that calendar torn off, the way they do in the movies, one by one, and the years change. And it wasn't April, 1934, it was May, 1934, then June, then July; and then '35, '36, '38. I slowly, gradually, systematically, brought her up to November 1951, and the event of her amnesia.

Some time later she developed another amnesia. It was 1943, and I used the same technique to bring her up to 1952. She became my patient and I learned a great deal about her history. She had had a tremendous number of traumatic experiences in 1934. I know who Eric was. He wore a moustache, had gray hair, and carried a cane. And she had good reason to fear anybody with gray hair who wore a moustache and a cane, and who had those syllables of Eric in his name.

That reversal of regression technique I have tried on experimental subjects many times without realizing its therapeutic situations with patients who suddenly get the needle stuck in a certain year and just can't get away from those events, keep repeating them in an obsessional, compulsive fashion. In such cases you systematically reorient them—a day, a week, a month at a time—until they come to the present age. And what happens? They know something about the control of obsessional, compulsive behavior.

In this same connection there is another exceedingly unpleasant experience that I had therapeutically. This patient came into my office. She had been my patient for some time, and I thought I was making excellent progress with her. That day she was wearing a brand-new dress and she said to me, "Doctor, would you like to have me model my dress for you?" She modeled it very nicely, and then she said, "You know, I'd really like to tell you about a dream I had." So I said, "Go ahead."

She sat down comfortably to tell me the dream, when a look of horror came over her face. She lost all contact with me, and I had to rush to the door to keep her from dashing out and dashing downtown until at least I could understand what was going on. My original diagnosis of her was acute paranoid schizophrenia, and she certainly looked and acted then like a paranoid schizophrenic. I had hypnotized her previously and made use of physical signs—lifting the arms, inducing catalepsy—because usually, with a therapeutic patient, where I use hypnosis I bring about some physical condition so that I can always get in contact. I finally managed to get close enough to her to get hold of her wrist and gently lift it so that she would go into a trance. She was, however, in one of those mute and unresponsive trances.

It took me about four hours, very painful hours, to find out how to handle that apparently deep paranoid episode. I finally hit upon this idea: She didn't like something, she wanted to escape from something. That something had happened at such-and-such an hour—four o'clock, on Tuesday, June 5th, and then of course it wouldn't have happened. And what was it that happened? Well, since it was before June 5th at four o'clock, nothing had happened—in other words, an absolute denial of everything. So I carried her back to May and reestablished relationships with her at the May level. She was friendly, agreeable; then I asked her what she thought about the possibilities of next month. We talked about the possibilities of next month, how she would feel about it, and what possible material might come forth next month. We speculated more and more; and as soon as I tried to approach Tuesday she started getting rigid, her face seemed molded, and so on.

It took four hours, as I have said, before I got her willing to admit the fact that on Tuesday, June 5th, at four o'clock she would come into my office and model a dress for me and then suggest the topic of dreams. The dream happened to be an incestuous dream, and she just couldn't tolerate it. By retiring her to May and then tracing up to June, it was possible to handle it. It was exceedingly slow, painful, and laborious, but the patient needed to get over it and to get an understanding of it.

Another patient was presented to me under rather difficult circumstances. Some people with a psychoanalytically oriented background came to me and said they thought hypnotherapy was without value, and they challenged me to give a demonstration of hypnotherapy. I told them I would be glad to do it and that we probably all would learn something. They said they would select a patient for me. Let's call him Harvey. I took one look at Harvey. He certainly was his mama's dishrag if ever there was one—colorless, coatless, discouraged. I found out that he had been under the treatment of another psychiatrist for a couple of years. He had a pain here—and then he had a pain here—and then he had another pain here. . . . He was wonderful—as a pathological specimen. But when you talked to Harvey, you wondered if underneath all of that there wasn't a nice guy.

I took Harvey into the seminar room and put him in a trance. He very willingly, very gradually went into a trance. He would do anything to please an authoritative figure. With him you could use the direct, forceful, hypnotic technique. One of the things I found out from his psychiatrist was that Harvey worked in an office doing clerical work far below his ability. He was usually sick about once a month and lost a day's work, and had a feeling of being unhappy in his work. One of the reasons was this: There was a pile of ashes outside his office, and there was a black man who came to carry away those ashes who was very resentful of white people. He would come into the office, open the window, and he would then shovel the ashes so that, when the wind was right, the ashes blew into the office. Poor Harvey would sit cowering at his desk and wish he could tell off that black man, who was only about 18 inches taller than Harvey and much more muscular.

Even though Harvey worked at a desk, he couldn't write his name legibly. The other psychiatrist had tried to get him to do that over and over again, but Harvey just couldn't write his name legibly. This poses the question as to where one starts in therapy. My feeling was that with

Harvey and the sort of situation presented I had an excellent opportunity to demonstrate the importance of the point of departure in therapy. I trained Harvey to be an excellent subject, so that he could hallucinate, both positively and negatively. I avoided the matter of writing. He could describe driving along the street and could bring forth childhood memories which, the other psychiatrist assured me, were not loaded with emotion. Finally, when I thought Harvey was a really good hypnotic subject, I took the opportunity of giving him a pad of paper and asking him, in the trance state, to write his name. His writing in the trance state was just as bad as it was in the waking state. I asked him to write, "This is a beautiful day in June," and it was barely legible.

I then had one of the group who had a beautiful handwriting write his name and "This is a beautiful day in June." When I praised that beautiful writing, Harvey simply cowered in his seat at hearing somebody else getting praised—a painful situation for Harvey. Then I asked Harvey, "How do you suppose Dr. Jones feels about what I said about his handwriting? How do you think he feels about that handwriting? How do you think the pencil feels in his hand? How do you think a pen would feel? How do you think his hand would feel against the pad of paper when he writes so beautifully? How do you think he will feel a year from now when he reads that?"

Harvey really started thinking about it. And then I asked him, "How much would you like to do that sort of thing?" Harvey said, "I'd give anything if I could write legibly, but I can't."

Having laid that foundation (which I have abbreviated very much), I had Harvey hallucinate in crystal balls—they're much cheaper than the kind you can buy in a magic store, and you can distribute them wherever you want all around the room. I asked Harvey to look into a designated crystal ball and to see a little boy, viewed from the rear. "That little boy must be pretty unhappy," I said. "I wonder why. He looks as if he's very, very unhappy. You look at him and tell me where he is."

Harvey said, "Why, that's a little kid about six years old, and he's sitting in his desk at school. The teacher just walked away. She's got a ruler in her hand. She must have been punishing him."

I said, "All right. Now look in that crystal up there [indicating another ball]. I think you'll see that same little boy at the age of 12. What's he doing?"

Harvey looked and, sure enough, there was a boy of 12 in it. "He's walking through the woods with his brother, carrying a gun."

I asked Harvey how he knew it was the boy's brother.

"I don't know. I just think that. The 12-year-old boy does not seem very happy. He doesn't like that gun, and he looks rather unhappy. I don't like the looks of that."

I said, "Why?"

"Well, there are the two boys. One's about 14 or 15, and the other boy is about 12. They have a dog with them. They are going hunting. But that 12-year-old looks just like that boy over there, and he's miserable. I wish I could see his face. Now he's left his brother, he's wandered off to that tree over there, and he's very miserable. He's practically crying."

"Well," I said, "what about that crystal up there? Can you see that same boy in that crystal about the age of 20?"

He looked, and he saw him there.

I said, "How does it seem to you that he's behaving?"

"Well, he's very, very unhappy. And you know, it's the same kind of unhappiness. They're the same boy at different ages, but they all have the same feeling. They're very unhappy."

"What about that crystal there? He's about 30."

Harvey looked. "The same sort of unhappiness!"

"Well, how does it happen that a six-year-old boy and a 30-year-old boy all have the same kind of unhappiness? At least you describe it as such."

"They're really the same boy—but how can that be? I don't understand. But they *are* the same boy, and it *is* the same kind of unhappiness."

So I asked him, as a preliminary, "Now, is there anything else in that crystal there . . . anything else in that crystal [indicating different crystals]?"

He said, "No, up there . . . but up there—and how did it get up there— there's a place for a doghouse, and it doesn't make sense. But there's a place for a doghouse down there too, and that doesn't make sense."

We discussed that for a while. The psychoanalyst questioned him about it, but Harvey was very limited in his replies. Then my question was "Now, suppose you look at this crystal and see if you can explain something—why there's dog here, a place for a doghouse there, and a place for a doghouse *there*. Just see something that explains it!"

Harvey looked into the crystal and said, "Why it's that six-year-old boy coming home from school. He's still got some unhappy feelings. I wish I could see his face, but I suppose it isn't important. He's still rubbing his face—at least, looking at him from behind, that's what he seems to be doing. There are some policemen there, and one of them is holding a revolver. The boy rushes in to see what it's all about, and the policeman has just shot his dog." He paused thoughtfully. "But he didn't know about that when he was at school. Then when he was 12 years old, he went hunting with his brother. . . . Why, there was an accident to his dog! And that boy has never dared to own a dog since then. *That's* why there's a doghouse there in that crystal and a doghouse there."

I said, "Well, maybe that does explain it. But the boy was crying in school, before he found the dog killed. Why was he crying in school?"

"I don't really know, but I've got the most awful feeling in my left hand. And I know just how that boy feels. It feels as if somebody took a ruler and rapped me on the hand for writing with my left hand."

So I quickly shifted the scene, dropped it right there. I awakened Harvey and had a social interview with the psychoanalyst, spending about half an hour chit-chatting about this and that, and then put Harvey into a trance. I wanted those ideas to soak into his unconscious.

When he was in a trance, I told Harvey, "I'm going to give you a piece of paper and a pencil, and I want you to write your name the way that six-year-old boy would have liked to write. But I want you to write with your right hand, just as the other psychiatrist told me he wrote with his right hand—and I mean that he *did write with his right hand.* I want you to have an idea that you can take over Dr. Jones's feeling about his excellent handwriting as you write your name. I don't want you to write it just yet. I'll put the pad of paper there and the pencil there, and after a while I'll have a cigarette and you'll pick up the pencil and you won't notice that you're doing it. You'll take it in your right hand, and you'll write your name and 'This is a beautiful day in June' right under Dr. Jones's handwriting. Then I'm going to awaken you, and you'll have no knowledge of having written. Anybody who tells you that you have written anything is nothing but a damned liar—and you tell them so. Make no bones about it. Just tell them they are damned liars."

He wrote his name and "This is a beautiful day in June." I awakened him and we chatted for a while socially. Then someone I had picked out took up the paper, looked at it, and said, "Well, Harvey, you certainly have a good handwriting."

"I have not!"

"Well, here's your name and here's where you wrote 'This is a beautiful day in June' . . ."

Harvey told him just what kind of a liar he was.

Somebody else told Harvey how good his handwriting was, and was informed as to his status and his veracity. We went through the entire group. Then I said to Harvey, "Well, they may be offensive liars, and cheats, and frauds, and so on, but if you watch that pencil there on the desk—if you just watch it, you're going to see something very interesting, because the hand that wrote your name and 'This is a beautiful day in June' in such good script is going to pick up that pencil. See if you can identify the hand."

"All right," Harvey said, "but nobody's really close enough, and it ought to be easy to identify the person who walks up to the pencil. So I'll watch the pencil . . ." He turned his attention carefully to the pencil. And then, "Why, that's *my* hand! But I can't write that good. I don't believe it! This writing here—'This is a beautiful day in June'—it's good script!" He paused a moment and then, very deliberately, said, "That *is* my hand and I *did* write it."

I said, "Then we're all agreed, and we're not going to dispute with you. That will be all for this session."

The next day—but it wouldn't have made any difference if it had been a couple of days later—the wind was blowing just right. The black man came in, opened the window, and started shoveling ashes. Harvey went out, stepped up to the black man, and said, "Listen, big boy. If you were working where I am, would you like all those ashes blowing in on you?"

"Well, no, I wouldn't."

"Then why did you open the window?"

"White boy, I think I was just being cussed, and I'm going to close it for you."

The window was closed by the black man. Harvey went home; the next day he went to his boss and said, "Listen, I've been working here for several years, and I haven't had a promotion or an increase in salary. Don't you think it's about time?"

The boss said, "Why, yes."

Harvey went to his psychiatrist and said, "I don't know what you've done to me. You know, I'm 32 years old and I think it's about time I got a girl. Don't you think so?"

The psychiatrist said, "Well, you know, I've got nothing to say about that. You'll have to consult Dr. Erickson."

And Harvey said, "To hell with Dr. Erickson! I'm going to get a girl."

Harvey's happily married. He writes legibly.

Now, where did that therapy take place? How much did I need to know about him? I started at the nuclear point—his handwriting. I didn't know what I would get in those crystal images, but I could see a succession of events there that I could investigate, one by one, and then give him that kinesthetic idea—that kinesthetic sense of a nicely written, right-hand script production—and allow him to vent all aggression by letting him call the members of the group damned liars. He had to call somebody a damned liar. He couldn't take out aggression against the policeman for shooting the dog: the dog was rabid, and he was just a six-year-old kid at the time. I didn't know about that either, nor did the other psychiatrist.

Harvey later gave a very nice account of this, when I gave him full recollection of the experience, at a medical group. Harvey is still getting along successfully, and this all took place back in 1945.

I should like to present at this point the use of hypnotherapy in an experimental fashion. I was very much afraid that one of my patients was going to develop schizophrenia. Her very best friend had. She was a very accomplished person, professionally trained, and she worked until 11 at night. As soon as she got off work, she would sneak home, cowering and shivering, because there were some peculiar figures that were following her. Her bedroom was peopled by monsters of some sort. I think you would call her a psychotic, although she had sufficient insight so that you could have some doubts about it. She wasn't quite certain whether she was having dreams or whether her experiences were real.

"How could I have a dream on the street? I've got the feeling, though, that there are monsters back of me in mid-air."

I asked Mary if it wouldn't be a very nice thing to see herself in a crystal ball. I produced one, and she described to me the little girl she saw there.

In some surprise she said, "Why, that's me! And I'm very happy there. I'm playing with my doll. Now I'm going to go over and swing. I certainly was a happy kid. And look at that blue-checked pinafore I'm wearing!"

She really enjoyed looking at herself at the age of six.

So I conjured up another crystal for her. She was several years older. She described herself with a great deal of pleasure.

I said, "Don't look at that crystal over there yet. Let's look at the crystal here."

Slowly, carefully, I carried her through a process of fourteen crystals. The thirteenth crystal was her present state, in which she was walking home from the hospital in fear of those hideous monsters and evils. Were they real or unreal? When she got to the tenth crystal, I told her that she wouldn't know who the girl was in the crystal ball.

She said, "That's a ghastly thing to have me look at."

"Well, you just describe it to me thoroughly, completely, and adequately." We went through the tenth to the twelfth, and they were very, very painful. I said, "Now, I want you to forget the identity of the person in all of these crystals. Just tell me what you think about them—and never mind that crystal over there."

She said, "Well, she was a happy little girl. Then she was a little bit older. There she's going to school—she looks as though she might be in such-and-such a grade. There she's in high school, and there she's going to a Christmas party." And so on. "My heavens! What's happened to that girl? Why should she have such horrible feelings?"

I said, "Well, I don't know—you don't know—but I've got a very pleasant surprise for you. If you'll look in that crystal there, and then look in that crystal over there, you'll discover that they're the same girl. And in that crystal over there, you'll see the picture of a girl who is acting and behaving very real. It isn't really a living picture—it's just a girl in that picture, and she's happy, and she's pleased, and she's going to be doing something that she really wants to do and she's really going to be enjoying it. Now that girl and this girl are the same girl. But the process of growth and development, the changes that occur in life, the accidents in life, and so on . . . You know, every story should have a good ending."

She looked, and she said, "Well! That six-year-old kid grew up to be a very pretty girl, didn't she? And look at her. She's on a diving board, and she's got on a blue bathing suit with a yellow dragon or something on it, and she's having a wonderful time, she's really enjoying herself. I can hardly believe it. That girl is enjoying herself—she really is!"

I said, "This is only June, but that girl up there is going swimming in August."

Mary went swimming in August. She went swimming in a blue bathing suit with a yellow figure on it—I don't know whether it was a dragon or not. At all events she went swimming. I found out afterward that she had learned to swim and then had developed tremendous fears and anxieties and distresses. She had developed all these other agonies, in spite of the fact that she actually had had professional training, and she had a very difficult time.

She is the head of a professional department at the present time, so I think that experiment was successful. I had a letter from Mary the other day, and she's very happy. She's married—happily married—and getting along very nicely.

What did I do when I started experimental therapy? I let her identify herself in a safe and sure fashion by putting her in a crystal.

There's another item that I want to mention, and that is the idea of time distortion. What do I mean by time distortion? It's been mentioned previously how time can pass very rapidly in the trance state. Lynn Cooper, I think in 1945, published the first article on the subject. Then a couple of years ago Lynn Cooper came to Phoenix, and we worked together on time distortion. Pell reported on that. Lynn Cooper was very much interested in knowing whether you could employ time distortion in therapy, and I agreed that I would try it out. I tried it out with two patients and with very nice results.

How long is time when you're asleep? I can remember the doctor who volunteered for some experimental work at the staff dining room, and I agreed to meet the doctor in the psychology laboratory at one o'clock. She came in. I picked up a book, and we got to discussing psychology and this particular book. I took advantage of that situation to put the doctor into a deep trance. I did the experiment, brought her out of her trance, sat her down, put the book in her hand, and renewed the conversation where I had interrupted it to put her in a trance. We concluded the discussion, and all of a sudden she noticed that it was five o'clock. She expressed her regret that she had allowed her interest in that book to distract me from my experiment.

I said, "Well, it's all right. Tomorrow's another day." She met me again the next day at one o'clock, and I used exactly the same technique, except that I had established a posthypnotic cue for her, saving both time and labor.

After three weeks of that sort of performance the doctor was a little bit irritated with me, and she really castigated me at the staff dining room table.

"Three weeks ago I volunteered to act as a hypnotic subject. All you've done has been to meet me in the psychology laboratory, utter a few inanities about psychological textbooks, and waste my afternoon for three long weeks. I'm sick and tired of that. Either you're going to use me as a subject or you're not. That's all there is to it." (She was downright unpleasant about it.)

Nevertheless, she went up to the psychology laboratory at one o'clock, and I met her there and used the same technique. When the experiment, which required that the subject not know what the experiment was, was completed, I told her that she had been a subject all that time; but I had to tell her in both the trance state and the waking state.

What did time really mean to her? I don't know how many times my patients will tell me, "I've been in here fifteen minutes, five minutes, three minutes." One of my subjects has a neat little trick of checking on a wristwatch, and never allows me to take that wristwatch off. Time perception in hypnosis is one thing; in the conscious state it is another. Cooper has been interested in that for a long, long time. With regard to different kinds of therapy, one of Cooper's subjects, for example, picked some irises, some 150. The actual time spent in that hallucinatory activity was 10 seconds. After the subject was awakened, the subject was told to remember and was told to demonstrate the rate with which the irises were picked. The rate was essentially the same as if it had been half an hour, which the subject had estimated.

The question came up: How could I use that therapeutically? I had a patient—and I'll give you just one miserable detail of that patient's history, so that you can appreciate why it was difficult to handle the patient. At the age of six a foster uncle decided to take the little girl for a visit. He took her to an isolated cabin, bound her hands and feet to the bed in a spread-eagle fashion, took a jackknife, and really carved up her body in a horrible manner. I've seen the scars.

The physician who referred the patient told me, "I had to fight like a madman to do a physical on this patient. She needs psychiatric care. She isn't an internal medicine case at all. I can't understand those scars. I wasn't able to do a complete physical examination because she fought so fiercely, yet she would apologize and then fight so madly."

It took quite a long time for me to do a physical examination on her. But the scars on her abdomen, and on her thighs, all over her body, were deep and vicious ones. Those of you who have had prison experience in psychiatric treatment know that sort of thing is possible.

I wanted to get from her an account of her past life. She was a good hypnotic subject, and I asked her first to describe a childhood birthday party. I had my stopwatch readily available. The stopwatch was no use. It took her just as long to describe the birthday party that she had hallucinated in a crystal ball as it took for the party to occur. I then tried an auto ride she had experienced when she was a little girl. The time was equivalent. She described things very nicely, very thoroughly, very consistently. If a birthday party took three hours to occur and the psychiatrist didn't know about it, it took three hours of his time to discover the fact. We didn't get very far until fall. It took from July until October to get a history from her. In every instance she gave me only pleasant things, good memories, but in such elaborate detail that they consumed as much time as the original experience.

I therefore carefully explained to her that in a hypnotic state, "just as you are now, time is going to change. Everything is going to speed up with tremendous rapidity, and by the time I drop my pencil you're going to remember everything that happened to you in the first eight years, going to school, things of that sort." I went over and over the idea of speeding up memory. I never got any really traumatic memory except the one relating to the scars that I had discovered. That was the only one. Apart from this I could only obtain from her a dully repetitious, "I got stabbed. I got stabbed. I got stabbed." My knowledge of psychiatry and criminology led me to the conclusion as to what kind of stabbing it was. After I had inculcated the concept of distorted time, rapid time, experimental time, or whatever you want to call it, I told her to look at a crystal ball. I said that I would give her all the time she needed; but in that crystal ball—where she had previously seen a birthday party, an automobile ride, a train ride, some horses, some trees, and things of that sort—she would see everything that had happened to her in a certain period of her life that covered 16 months. I didn't say 16 months. What I said was "Everything that happened to you from 1930 to 1933, roughly speaking. I don't know, maybe it's the wrong period; but somehow we're going to select the period you should tell me about."

She agreed that she would look in the crystal, and then I explained the distorted-time idea. I told her that when I said, "Start," she would see in the crystal everything in slow motion so that she could memorize and recall and understand everything so that she could remember and tell it to me. I further indicated that although she would be seeing things in slow motion, it wouldn't take very much time for her to describe what she saw. This was rather a contradictory suggestion, but she understood that. At the proper signal I set my stopwatch; 20 seconds later she had covered 16 months of the most traumatic material imaginable, and did a thorough job of it. The death of her father, the death of her mother, the death of several other people—it was just incredible. It was as if she were held immobile, as if she were fascinated by the terrible procession of events in the crystal. She just couldn't stop, as that chain of slow motions with such extreme rapidity took place.

After 20 seconds' time I noticed that I was fatiguing that poor woman much too much. I put an end to the session, awakened her, and then said to her, "You know, I've never been able to get you to tell me the facts of your life. I've been working through July, August, September, and now it is October. I really don't know very much about you. I do know that you've been stabbed—that's essentially all I know."

She said, "I couldn't stand to tell you."

"Well, we've got the rest of the day. Suppose you tell me."

The rest of the day and a good share of the next day were spent for her to tell the series of events and to bring forth corroborating evidence. I corroborated item after item. I had to write to various sections of the country to get proof. For example, did a certain person and the patient, on such-and-such a day, in such-and-such a year, have an automobile accident? You can get such information from vital statistics, police departments, and public records. I wrote to five different states and found she had given me reliable information. It had taken just 20 seconds to secure the impetus of events. The momentum seemed to carry her along with such impelling force that she was unable to stop. I will agree that I had a difficult time with the patient, for she said, "You have no right to know these things." It took quite a long time for her to recognize that I did have the right to know those things. I explained that she had been hospitalized for severe headaches that would last for three weeks at a time, with nausea and vomiting that couldn't be touched by morphine or anything else. There were other details, but I will not relate them here.

Whether 20 seconds, or 10 seconds, periods increased to obtain information about some other aspects of her life. It took me 10 seconds to get a completely repressed memory. She didn't know why, when she came to my office, she didn't like my six-year-old son. I think he's adorable; but he is the most awful, hateful pest—a nuisance—she would shake and tremble at the sight of him. I did everything I could to try to find out why. I gave every association test that I knew. Why did she hate poor little Bobby? He's just an ordinary kid. What could I do about it? Nothing. She had complete repression. In 10 seconds' time I found out by the same process I had used earlier. I had her look in a crystal, and I said to her, "Somehow or other Bobby's in that crystal over there . . ."

"Oh, no! Bobby *isn't* in that crystal!"

"Now, why should Bobby be connected with that crystal in any way?"

She told me that what I was saying to her didn't seem to make sense. I said, "No, but it's your job to make sense out of it. So let's put Bobby out of it and put the sense in."

In 10 seconds' time she recalled that in the early 1940s her husband had brought home a girl and announced that this girl was his mistress and that she would have to wait on this girl. There weren't to be any ifs, ands, or buts about it; and he slapped her down. The girl demanded a cup of tea, just to show her power. My patient said, "But the baby's just started crying." (That was the first I knew about that.) Her husband slapped her down again, and she got the cup of tea for the mistress. She then went in to the baby.

The autopsy reported that the baby had strangled to death on a ribbon in his nightie.

Another patient who had been suffering from asthma came to my office and told me she couldn't understand why she had asthma or why she had it only at certain times. I said, "Well, we'll try to diagnose it in this interview."

She said, "You must have a pretty good opinion of yourself."

I said, "All right. It's now two o'clock. At 2:36, by that clock there, you will have an attack of asthma."

She looked at me as though she thought I ought to have my head examined. We chatted on and on very casually about various things, including her childhood. At 2:36 she had an attack of asthma. Why? I guided that conversation very carefully. It seemed to be just an ordinary social conversation, but actually I kept loading it progressively, and at 2:36 I asked her how often her father wrote her letters? As soon as I mentioned her father's letters, she developed an attack of asthma.

I had already learned in her previous history that her father never wrote her during the summertime, but always wrote her in the fall, the winter, and the spring. What had her father done to her? Her father had really mistreated her mother in a most outrageous fashion. The mother had left her share of the property to the daughter out of that property. Moreover, the father had written a lot of very disagreeable letters to his daughter every fall, winter, and spring. I was quite safe when I said 2:36, because I knew I could mention her father's letters at 2:36 and that she would get an attack of asthma. I felt sure of this because in her previous history taking I had had her describe when the attacks of asthma came on, where she was sitting, whether by this window or that window, and what she had happened to be doing. The mailman intruded into that situation too many times. Therefore, I wondered about the letters. Yet she had told me about her father not being fair, about his being unjust to her mother and unjust to her; but that wasn't sufficient knowledge. I had to mention the specific item—the father's letters.

She hasn't had any asthma since we discussed her father's letters, and I helped her compose a few replies to her father. I think that perhaps I may have done some psychiatrist in that state a favor by giving him a patient.

One of the psychosomatic problems that I want to mention now concerns the matter of stuttering that so often constitutes a serious problem. In every psychiatric case you have to take the individual personality into consideration if you're going to handle stuttering. The psychotherapeutic approach and the hypnotic approach, in my experience, are most effective if you recognize one general factor. Stuttering is a form of aggression against society and people in general. You know the old joke about the great big man who asked the small-sized man how he could get to the Union Station in Chicago, and the small-sized man looked at him blankly and didn't answer. The large man went on and asked someone else. Someone went over to the small-sized man and said to him, "Why didn't you tell that chap how to get to the Union Station?" The small-sized man said, "D-d-did you th-i-nk I wanted to get my b-b-bl-o-o-ock knocked off?"

Stuttering is a form of aggression. Why should the patient aggress in a way that is uncomfortable to the patient? I had a patient, a physician, who had stuttered all of his life. When he came to me as a patient, I told him very frankly that his stuttering was an aggression and that I would be very glad to take care of it, if he were willing. I stated also that it would not be a pleasant sort of thing. He asked me if I thought stammering or stuttering were very pleasant things. I put him in a trance and worked quite a while with him on the subject of how he felt about speech and how he felt about people in general. I then built up a negative attitude and aggression toward me, which serves the purpose of allowing the patient to vent his aggression on me individually.

As a result the doctor is in a difficult situation. He speaks clearly and lucidly, has no stammer or stutter. He never fails to send me a Christmas card, but he always writes: "I hate your guts and I'm going to keep right on." Nevertheless, he sends me a Christmas card, and he sends Christmas presents to my children, but he always has a nasty crack for me. When we meet, we laugh and talk and exchange stories. The one I just told about the big man and the little man I've told him, and we've both laughed about it; he thinks it's funny. "But," he has told me, "it seems to me I've got a need for a lifelong hatred of something—I don't know what it is. You're convenient, and you're a nice guy to hate."

I said, "That's right, and it's solved your stammering problem."

Another one of my patients decided that he would get psychoanalyzed. He spent five years in the process to find out what had caused his original stammer. After five years he said, "You know, I've learned a lot about psychoanalysis and the treatment of patients by psychotherapy, but actually, you corrected my stammer. You gave me a certain hatred that was very, very useful, and my psychoanalyst tried to take it away from me."

The hatred I gave him was that trees should not be less than 18 inches from the sidewalk. I thought that was a fairly harmless hatred. He didn't have to do anything about it. He could ignore it, it shouldn't cause him any kind of distress; but at the same time he could really hate it.

"My psychoanalyst," he went on, "tried to take that away from me. He almost succeeded, and then I started to stammer. I decided I was going to keep right on. That hatred was some sort of crutch that I was really using."

He still doesn't stutter. What did I do? I don't know. It was an experimental case, and he came to me on that basis.

There is still another instance that I would like to cite. Chester Garvey came to Worcester, where I was working, and said that he had seen Hull induce hypnosis but didn't quite believe it. Would I please demonstrate hypnosis for him? He was rather antagonistic and hostile toward the idea of hypnosis.

I called in Art and Hulda, who were psychologists working for their Ph.D.s and who were good hypnotic subjects. I explained Dr. Garvey's desire and his disbelief in hypnosis. I asked them if they believed in it. They said they certainly did. I then said, "I've got to go downstairs and do an experiment on the ergograph. So I'm going to hypnotize you, Art, so that hypnosis can really be demonstrated."

Art said, "Okay," and went into a very nice trance, and I promptly left. I wondered what would happen as I left Garvey there with those two Ph.D. candidates. Garvey walked over to Art in the trance state, because Art was in a somnambulistic state, and Art said, "Well, Dr. Erickson has left, and you wanted a demonstration of hypnosis. Both Hulda and I are good subjects. Suppose I put Hulda into a trance." Hulda, assuming that she was going to demonstrate Art, found herself going into a trance! This was a very confusing thing for Garvey. Art put Hulda into a trance and demonstrated a great variety of hypnotic phenomena.

When I came back from the ergograph experiment, I walked into the room and spoke to Art. He said, "I think we're through demonstrating hypnosis." I turned to Hulda to speak to her and realized that she was in a trance state. So I said, "How do you mean?" Art replied, "Well, I put Hulda in a trance to demonstrate to Dr. Garvey what hypnosis is."

I thought that I would add a little more confusion to the situation. I awakened Art. He was still in rapport with Hulda, but I was not in rapport with Hulda. I had him awaken Hulda, and I asked him if she would demonstrate hypnosis to Dr. Garvey. She, not knowing that time had elapsed, proceeded to try with Art in the waking state to demonstrate catalepsy and a few other phenomena. Art kept telling her, "But I'm awake!" Hulda insisted, "No, you're not. I saw Dr. Erickson put you in a trance, and I know you're in a trance."

Of course, that settled it for Garvey. He didn't expect it, I didn't expect it, and it certainly is in contradiction to White's theories of goal-directed behavior, no matter what qualifications you put upon it.

What bearing does that have upon therapeutic approaches? It has a bearing on indirectness of approach. Art was thoroughly appreciative of the fact that Garvey was hostile and antagonistic and resentful. Consequently, he contrived a situation that would overcome it in a way that

Garvey could not possibly resist. I use that approach therapeutically quite often. I have an Arizona State College student that I have used a number of times. A patient will come into my office, sit down, and say, "Well, I'm here. What are you going to do about it?" Frankly, I can't do a thing about it because of his attitude. Yet such patients honestly want therapy, but they are antagonistic and resentful. It is very easy to chat with them socially for a while, then bring in a student that they might like to meet and have the student put them in a trance for me. They have no resistance toward the student; it's all channeled and directed toward me. Resistance should be channeled toward the therapist. The student puts them in a trance and then I supplant the student.

Sometimes I have to put the student in a trance first, just to demonstrate that I do know how to produce hypnosis. The patient watches and says, "Well, there's no question about it. You can hypnotize that person." The patient has no resistance against a hypnotized person hypnotizing him. It is a very simple, easy method of overcoming some of the tremendous resistance that psychiatrists meet over and over again.

Yesterday I mentioned a color-blind girl and her reaction to the fact that somehow I had changed her dress on her, and what explanation could I give for that. She was entitled to ask a qustion like that. I've had that happen more than once, when I've changed a situation. What excuse did I have for taking her out of my office and taking her into her own bedroom? Physically she was still in my office; psychologically she was in her bedroom, and what business did I have there? There is a tremendous need for protecting patients in ordinary psychotherapy. How often is the resistance the result of the therapist's intruding upon intimate memories, intimate ideas? This accounts for a great deal of resistance, and in hypnotherapy one can reach that sort of situation by stating to the patients very definitely your intention to protect them. Patients should understand that, and you should not overlook the possibility that you can unwittingly intrude upon the legitimate privacy of a patient.

There are certain frightened reactions that patients show. I remember getting in trouble with an adult male whose legs I had anesthetized to test for the knee-jerk. He showed an excellent anesthesia; but he decided to shift in his chair, and as every anesthetist knows, with a spinal block you don't move your legs around very much, depending, of course, upon the level of the block. In hypnotic anesthesia, where is the level of the block? In hypnotic anesthesia, you get a motor block also. The patient isn't aware of that. This patient of mine discovered that he couldn't walk, and he was infuriated. I had no business paralyzing him! You'll find, in producing catalepsy in a patient, that he can resent that with tremendous force. Usually, when I find that sort of thing, I use it as a center for localizing hostility, resentments, antagonism, and aggression. It's a convenient one that the patient has picked out for me, rather than making it necessary for me to produce it.

I was asked yesterday by someone about the problem of phantom limbs. "How do you handle that in hypnotherapy?" A friend of mine who had suffered an amputation had a discussion with me one night. He was also a psychiatrist and psychologist. He had written out his ideas, and he started quizzing me on the subject because he had experienced a great deal of difficulty with his phantom limb. We both had worked out essentially the same method. I suppose you would call it reconditioning.

I will give an illustration. The amputation is here on the arm—the index and second fingers get crossed, you can't straighten them out, and they are painfully tired. How are you going to approach that sort of thing hypnotically? The thing I do is to put the subject in a trance, try to reorient to a time previous to the amputation, which is a very difficult thing. He has only got one arm, and he can't balance his body properly. You reorient, however, certain memories, then you raise this question of crossed fingers. "Now, where do you feel that? Do you feel pressure here, or do you feel it in the joint? Or perhaps your wrist gets tired?" I am speeding up the procedure; but you discuss such matters, and you slowly move up the locus of the feeling to the stump. Get the patients to understand the progressive upward movement, so that they can't be certain it's their fingers, or just exactly where it is.

A patient came to me with very serious neurotic complaints of heart pains. Most medical practitioners will explain to you that you don't get heart pain in the chest wall. But this man knew that he got heart pains in the chest wall, and I became very much interested. Was it on the left side of the sternum, in the middle of the sternum, the right side? Was it between this rib and that rib? I slowly had that pain migrate to his shoulder and migrate down his arm. As it migrated, the pain decreased more and more until it finally vanished.

That isn't the end of the problem, however; because the question is, why does he have heart pains? As long as that chap had heart pains, that is what he talked about. I didn't want to hear about those heart pains; I wanted to hear about some of the reasons why he had heart pain, and I didn't want him wasting his hours describing that pain endlessly, re-petitiously, and in tremendous detail. We erased the pain so that we could get down to brass tacks. How did he feel about this person, that person? How did he feel about himself? What was his attitude? The removal of symptoms with which the patient was preoccupied enabled the patient to enter into the causality of the symptoms.

II. Indirect Approaches to Symptom Resolution

The papers of this section illustrate a variety of Erickson's indirect approaches to symptom resolution. He rarely makes direct suggestions because too often they tempt the patient's ego (the patient's conscious, voluntary abilities) to do something: the ego usually makes a conscious effort to carry out the suggestion. In hypnosis, however, Erickson prefers that autonomous response systems, which bypass the patient's conscious, voluntary intentionality, carry out the suggestions. If a patient's ego were able to solve the problem, the patient would not require a therapist. The therapist is needed to facilitate the emergence of untapped potentials and response systems that the patient's own ego has not been able to utilize in a voluntary and intentional way. Thus, the basic purpose of Erickson's indirect approaches is to circumvent the patient's learned limitations so that previously unrealized potentials may become manifest.

The following dialogue between Erickson and the editor illustrates the natural relation between indirect suggestions and the utilization approach in dealing with performance problems and maximizing human potentials. The papers of this section all illustrate the manner in which these principles can be applied to symptom resolution.

E: In 1959 I was asked by the Army to help teach the American rifle team. In teaching marksmen, you first have to get them to relax their feet, their knees, their hips, the entire body. Let your hand be comfortably placed. Let the butt of the rifle be placed against your shoulder just right. You slowly lean your cheek against the butt until it feels very comfortable. Then you let the gunsight wander up and down and back and forth across the target, and at the right moment you gently squeeze the trigger.

R: You gave the men those suggestions rather than what? What would have been the wrong way?

E: "Keep your eye on the target!" That tense and rigidly direct, forced focus is the wrong way.

R: We know the body is always in a natural equilibrium of constant movement. The demand to keep your eye on the target interferes with those natural micromovements of the body, and that puts the person under tremendous strain.

E: You try to keep the body in natural movement with a sense of comfort. They are to coordinate their whole body along with their eye fixation—

R: —rather than treating themselves as inanimate mannequins that must be exactly and rigidly fixated on the target in a motionless manner.

E: That year I helped the Army rifle team to beat the Russians for the first time. Instead of selecting just one part of a total picture (trying to focus on the target only), you take the entire picture of total body functioning.

R: I wonder if this is a general principle we can use in maximizing human potentials. When people have performance problems, it's because they are functioning *within a restricted part of themselves*. You help them deal with a *broader frame of reference* in which they utilize more of themselves. This is also the essence of your indirect approach: The members of the rifle team did not know that your suggestions about body comfort and natural movements were actually helping them use more of their innate abilities.

E: You let them know that they do know a lot more than they realize. They have that knowledge in their unconscious.

R: Indirect suggestions let their unconscious potentials be utilized without any interference from rigid and limiting preconceptions of their conscious frames of reference.

8. A Clinical Note on Indirect Hypnotic Therapy

Milton H. Erickson

A young couple in their early twenties, much in love and married for a year and close friends of several of the writer's medical students at the time, sought psychiatric help. Their problem was one in common—lifelong enuresis. During their 15-month courtship neither had had the courage to tell the other about the habitual enuresis.

Their wedding night had been marked, after consummation of the marriage, by a feeling of horrible dread and then resigned desperation, followed by sleep. The next morning each was silently and profoundly grateful to the other for the unbelievable forbearance shown in making no comment about the wet bed.

This same silent ignoring of the wet bed continued to be manifested each morning for over nine months. The effect was an ever-increasing feeling of love and regard for each other because of the sympathetic silence shown.

Then one morning, neither could remember who made the remark, the comment was made that they really ought to have a baby to sleep with them so that it could be blamed for the wet bed. This led at once to the astonishing discovery for each that the other was enuretic and that each had felt solely responsible. While they were greatly relieved by this discovery, the enuresis persisted.

After a few months discreet inquiry of the medical students by the couple disclosed that the writer was a psychiatrist and a hypnotist and probably knew something about enuresis. Accordingly, they sought an appointment, expressed an unwillingness to be hypnotized and an incapacity to meet the financial obligations of therapy, but earnestly asked if they could be given help.

They were informed that they would be accepted as patients on a purely experimental basis and that their obligation would be either to benefit or to assume full financial responsibility for the time given them. To this they agreed. (This reversal of "cure me or I won't pay" is often most effective in experimental therapy.)

From the 1954 *Journal of Clinical and Experimental Hypnosis* (*2*, 171-174).
Copyrighted by The Society for Clinical and Experimental Hypnosis, 1954.

They were then told that the absolute requisite for therapeutic benefits would lie in their unquestioning and unfailing obedience to the instructions given to them. This they promised. The experimental therapeutic procedure was outlined to them, to their amazement and horror, in the following fashion:

You are both very religious, and you have both given me a promise you will keep.

You have a transportation problem that makes it difficult to see me regularly for therapy.

Your financial situation makes it practically impossible for you to see me frequently.

You are to receive experimental therapy, and you are obligated absolutely either to benefit or to pay me whatever fee I deem reasonable. Should you benefit, the success of my therapy will be my return for my effort and your gain. Should you not benefit, all I will receive for my effort is a fee, and that will be a double loss to you but no more than an informative disappointment to me.

This is what you are to do: Each evening you are to take fluids freely. Two hours before you go to bed, lock the bathroom door after drinking a glass of water. At bedtime get into your pajamas and then kneel side by side on the bed, facing your pillows, and deliberately, intentionally, and jointly wet the bed. This may be hard to do, but you must do it. Then lie down and go to sleep, knowing full well that the wetting of the bed is over and done with for the night, that nothing can really make it noticeably wetter.

Do this every night, no matter how much you hate it—you have promised, though you did not know what the promise entailed, but you are obligated. Do it every night for two weeks—that is, until Sunday the seventeenth. On Sunday night you may take a rest from this task. You may that night lie down and go to sleep in a dry bed.

On Monday morning, the eighteenth, you will arise, throw back the covers, and look at the bed. *Only as you see a wet bed, then and only then* will you realize that there will be before you another three weeks of kneeling and wetting the bed.

You have your instructions. There is to be no discussion and no debating between you about this, just silence. There is to be only obedience, and you know *and will know what to do.* I will see you again in five weeks' time. You will then give me a full and amazing account. Goodbye!

Five weeks later they entered the office, amused, chagrined, embarrassed, greatly pleased, but puzzled and uncertain about the writer's possible attitude and intentions.

They had been most obedient. The first night had been one of torture. They had to kneel for over an hour before they could urinate. Succeeding nights were desperately dreaded. Each night they looked forward with an increasing intensity of desire to lie down and sleep in a dry bed on Sunday the seventeenth. On the morning of Monday the eighteenth, they awakened at the alarm and were amazed to find the bed still dry. Both started to speak and immediately remembered the admonition of silence.

That night, in their pajamas, they looked at the bed, at each other, started to speak, but again remembered the instructions about silence. Impulsively they "sneaked" into bed, turned off the reading light, wondering why they had not deliberately wet the bed but at the same time enjoying the comfort of a dry bed. On Tuesday morning the bed was again dry, and that night and thereafter Monday night's behavior had been repeated.

Having completed their report, they waited uncertainly for the writer's comments. They were immediately reminded that they had been told that they would give an "amazing account" in five weeks' time. Now they knew that they had, and that the writer was tremendously pleased, *and would continue to be pleased,* so what more could be asked?

After some minutes of carefully guided, desultory conversation they were dismissed with the apparently irrelevant statement that the next month was May.

About the middle of May they dropped in "spontaneously" to greet the writer and to report "incidentally" that everything was fine.

A year later they introduced the writer to their infant son, amusedly stating that once more they could have a wet bed but only when they wished, and it would be just "a cute little spot." Hesitantly they asked if the writer had employed hypnosis on them. They were answered with the statement that their own honesty and sincerity in doing what was necessary to help themselves entitled them to full credit for what had been accomplished.

COMMENT

To understand this case report it might be well to keep in mind the small child's frequent demonstration of the right to self-determination. For example, the child rebelling against the afternoon nap fights sleep vigorously despite fatigue and will repeatedly get out of the crib. If each time the child is gently placed back in the crib, it will often suddenly demonstrate its rights by climbing out and immediately climbing back and falling asleep comfortably.

Concerning the evasive reply given to the patients about the use of hypnosis, by which they were compelled to assume fully their own responsibilities, the fact remains that the entire procedure was based upon an indirect use of hypnosis. The instructions were so worded as to compel without demanding the intent attention of the unconscious. The calculated vagueness of some of the instructions forced their unconscious minds to assume responsibility for their behavior. Consciously they could only wonder about their inexplicable situations, while they responded to it with corrective, unconscious reactions. Paradoxically speaking, they were compelled by the nature of the instructions and the manner in which these were given to make a "free, spontaneous choice" of behavior and to act upon it in the right way without knowing that they had done so.

Favoring the therapeutic result was the prestige of the writer as a psychiatrist and a hypnotist well spoken of by their friends, the medical students. This undoubtedly rendered them unusually ready to accept indirect, hypnotic suggestion.

The rationale of the therapy may be stated briefly. Both patients had a distressing, lifelong pattern of wetting the bed every night. For nine long months both suffered intensely from an obvious but unacknowledged guilt. For another three months they found their situation still unchanged.

Under therapy, during a subjectively never-ending two weeks, by their own actions they acquired a lifetime supply of wet beds. Each wet bed compelled them to want desperately to lie down and sleep in a dry bed. When that opportunity came, they utilized it fully. Then, the next evening, understanding unconsciously but not consciously the instructions given them, they used their bed-wetting guilt to "sneak" into and enjoy a dry bed, a guilty pleasure they continued to enjoy for three weeks.

The uncertainty, doubt, and guilt over their behavior vanished upon discovery at the second interview that they had really been obedient by being able to give the "full and amazing account." Yet, unnoticeably to them, the therapist's influence was vaguely but effectively continued by the seemingly irrelevant mention of the month of May.

Their final step was then to bring into reality a completely satisfactory solution of their own devising, a baby, the solution they had mentioned and which mention had led to an open acknowledgment of enuresis to each other. Then, at a symbolic level, they dismissed the writer as therapist by introducing him to the infant, who in turn represented a happy and controllable solution to their problem. This they almost literally verbalized directly by their amused comment about having a wet bed any time they wished and that it would be only a pleasing thing of adult and parental significance.

9. The Hypnotic and Hypnotherapeutic Investigation and Determination of Symptom-Function

Milton H. Erickson and Harold Rosen

With some emotionally sick patients symptom-function can be determined rapidly under hypnosis, in a therapeutic setting.

Symptoms and even syndromes, when emotionally based, may subserve the repetitive enactment of traumatic events; may reproduce, instead, specific life situations; may satisfy repressed erotic and aggressive impulses; or may at one and the same time constitute defenses against, and punishment for, underlying instinctual drives (Weisman, 1952). They may mask schizophrenic reactions or hold suicidal depressions in check (Rosen, 1953b, 1953c). They may serve all these functions concurrently, or none of these, or any specific one or combination of them.

Patients, it should be stressed, see psychiatrists because they have symptoms which cause them trouble. They frequently insist on symptomatic relief. This sometimes is possible: transference cures not infrequently may be effected; environmental manipulation may occasionally be sufficient; defenses may be strengthened; or, with selected patients, symptom site may be transferred (Erickson, 1954), or less incapacitating symptoms substituted for those which otherwise would invalid or hospitalize them. Such symptom substitution, however, can best be achieved if at least a few of the functions served by specific complaint symptoms are known. Once these are determined, the attempt can then be made, with better chance of success, to substitute under hypnosis less incapacitating symptoms which nevertheless serve the same underlying neurotic or even psychotic needs.

However, there are patients with whom this would be impossible. Some may occasionally, nevertheless, be helped—and helped rapidly. They see psychiatrists in the hope, not of ridding themselves of symptoms, but of imbedding them. This is a therapeutic possibility. Symptoms can be

Read in part (a) at the 107th annual meeting of the American Psychiatric Association. Los Angeles, California, May 4-8, 1953; and in part (b) at the Conference of Directors of Mental Hygiene Clinics of the State of New York, Pilgrim State Hospital, Brentwood, Long Island, N.Y., June 2, 1953. Quoted here from the *Journal of Clinical and Experimental Hypnosis,* 1954, 2, 201-219. Copyrighted by The Society for Clinical and Experimental Hypnosis, 1954.

narrowed down. A 59-year-old railroad worker,* for example, after a fall one year before he was eligible for pension, developed a hysterical paralysis of one arm. He was willing to accept seven days' hospitalization, but seemed grimly determined to retain his paralysis. The psychiatrist spent the first five of these seven days with another physician, "thoughtlessly" discussing the hopelessness of his case, examining and reexamining the patient while he was in a trance, and debating whether or not a specific syndrome was present. If so, he would wind up, they agreed, with a hopelessly paralyzed wrist but with free finger, elbow, and shoulder movement. On the sixth day these came back. Internist and psychiatrist both mourned his stiff wrist! The patient had his symptom. He became actually proud of his stiff wrist. He had all the trouble he wanted with it, and all the narcissistic gratification he desired from it, but he was now able to work, and he and his wife received their pension (Erickson, 1954).

Symptom restriction of this type constitutes an exceedingly important adjuvant hypnotherapeutic technique, significant enough to warrant detailed consideration. In this paper, however, we propose to limit ourselves, for the most part, to a discussion of our clinical experience in the investigation and evaluation of symptom-function, with various of the newer and more radical hypnotherapeutic techniques now under investigation. Dissociative states may be induced, for instance, or dream acting-out suggested; attacks may be precipitated and then blocked, either by direct hypnotic suggestion or by regressing patients to a period predating the onset of their disease, so that substitutive motor, vegetative, or other activity is precipitated out in a form accessible to therapeutic investigation; attacks may be precipitated in slow motion, so that individual components can be investigated therapeutically in detail; symptoms may be suggested away, while emotions back of symptoms are concurrently intensified, so that, again, underlying dynamic material will immediately become accessible for therapy; or still other techniques may be utilized (Rosen, 1953b).

To illustrate † a hypnotically precipitated attack in slow motion, a patient with what for years had been diagnosed as epilepsy began making, as part of her supposed epileptic symptomatology, forced sucking movements with her lips as she acted out the fantasy of trying to suck on—and to bite into—her mother's nipple. In another patient with what was originally diagnosed as psychomotor epilepsy, an attack was hypnotically induced and then deliberately blocked by direct hypnotic suggestion; at this she was intensely aroused sexually, begging her impotent husband, whom she hallucinated as present and whose flaccid penis she was digitally trying to stimulate, to attempt intercourse with her more than once every

* Patient of M.H.E.
† Patients of H. R.

three weeks. A patient with pruritus insisted that it was her itch, and her itch alone, which was responsible for her tension, her inability to sleep, and her general irritability. Once hypnotized, she was told that, if she really wished it to, her itch could disappear but that whatever it stood for, no matter what, would become so strong, so unbearably strong, that she would be unable to contain it any longer. She began shouting: "Don't let me dig her out! Don't let me dig her out!" And at this, although her itch had disappeared, she began digging her nails into her skin. Early aggressive and traumatic material, with specific reference to her mother, was then spontaneously abreacted. Her pruritus, among the various functions which it served, satisfied hostile and aggressive impulses on one level against her husband and, on another, against her mother. It served also to mask her underlying depression and to hold it in check.

At times a much more indirect approach than this seems indicated. A second patient with pruritus vulvate,* who had previously been treated by various allergists and dermatologists, was unwilling, so she stated, to be hypnotized if the psychiatrist was curious about her problem: it would, rather, be a question of her conscious strength of character to tell it. It was therefore suggested that she could go into a trance and while in it do something, no matter what, that she would have no hesitation letting the psychiatrist know about. She agreed, hallucinated playing tennis, became "hot and sweaty," and explained that she felt like taking a bath. She was told that, since she was a big girl, the psychiatrist could not let her really take one, but that, if she were a little girl in a big tub, she could. It was added that perhaps a bath by proxy might be even more satisfactory. So she watched and, because the psychiatrist was not wearing his glasses, described seeing a little girl bathing, playing with her genitals, being horribly punished by her mother, and then being forced to scrub the ring off the tub.

During the next session she stated without being hypnotized that she had a silly thing to tell: she had taken a bath the night before and washed the ring off the tub, and she knew that in telling him this the psychiatrist would undoubtedly understand something, although she did not know what it was.

Our approach may at times be, at first, direct and, later, indirect. One patient,† for instance, was a rather depressed 28-year-old truck assembler with spasmodic torticollis of almost six months' duration, who finally began drawing unemployment compensation because his wry neck had made it impossible for him to continue paying the close, detailed attention to his work which was demanded of him. Despite long-continued traction

---

*Patient of M. H. E.
†Patient of H. R.

his neck would twist immediately to the extreme left once this traction was discontinued.

During the anamnesis some of the defensive aspects of his symptom were hinted at. He had always been shy and embarrassed, had always been afraid of girls, had seldom had a date, and had never had intercourse. But one of his fellow workers had promised to "fix him up" with a girl, once he purchased a car with the $2,000 he had saved. "He said she's a sucker for a guy on a ride," he explained, "And he gave me a rubber. I've still got it. See! And I was just going to buy it [the automobile] when my neck started like this. So I'll have to wait till it's better now. I can't drive this way . . ."

"And for two years" before the torticollis started, "my hands'd shake, and I'd tremble. And sometimes my head would too, just like my hands when I'm nervous. That's because I'm so tight inside. I can't relax at all."

He was hypnotized under the pretext of testing his ability to relax. As long as his head remained twisted to the extreme left, he appeared placid, calm, and even serene. But when, on direct verbal suggestion, his head reverted to the midline, his right hand seized his penis through his clothes, and he began to masturbate. When given permission for his head to revert to the extreme left, he again became the same motionless, placid, and apparently serene individual. At the suggestion, "Your head can remain unturned," his masturbatory activity resumed. "You can, you know," so he was then told, "remain motionless, if you wish, while your head is unturned." At this, his hands fell to his sides and he again became motionless, but this time all the physiological concomitants of acute anxiety appeared. He began perspiring profusely, seemed drenched in perspiration, and became visibly tremulous.

Since it was not thought that at this point he could tolerate the anxiety attendant upon realizing what at least one of the functions served by his torticollis was, amnesia for this particular part of the hypnotic session was suggested, *provided he would rather not remember it.* Symptom substitution seemed possible. He could, for instance, have been allowed to squeeze a hallucinated rubber balloon and, later, to hallucinate watching someone else doing this. Instead, as a temporary expedient on his new job, he found it possible to hold an oversized pencil rigidly against the steering wheel as he drove a truck.

It should be emphasized that while he hinted during the anamnesis at some of the defensive and perhaps adaptive aspects of his symptom, these did not appear during the hypnotic investigation. Instead, perhaps as a result of the specific hypnotic techniques utilized, one symptom function—that of substitutive satisfaction for autoerotic activity—became obvious. Ferenczi (1950), it will be remembered, believes that tics constitute masturbatory equivalents. This patient's torticollis can under no circumstances be considered a tic, but nevertheless, because of his behavior during the hypnotic investigation, Ferenczi's discussion immediately comes to mind. So does that of Melanie Klein (1948), whose 13-year-old Felix's tic had appeared when homosexual and masturbatory impulses were repressed. However, it should be remembered that with our patient this material came to light specifically as a result of whatever was going on between him and the therapist within, rather than because of, the hypnotic interpersonal relationship. If other hypnotic techniques had been utilized, or if the investigation had proceeded in some other way, the results obtained might in all probability have been different.

One of our patients was a miner's wife* in her mid-thirties who was hospitalized for further gynecologic study after having had a hysterectomy three years previously. The abdominal pain of which she still complained and for which she had wished further surgery was thought by her present surgeon to be on an emotional basis. Because of her 20-year history of "nervous spells," a psychiatric consultation was requested.

These "spells" turned out to be, for the most part, anxiety attacks. She would feel as though she were trembling inside; become "horribly frightened" and convinced that she had heart disease; wake screaming from nightmares in which she would see her father in a casket or her husband and son killed; and frequently sigh without knowing why. She was not articulate, gave practically no meaningful details about her developmental history, and characterized herself as a fairly happy, well-adjusted, and socially not incapacitated person, with everything she really wished for. She was able to talk spontaneously only about her "spells," but no additional factual information was elicited about them. X-rays had previously shown a nonfunctioning gallbladder with stones, and a cholecystectomy had been recommended. She knew that the operation was necessary. In addition, she wished treatment so as not to feel compelled to toss and squirm half the night through, night after night, before falling asleep.

It was suggested that she concentrate on this trembling inside herself of which she complained so much. However, so it was added, with every breath she drew, with every second that passed, she would grow more and more relaxed, more and more relaxed, so relaxed, so completely relaxed that, if she wished, she could fall asleep. "With some patients," the therapist added, "this takes two or three minutes—and with some, much more. Just breathe on, just breathe on, thinking only of this trembling inside you; breathing deeply and gently, deeply and gently, deeply and gently." No other suggestion was made. Lid-paralysis was not suggested. This was repeated over and over again, and the cadence of the hypnotist's statements was timed to her respiratory rhythm. Within four minutes her eyes had closed. She looked as though she were sound asleep.

* Patient of H. R.

The therapist began to speak in a low, relaxed tone. "You've had a number of symptoms, Mrs. G," he stated. "You've come here with female trouble, and with what seems to be a bad gall bladder, and with what you think is heart disease. Think only of these symptoms, of nothing but these symptoms. . . . Begin feeling them now. . . . There's something that's common to them all. There's something that's common to them all. Try to feel it. Try to feel it. Feel it, *FEEL IT,* feel it more and more intensely, more and more intensely, until you feel it so strongly that you know it for what it is. This symptom of yours, this main symptom of yours, is getting stronger and stronger now, stronger and stronger, stronger and stronger still. Feel it, *FEEL IT,* FEEL IT now."

At this she began to tremble. "I'm shaking and I'm trembling" she almost stuttered, but in a low voice, "I don't know why. And that's how I feel all the time." Tears began to flow silently from her eyes. There was no audible sobbing on her part.

"If you'd like to stop trembling now," the therapist stated, "you can. Your symptom will disappear, if you really wish it to, but whatever it stands for, whatever is back of it, whatever it covers up, whatever it's really about, will come to the surface right now. You're strong enough to face it, whatever it is. If you really wish it—it's up to you to decide—your symptom will disappear, but whatever emotion it covers, whatever it's really about, will come to the surface now. You'll know it for what it really is. As I count to three, if you really wish to, if you really wish to know, if you really wish to get treated for it, your symptom will disappear, but whatever it covers up, whatever it stands for, will come to the surface—and we'll see it, we'll see it for what it really is."

At this she was 10 years of age, extremely frightened, nauseated, afraid she was bleeding to death, not realizing that her periods were starting or what they were. A moment later, she was spontaneously abreacting a rape, extremely frightened again, nauseated, and, again, afraid that she was bleeding to death. It was "this same sensation," so she later explained, that she invariably felt not only on intercourse but also whenever her husband seemed to be growing "tender" toward her.

It should be noted that her anxiety manifested itself when it was hypnotically suggested that she concentrate on whatever was common to her cardiac, digestive, and urogenital symptoms. When her underlying emotion of the moment was then hypnotically intensified, it gave rise to the enactment of what emotionally to her was the same repetitive traumatic event. Much more than this was involved, however.

Other factors and other problems will become apparent from even a cursory study of that part of her case protocol which has been abstracted. We feel that in the hypnotic interpersonal relationship, full-blown transference phenomena may develop rapidly, at times within hours or even minutes (Fisher, 1953; Gill, unpublished article; MacAlpine, 1950,

Nunberg, 1951). This will be developed in detail in another paper now under consideration. When this patient, however, was told, "Feel it, *feel it,* FEEL IT, more and more intensely," we were obviously on a "fishing expedition," working in the dark, not knowing what was involved, and hoping that something meaningful, no matter what, that could be utilized, would be stirred up. This technique can be exceedingly effective with some patients. Others may be told that, in addition to feeling "it" more and more intensely, they will be interested and curious about knowing what "it" is, but they will not know this until at a time and in a place, no matter when or where, that they wish to and which will be most helpful, therapeutically, to them. One patient,* for example, stated that she could not tell us, either in the trance state or on a conscious level, what her trouble was. The history which she gave seemed barren of any lead. She was therefore told, while in a trance, that whatever her problem was, she would feel it with increasing intensity, but only at what for her would be both the right time and the right place. This was repeated during half a dozen trance sessions, after which she stated, "I have something utterly silly to tell you. I do my own washing. But my living expenses have been terrible because I never wear a pair of panties more than once. I always take them off in the dark and throw them in the trash can. I never look at them again. The other day I felt the need for a bowel movement, and I felt it very strongly."

"I was in the bathroom at the time. While I was sitting on the toilet, I suddenly realized that I used the bathroom very little. Since childhood I have been soiling my pants and hiding it from myself, and that is silly. Now I can feel it in the right place at the right time, and I wonder what I will do with the three or four dozen pairs of panties I have in stock." It later developed that she took from one to three baths each day. This had always been a nuisance to her. Her bath compulsion has now disappeared.

Even when the psychiatrist goes on such "fishing expeditions" in the dark, if his words be well planned and carefully chosen, his patients will understand and relate their meaning specifically to their own problems. It is not necessary to know what it is that the patient knows. Somewhere in the patient's unconscious there is understanding, just as there is understanding of—and at the same time resistance to the recognition of—the meaning of even the most anxiety-ridden dream. The therapist's permissive attitude, of being willing to let his patient know but without himself knowing until and unless the patient is ready and wishes him to, serves to make it possible for some patients to place whatever meaning to their symptoms seems to them at the time therapeutically necessary. However, it is of prime importance for the therapist to make it clear, somehow, to the patient that the right, the correct, the concrete, the specific meaning,

---

*Patient of M. H. E.

applicable at that particular time, be placed on his generalities.

If this be done, the psychiatrist does not fall into the trap, so frequently set—and not only by patients poorly motivated for treatment—of trying to do too much for the patient too quickly. The patient can be relied upon to fit the jigsaw puzzle together and, in point of fact, should have joint responsibility with the therapist for doing so.

Occasionally, when specific investigatory procedures are decided upon, the adaptive aspects of the patient's symptom or symptoms may be emphasized. Or their defensive functions may become apparent. Disguised acting-out frequently takes place. With the unmasking of symptoms, the basic conflict or even personality structure may at times be apparent. This is especially true of those patients whose neurotic symptoms make it possible for them to keep their underlying psychosis in check so that, as a result, they are enabled to continue making, at least at times, a not too inadequate social adjustment.

To illustrate:

One of our patients with torticollis* could not meaningfully be investigated by any of the techniques so far described. During the consultation session he answered questions almost monosyllabically. He made no spontaneous comments. According to his referring psychiatrist, he had been inaccessible to therapy because of the narcissistic gratification which he gained from his apparent organic disease. Since he had been referred specifically for investigation and, if indicated, for treatment under hypnosis, he was hypnotized by an eye-fixation method. Direct suggestion to the effect that, if he wished, his neck could—it will be noticed that the word *"would"* was not used—revert to the midline, was ineffective. At this he stated that he felt "disappointed, frustrated, hopeless," and with nothing any more that he really wished to do.

"That seems to be your feeling here," the therapist agreed, "frustrated and hopeless. And yet, there must have been a time when there was something you really wished to do—and enjoyed doing. As I count from one to ten, you'll pass back through time, back through time, to that other time when there was something you really wished to do—and enjoyed doing. One—back through time, back through time, to that other time when there was something you wanted to do, something you very much wanted to do—and enjoyed doing. Two—back through time, back through time, to that other time when there was something you very much wanted to do, something you exerted your every energy to do—and enjoyed doing. Three—" etc. The suggestion was reinforced in various ways until the count of ten had been reached.

At this he rose from the chair, strode to the middle of the room, nodded to left and right, smiled, lifted his right hand, and made an impassioned

*Patient of H. R.

plea for blood donors to the local Red Cross. This, as it developed, was an actual speech which he had made five years previously. It was, in fact, rather good. It lasted about 15 minutes. During this, his head turned at times toward both the right and the left. It frequently was in the midline. After he had finished, he seated himself, smiling, pleased, obviously enjoying the applause. His head remained in the midline. He was then hypnotically progressed through time (with the one suggestion, however, that his head remain in its present position), at first year by year, then month by month and finally week by week, into the present. His head stayed in the midline, not fixedly but naturally so, without obvious effort on his part.

After he had been hypnotically returned to the present, he remained silent for about five minutes. The therapist remained silent also. He then began whispering, "That c.s. bastard's been telling everybody I'm a c.s. I'd like to kill him. But he's pushed invisible wires into me. So if I do, I'll turn into a c.s. myself. But if *you'll* suck him off, they'll melt away—and I'll be free to kill him. Won't you? *Please!*"

So long as his neck remained in the midline, he was clinically paranoid and psychotic. His productions remained on this level. When, however, on direct hypnotic suggestion his neck again twisted to the extreme left, this paranoid material was no longer evident and he became amnestic for it, even though he was still hypnotized and no suggestion to this effect had been made.

Although his torticollis made it impossible for him to continue practicing his profession, it seemed inadvisable at this particular time to attempt to deprive him of his symptom, since it appeared probable that, if this were done, he would develop in its stead a clinically paranoid psychosis for which institutionalization might be mandatory. This patient, incidentally, after leaving Baltimore saw a surgeon who "cured" his torticollis by operating on him. According to Garnett and Elberlik (1954), who have seen and followed this patient, he did not become psychotic, as we could have expected, although he no longer, at least at first, was able to take recourse in this wry neck of his. The symptom, incidentally, was reprecipitated a few months later. An attempt will be made to get a meaningful follow-up on the type of adjustment which he later on finds it possible to make.

Whether with a patient like this it might, in the last analysis, be most helpful to rob him hypnotically of his defenses so that he could be treated, if he could effectively be so treated, by the type of technique developed by John Rosen (1953), is something about which, without such a follow-up, we at this stage of our research are not qualified even to hazard a guess, nor did we feel it indicated to make the necessary investigation at the time we saw him. The danger to this patient in circumventing symptom-formation by acting-out seemed much too great. What his surgical "cure" involved, and what it had meant to him in fantasy, can only be surmised.

With another type of patient, however, and especially with the patient whose drug addiction is on a schizophrenically depressive, potentially suicidal basis, we think that research in this particular direction may well be warranted, since the symptom of drug addiction may be much worse in its effect than the disease process which it masks and perhaps holds in check, and since with its removal the underlying disease process itself may become accessible to treatment. We feel, at least, that this warrants investigation.

It would seem impossible to overemphasize those dangers which potentially could be involved in the use of investigatory techniques like these. If they are utilized, the patient with a "neurotic schizophrenic" reaction must be given enough concurrent support to abort or, rather, to prevent a clinically psychotic shattering of his ego. And for patients with organic or so-called psychosomatic disease, it seems necessary to proceed at an exceedingly slow and cautious pace: the possibility of precipitating a psychotic episode at times is so pronounced, even if insistence be only on the recall of forgotten memories, that many psychiatrists hesitate or refuse to accept such patients for treatment—and unless an eventuality such as this is anticipated and adequate safeguards taken, such patients can become much more seriously ill emotionally if they are investigated by the hypnodiagnostic techniques described in this article. On the other hand, if the psychiatrist is well-trained and if adequate precautions are taken, these dangers can be circumvented and patients who otherwise would receive no help can be helped—and perhaps helped a great deal.

One of our patients was a veteran in his mid-twenties* who had developed a rather severe ulcerative colitis. He was first seen four years ago. We felt that his colitis was serving as a suicidal equivalent, and therefore recommended that he make arrangements for comparatively intensive psychotherapy. Instead, he decided on supportive medical treatment from his gastroenterologist. His colitis went from bad to worse. It ultimately reached the point of necessitating V.A. hospitalization, five months later, for an ileostomy. His gastroenterologist and his surgeon both felt that the operation was mandatory. His colon, they stated, looked like a "red hot" appendix.

The problems involved were discussed with the chief of the medical service and the surgeons, and it was agreed that during the following month our total consultation time at the hospital would be devoted to an attempt to help him desire psychiatric treatment. This was the only psychotherapeutic goal set. Surgery was therefore postponed, although outside consultants were called in to help residents sales-talk, bludgeon, and threaten him to request it. They were unsuccessful.

*Patient of H.R.

Within six weeks he reached the point of being ready and willing to accept psychiatric treatment. He was therefore transferred on voluntary commitment, and at his own request, to another V.A. hospital, where for several months he received fairly intensive psychotherapy. He became well enough to leave the hospital, was seen on an outpatient basis for several more months, was not thought to have sufficient motivation for actually intensive psychotherapy, and was therefore carried supportively for some time.

Three and a half years later he requested an emergency appointment. "I am," so he stated, "losing control of my bowels and soiling my underwear almost every day." He explained that since he was a salesman making only $75 a week, he wished just treatment enough to make it unnecessary for him to continue losing bowel control while outdoors. "I don't wish to let it come out!" he emphatically stated.

He was rapidly hypnotized by an eye-fixation method to a trance state deep enough for amnesia to be suggested, and then told that he had the choice of keeping "it" in or not as he himself wished; but that the choice was his, and his alone, of letting "it" come out or of holding "it" in. So far as possible his exact words were used. It seems obvious that when he used the word "it," he was referring to his bowel movements; but it seemed worth probing in the direction in which probing was being attempted, since otherwise, so far as could be judged, we would be stymied.

Immediately after this suggestion had been made, he began squirming around and, while crying convulsively, shouted at the top of his voice, "I won't! I won't!"

"You don't have to, if you don't wish to," the psychiatrist agreed. "It's entirely up to you." At this he began swallowing rapidly. He then got on his knees in the middle of the office floor, made movements which could be interpreted as pulling down a zipper, went through the motions of taking something in his hand, pulled his mouth over to it, and began sucking rapidly and forcibly. He suddenly again began shouting, "Blow storm! Blow storm!" went over to the couch, lay upon it, kept moving his lips in forced and pronounced sucking movements, laughed and sobbed alternatively, became silent, and then gradually grew relaxed. The session came to an end after he was told that he could remember what had transpired or not, as he himself wished, but that the choice was his and his alone. He became amnestic for this abreaction, and, incidentally, still has no memory of it.

He was seen twice the following week. On both occasions he lay on the couch, was hypnotized by the same eye-fixation method but to a light trance only, and was told that the psychiatrist would remain silent as he stated whatever came into his mind. He was also told that he would remember everything that took place, and everything that he said, during these two sessions. He was able to think only of "Blow storm! Blow storm!" For months he had had a "terrific desire" for cunnilingus, but had never had courage enough to try it. But that had had nothing to do with his symptoms, or so he stated. What he most wanted out of treatment was to get rid of them, and to be able to lead a normal life with marriage and with children, even though he didn't know any girl he'd like to marry. By now, incidentally, he was no longer soiling his clothes.

He was scheduled to be seen twice the following week, but unfortunately contracted one of the "virus flu's" that were so common at the time. Previously, whenever he had had a cold, so he explained, he would lose complete control of his bowels. For some reason, perhaps related to therapy or perhaps not, he was now able to control them. This was discussed with him in detail two weeks later when he was next seen.

This session was completely on a nonhypnotic level. Immediately after entering the office, he wished to know what the therapist would do himself, if he had his symptoms—I would wish intensive therapy, probably analytic but most certainly analytically oriented (Cushing, 1953). He wished this but could not afford it. He would have to ask his uncle for that much money, and he'd rather die than do that. He could get it, of course, if he really needed it, but he'd rather die. Anyhow, he was no longer that sick! And he had just bought a $3,000 automobile. If it came to a choice between paying a psychiatrist or buying a car, he preferred the car. All that he really wished, and he was exceedingly frank about it, was to be seen on a twice-a-week basis for the next month, so that he could get his symptoms completely under control. If it became necessary to have treatment every once in a while, in the future as in the past, he would feel satisfied. It was therefore agreed that he would be seen on a twice-a-week basis during the following month.

The next session was an exceedingly dramatic and even melodramatic one. Once hypnotized and in a light trance state, he began panting, gave every overt evidence of pronounced anxiety, and then breathlessly exclaimed, "I'm thinking of a blow storm." He made no further comment about this, however, but stated instead that he was now thinking about a friend's wife, then about the wife of the psychiatrist who had previously treated him, and then about John, an effeminate acquaintance of his whose nose was the same shape as hers. He then began gagging, felt as if he had to rush to the lavatory to keep from vomiting over the office rug, and leaped from the couch in order to do so, only to find that his gagging had ceased. "I came in John's mouth," he explained, "and that's what made me gag." In the discussion which followed it became obvious that he knew he had not been having this particular acquaintance perform fellatio upon him, even though "it seemed real while it happened." This led to a discussion of the fact that when in the street in the course of his daily work he not infrequently experiences exactly the same reaction, but without the conscious homosexual fantasy, although nevertheless "I go through the exact same experience." And, so he continued, "Here's the angle—either I get a cramp or I gag. These are the two forms it takes. In conscious life, if I think I'm coming in John's mouth, I spit—and the moment it's out, I get release."

The session had practically come to an end by this time. He was therefore told that if he wished to remember this material, he could; but that if he did not, he need not. He was then dehypnotized on signal, and the material elicited during the session was briefly discussed with him on the conscious level. He remembered it completely and was able to discuss it in a meaningful way. He had now come into what seemed on the surface a fairly good treatment relationship.

This patient's underlying anger and rage did not come to the fore until later, at least not in a form accessible to therapy. It nevertheless was hinted at during the course of his rather melodramatic sexual acting-out.

This acting-out itself seems worthy of comment. It will be noted that his originally articulated conscious fantasies were those of cunnilingus. Under hypnosis the fantasy which, incidentally, he could remember, was that of fellatio performed upon him. His fantasies on a still deeper level, as evidenced by the acting-out for which he spontaneously became amnestic, were those in which he himself orally and actively engaged in the practice. And all of this, even in the early sessions, he somehow tied in with his colitis symptoms. The orality emphasized by Mary Cushing in her discussion of the psychoanalytic treatment of a patient with ulcerative colitis (1953) immediately comes to mind.

In our experience acting-out of this type frequently concerns itself with suppressed, as well as with repressed, desires. This seems especially true when masturbatory activity manifests itself. Examples have already appeared in the literature. Apparent epileptic or asthmatic attacks, for instance, can be deliberately precipitated during hypnodiagnostic consultant sessions, and then blocked, after which the inevitably resultant anxiety can be repressed by direct verbal suggestion, so that underlying fantasies may erupt into conscious awareness even to the point of being acted out. As one would expect, attacks investigated up to the present in this way seem to consist of partially repressed erotic or aggressive drives with actual or substitutive motor defenses against their appearance (Rosen, 1953a, 1953b).

One patient, for instance, was a 20-year-old miner's wife* with a two-and-a-half year history of what had been diagnosed as "psychic epilepsy." She was referred for intensive neurological and neurosurgical investigation. No studies, however, yielded clear-cut results. A psychiatric evaluation was therefore requested. Because she had been "snowed under" by drugs during electro-encephalography, she was almost an hour late for the

* Patient of H. R.

appointment. Her nurse at first had been unable to awaken her. Since she was groggy and all but asleep when she reached our office, hypnotic suggestion was utilized to awaken her to the point of making possible a meaningful psychiatric investigation. She then began to explain what her "periods" were like. It was obvious that by this slip of the tongue she was referring to her attacks. They had started, so she stated, "right after I graduated and was looking for a job. I'd feel like I was grinning—just a *silly* grin—and I couldn't control it, but I tried hard. And I always felt somebody was laughing at me, or looking at me. And that made me embarrassed. I always feel embarrassed with these attacks. But if I cough or laugh, I get over them. That's how I stop them. They wake me up, and I start hollering and trying to cry. And they're getting worse, so I get them four or five times a night now."

One of her attacks was then precipitated by the direct hypnotic suggestion that she have it. She opened her mouth, her whole body seemed to quiver, and she moaned. Her right hand went over her mouth, she began to cough, and the "attack" was aborted. She was next told that, at the count of 10, she would have another attack, but that there would be no coughing this time. She moaned; her body quivered, and her legs drew up under her. Both arms became stiff and rigid, and both fists were clenched and held in midair. Her head shook back and forth, as though in negation. Her eyes closed, and she seemed to frown. Her lips were so widely parted that one could see her tight-clenched teeth. After some eight minutes she suddenly went limp, seemed completely relaxed, and showed the "silly" grin she had previously described.

("You seem relaxed. Could you tell me what it is you're feeling?") She had had no feeling at all, either during the attack or after it, or so she said. At this, she was told at the count of five she would have another attack, and that this time she would feel, *really* feel, whatever emotion, whatever feeling, was *really* connected with it. The psychiatrist slowly counted to five. She became rigid, arms bent on elbows, hand and arms jerking rapidly back and forth, head jerking from side to side as though in negation, legs stiff but trembling.

("The attack will cease now as I count to five. It will cease when I count to five. One, two, three, four, five.") She suddenly relaxed, then began to tremble. She seemed fearful.

("As I count to five, your trembling will cease. There's no need to be afraid now. You can face it, whatever it is. One, two, three, four, five.") She seized one hand with the other. Her abdomen began heaving more and more rapidly and more and more violently. She suddenly put her right hand between her legs and for perhaps a minute and a half masturbated herself rapidly through her dress. This was followed by a long drawn-out sigh, after which she lay back on the couch, apparently completely relaxed, and with the same "silly" grin on her face.

After several minutes the psychiatrist asked, "We both know what this is now, don't we?" She nodded. So this meant that every time she had one of these attacks, she was playing with herself. . . . She remembered when she was very small and her brother was putting a snow suit on her. She had asked him if she could play with herself first, if he wouldn't tell her mother. He said he wouldn't. But he did. So her mother told her she would go to hell for it. . . . And now, every time she has one of these attacks, was that what she was doing? . . . She was a Catholic, and it was a sin. What should she do? The subsequent discussion centered on her need for psychiatric treatment, and the advisability of her making the necessary arrangements to receive it.

With another patient* with a "silly grin," such acting-out was neither indicated nor necessary. This patient explained that these silly grinning periods of hers would come on at certain irregular intervals. While she was in a trance state, the psychiatrist discussed the duration of smiling, how it begins slowly and ends slowly, and how the person who smiles is pleased and feels better, as does everybody else. Since it is a very natural thing, so it was stated, it should never be called a grin, nor should it be termed silly, nor a dirty look, but it should be appreciated as one of the normal functions of the expression of the person, whether male or female. Somehow or other, the therapist added, there is an expression that is meaningful.

In her next trance this girl asked the psychiatrist to explain menstruation to her. She was asked if she wanted this on conscious or hypnotic levels. The girl's simple statement was, "I think probably I ought to know in both ways, so tell it to me now, and then awaken me and tell it to me again." Her "silly" grinning periods are now over. Her menstrual pain has disappeared. She no longer stays in bed three days each month with severe cramps. Her statement during her next period, when she walked into the office, was, "Doctor, I am a queen today."

During the past five years one of us has seen masturbatory responses, like the one shown by the first of these two patients with the so-called "silly" grins, in three other nonpsychotic hypnotized patients† (Rosen, 1953b). He has, in addition, seen on the medical wards during the same period of time three patients whose psychoses had previously not been recognized, and who, during the consultation session, touched or otherwise digitally manipulated their genitals. Needless to say they were not hypnotized. Psychiatric hospitalization was recommended in each case.

It seems of parenthetic interest that patients with borderline schizophrenic reactions are applying more and more frequently for treatment

---

*Patient of M. H. E.
†Patients of H. R.

under hypnosis. One patient,* for example, stated that she had no symptoms but was applying for psychiatric treatment under hypnosis because she wished to become even better adjusted and even healthier emotionally. Immediately after entering the office, she lay on the couch, bent legs over thighs and thighs over abdomen, and began moaning while making what to all intents and purposes seemed convulsive abdominal movements. She was at no time hypnotized. On questioning, it developed that she was spontaneously abreacting—without any suggestion by the therapist and without being hypnotized—the delivery of a child. When this was further investigated, it developed that she was fantasying going through the birth canal herself and being "reborn." She was showing, as it further developed, a catatonic reaction.

The schizophrenic patient can be said to have ready access to his unconscious. This is amply illustrated by the case material published, for instance, by Frieda Fromm-Reichmann (1950), by John Rosen (1953), and by others. The hypnotized neurotic patient, on the other hand, so we feel, may at times have ready access, not so much to his unconscious as to his preconscious. It is because of this that with selected patients symptoms and syndromes can readily be investigated by hypnotic techniques of the type described. Symptom origin occasionally may be rapidly correlated with life situations or traumatic events. Their symbolic significance, especially when homosexual, masturbatory, aggressive, or homicidal impulses are repressed, may become apparent (Seitz, 1953). Isolated affects, thoughts, or emotions, especially if phobic material is being dealt with, can be appropriately fused even in the conscious acting-out of a previously traumatic event. Or specific fantasies, likewise, may be acted out.

One patient,† for instance, with pseudocyesis was seen in emergency consultation after having wired mother and mother-in-law, both of whom lived in other states, to come immediately, since labor had started two weeks earlier than she had expected, and since she was now leaving for the hospital.

She came to the office under protest, walked over to the couch, and lay upon it, drawing both legs up under her. Because of her abdominal protuberance, she could easily have been taken for a pregnant patient.

The therapist remained silent. After three or four minutes she spontaneously began sobbing: "I don't want to kill myself! I'm not too unhappy at not having a child. But I don't think that I can live without one. . . .

"I thought I was pregnant. I felt those movements, and I was so happy. I'd throw up my food and laugh about it. I went to a doctor—almost nine

---

* Patients of H. R.
† Patients of H. R.

months ago—and he told me I was [pregnant]. Then I started spotting. So I went to Dr. A. He said, 'If you are, it's too soon to tell!' I wondered why he didn't tell me, so I went to Dr. B. He said I was. Then, two months later, he gave me a test and said I wasn't. But I knew I was. So I watched my diet and took care of myself. I feel life. I'm pregnant. I know I am!" And at this, she began sobbing convulsively.

As it developed, she had told her neighbors, her friends, and her relatives that she was pregnant. She had even told everybody the date on which she expected to enter the hospital for delivery. "I feel life inside me now," she insisted, "I'm about to have the baby. It won't be long now."

"And yet, every physician has told you you're not pregnant. Why do you think they've said this?"

She was silent about five minutes and then, very slowly, began to speak: "These past months I've been living in a dream world. I've planned and I've talked. I wish I were dead now. I couldn't do anything to myself—I'm Catholic—but I keep thinking of stepping in front of a car . . . It's been four years ago last May, when my father died, and that's when I cried too much. And ever since *I've kept everything inside.* I didn't want to worry my Dad. We didn't have no mother. It's never borthered me, being so bottled up all my life, but I never really cried because my Dad would worry—except when the doctor said he had only 30 days to live. And he was buried on my first wedding anniversary." She was now sobbing convulsively. She then began to scream, "I'm going to have my baby! I'm going to have my baby!" And at this, she ceased speaking.

She was hypnotized at this point. Her legs spread apart on the couch; her knees bent; her thighs drew up over her abdomen; she began moaning and groaning; and then, during the next ten minutes, her buttocks and abdomen heaved up and down, back and forth, almost rhythmically. When asked what she was doing, she answered, "Having my child." The psychiatrist repeated, "Your—child? Are you sure?" Her body movements stopped at this point, she ceased groaning and moaning, and in an almost inaudible voice exclaimed, "No—not my child. It's my father I'm giving birth to—I need him so much." And at this, she became completely silent and motionless.

She then spontaneously added, while still hypnotized, that she knew intellectually she was not actually pregnant, but she felt she was. . . . However, she had now delivered—so she was no longer really pregnant!

Before the hypnotic session was terminated, this patient was told that she could remember everything that had taken place and everything she had said, provided she really wished to; but if she wished to, she could forget anything she had said or done while she was hypnotized, either in whole or in part. The hypnotic session was then terminated.

Actual acting-out of this type can not infrequently be circumvented by having the patient dream, while in a trance, whatever it is she really wishes, dreaming it very freely, very vividly, without need for inhibition, so that it becomes real to her. This dream method of acting things out can also be exceedingly effective. Because of the length of this article, and the simplicity of this technique, examples will not be given here.

DISCUSSION

In this paper we have stressed and illustrated various of the hypnotic techniques whereby symptom-function in both neurotic and psychotic patients can be evaluated. Parts of hypnodiagnostic sessions were quoted almost verbatim. Basic conflicts and even personality structure at times became apparent. No attempt has been made, however, to describe the course taken later in therapy by these patients. This will probably be done in a number of clinical papers dealing specifically with the individual patients involved. In this paper we have attempted to limit ourselves to a discussion of hypnotic and hypnotherapeutic investigatory techniques in the determining of symptom function.

With some patients functions served by neurotic symptoms seem almost conscious. They become obvious almost immediately on trance induction. No specific specialized hypnotic techniques seem necessary. One patient* with severe pruritus, for instance, who stated that she wanted nothing so much as the intercourse which nevertheless caused her intravaginal itch to become unbearable, was convinced that her only "cure" lay in obtaining a divorce. With other patients, on the other hand, this material is, of course, preconscious. This nevertheless may be elicited or acted out, again, merely on hypnotic induction. Our patient with pseudocyesis is a case in point. But with some patients, like the one with ulcerative colitis, specific key words must be seized upon and repeated before dynamics or function become experimentally clear. And with still other patients specialized hypnotic techniques must be utilized. These have been illustrated in detail during the preceding discussion.

When these techniques are utilized, however, a word of caution seems necessary. Regression, as Kris has stated, under certain circumstances can be in the service of the ego. However, the inept use of these techniques by diffidently trained or untrained psychiatrists, psychologists, or even self-ordained family counselors, who neither know nor realize what they are dealing with, can result in pronounced harm to the patient. Fantasy formation may be encouraged with psychotic patients, or the patient may, either by direct suggestion or by the mishandling of dynamic material, be enabled and pressed to consolidate defenses when such consolidation would be contraindicated. This does not constitute an objection per se to

* Patient of H. R.

the use of radical hypnotic investigatory techniques. We do object, however, to the unlicensed and uncontrolled use of hypnosis by inept and untrained individuals who consider it a parlor trick and who utilize it either as a cloak for their own lack of adequate training in dynamic psychiatry or as a means of obtaining substitutive gratification for some of their own unresolved personality problems (Rosen, 1953c).

It can readily be seen, for instance, that if specific precautions were not taken, some of our schizophrenic (preschizophrenic or psychoneurotic schizophrenic) patients who were making a fairly well-compensated social adjustment could utilize such techniques for the precipitation even of a catatonic state. Reality testing, with preservation and strengthening of the ego, rather than merely the abreactive induction of aggressive phenomena, must always be the desideratum. On the other hand, with some psychotic patients this may, paradoxically enough, be of value.

To illustrate: the husband of one of our patients* thought, so he stated, that his wife was catatonic. He turned out to be a petty criminal, a voyeur, and a sexual exhibitionist. Shortly after he was arrested and sentenced, she asked why we kept roses floating up in the office. She knew that the psychiatrist was a hypnotist and, on entering the office, she had gone into a trance. She was told to let the roses float into a vase. They were then made, first to change color, then to change into a rosebush, but a rosebush which the psychiatrist had never seen. As a result of this, our patient described a little girl watching her father cut roses. After some months of treatment she would exclaim spontaneously, "Let me sit over there, and I will tell you what to do with those roses and with that little girl who is growing up." The roses dropped out. Her varied ways of spelling her name at different age levels came up. She would often discuss that hallucinated figure of hers, which bore different names, wore different clothes and was in different places according to the particular event described. High school adjustments ultimately came into play, and then college adjustments followed. She is no longer clinically psychotic, and is now able to hold a responsible position.

In a field as complex as that of human behavior it usually is extremely difficult and sometimes impossible to set up satisfactory experimental conditions for the investigation even of what may be assumed to be relatively simple phenomena (Wolberg, 1945). When behavioral patterns come under investigation, hypotheses can frequently be advanced but seldom validated (Brennan, 1949). Determination of symptom-function, unless the patient is under long-term therapy, is usually impossible. Nevertheless, with selected patients hypnotic techniques have already been utilized as potent therapeutic and experimental tools in the validating of previously described dynamic concepts. The most significant of

---

* Patient of M. H. E.

these, in all probability, are Erickson's hypnotic experiments on the psychopathology of everyday life (1939c), Erickson and Kubie's translations of the cryptic automatic writing of one hypnotic subject by another when in a trancelike, dissociated state (1940), Farber and Fisher's investigation of the interpretation of dreams not their own by hypnotized college students (1943), Wolberg's direct suggestions for material to be incorporated symbolically into dreams by his hypnotized patient (1945), and Rosen's studies of hypnotic fantasy-evocation and dramatization techniques, especially in a patient with severe pruritus vulvae (1953b). Seitz' experiments, in addition, warrant careful study (1953).

It will be noted that a number of our patients abreacted spontaneously, occasionally in the present but at times by regressing to earlier life situations and behavioral patterns. In most of the illustrative cases this seemed to be on a compulsive basis.

While we feel that abreaction of this type may serve to make evident at least some of the functions which symptoms and symptom-complexes serve, nevertheless even here a word of caution seems necessary. These patients may somehow, perhaps not too rarely, find it possible to seize on the hypnotic relationship to rationalize to themselves their acting-out of suppressed or repressed desires. With a number of patients, this in all probability constitutes a sexual advance toward the therapist, and must be considered as both an attempt at seducing him and an expression of unconscious sexual impulses which nevertheless are being utilized to mask, but without effectively disguising, pronounced underlying hostility and aggression—on one level against him, and on deeper levels against key figures in early childhood and infantile environments (Rosen, 1953b; Wolberg, 1945).

Such acting-out, although for the moment serving to release tension and thereby provide emotional relief, solves no personality problems and as a result cannot be considered curative. It does to some extent, however, involve dynamic participation on the part of the patient, and may make— or help make—possible his active participation in the setting of the therapeutic goals to be attained, as well as his active collaboration later during the treatment process itself. A discussion of this, nevertheless, would be beyond the scope of this paper.

SUMMARY

1. Symptoms and even syndromes may subserve the repetitive enactment of traumatic events; may reproduce, instead, specific life situations; may satisfy repressed erotic and aggressive impulses; or may at one and the same time constitute defenses

against, and punishment for, underlying instinctual drives. They may mask underlying schizophrenic reactions or hold suicidal depressions in check. They may serve these and other functions concurrently, or none, or any specific one or combination of them.

2. With selected patients under hypnosis symptom-function may be determined rapidly and in a therapeutic setting. Various techniques can be utilized. Attacks may be precipitated and then blocked, either by direct hypnotic suggestion or by regressing the patient to a period predating the onset of his disease, so that substitutive motor or other activity will be precipitated in a form accessible to the therapeutic investigation; attacks may be precipitated in slow motion, so that individual components can be therapeutically investigated in detail; dissociated states may be induced; dream acting-out may be suggested; or symptoms may be suggested away while emotions back of symptoms are concurrently intensified, so that, again, underlying dynamic material will immediately become accessible for therapy. Still other techniques may be utilized.

3. If treatment, as well as evaluation, is through these techniques, and if treatment is successful, it may be that the analogy of a log jam will be of value. The jam can usually be broken by pulling out one or two key logs. The rest then start falling into place—and the whole log jam disappears. This may be what happens, although to a limited extent, during therapy of this type.

4. Various of these techniques have been illustrated throughout this paper. Case histories however, have at times been distorted in order to maintain the anonymity of the patients involved.

10. Experimental Hypnotherapy in Tourette's Disease

Milton H. Erickson

Two patients, both in their mid-thirties, one a married woman with three children, the other a married man without children, much to his regret, presented themselves for treatment for Tourette's Disease. Both had a history of a sudden acute onset, and both required therapy over a two-year period, the therapeutic sessions becoming progressively more infrequent as therapy continued. Both insistently demanded hypnotherapy and were convinced that it would be their salvation. For both the onset of the condition was acute and circumscribed and remarkably similar.

FIRST PATIENT

During the course of listening to a sermon one Sunday, this patient, the woman, had become horribly distressed to find herself unaccountably impelled to utter a variety of obscenities, particularly vulgarisms concerning body functions and sexual activity, all being ascribed to Jesus. She fought the overpowering vocal impulses desperately along with compelling desires to grimace, to gesticulate, and to posture. Her husband, noticing her distress, tried to make whispered inquiries, and this intensified her symptoms. She finally resorted to the measure of covering her mouth with handkerchiefs and shoving her fingers as far as she could into her throat. This resulted in retching, and she hastened to the ladies' lounge, shouting "Get out" to those who sympathetically came to her assistance. By turning on a faucet and a continuous flushing of the commode, she managed to cover-up a half-hour's exhaustive repetitious vulgar vocalizations. Fortunately, since she had the keys to the family automobile in her handbag, she managed to get to the car and then to drive a mile to reach home, racing the car engine in first gear to cover-up her continuous vocalizations. She locked herself in the bedroom and spent an exhausting afternoon in vocalizations, grimacing, and posturing,

Reprinted with permission from *The American Journal of Clinical Hypnosis*, April, 1965, *7*, 325-331.

interrupting herself only enough to yell at her husband that she was all right, that she wanted solitude, to let her alone, that she would see him on the morrow. That evening, without having eaten lunch or dinner, she took a heavy dose of sedatives and managed to sleep.

The next morning she awakened in acute fright, wondering if she had developed a sudden psychosis. The compulsive vocalization was still present as well as the need to grimace, to gesticulate, and to posture. She yielded to these and desperately reviewed mentally possible measures of concealing, distorting into more acceptable forms, and passively yielding to the impulses so that she could pattern her symptomatic behavior into some less distressing form. Since she had met the author socially on a previous occasion, she made use of her bedroom telephone extension to solicit his aid. The content of her telephone call was practically diagnostic in its character.

A house call was made, and the husband was reassured after a fashion to permit some reasonable provisions to meet his wife's condition. He was distressed by the secrecy being maintained but yielded to the extreme violence of her demands issued through the bedroom door in halting phrases because of interspersed whispered obscenities.

She demanded hypnotherapy, about which she had read various glowing lay accounts. Despite the adverse nature of the situation the author agreed, but emphatically demanded that she yield completely in utter submission to his choice of procedure. Approximately two hours were spent because of her involuntary interruptions of the author in making certain that she agreed without any reservation to any therapeutic procedure the author had in mind. Innumerable seemingly outrageous possibilities were outlined to her to make certain that she understood that the psychotherapy in mind was by no means even remotely orthodox. As soon as she understood this fully, hypnotic induction was undertaken. All appropriate and fitting hypnotic suggestions were offered in the proper sequence and progression that the author's experience had disclosed to be most reasonably effective. However, those suggestions were embellished, interlarded, couched, and elaborated with obscenities, vulgarities, and profanities that far exceeded the worst she had uttered.

She was utterly appalled, horrified, and what was most important, completely silenced with a rigid fixation of her attention upon the author and the hypnotic suggestions being offered to her in such a peculiar emphatic fashion. (The fact that she knew the author well socially undoubtedly constituted a highly significant but not measurable factor in the total situation.) At all events, within 10 minutes she developed a profound somnambulistic hypnotic trance in which silence, passivity, and abject obedience were demanded and received. With urgency and calculated haste she was disoriented for time and place, suggestions of a state of fright, of complete obedience to, and of utter dependence upon, the author as the representation of all that was good, reliable, comforting, and helpful were emphatically given to her. Thereupon she was reoriented with extreme care to avoid any possible traumatic event to a time two years in the past with emphatic instruction to remain so oriented or regressed after awakening from the trance despite all disturbing and wonder-provoking stimuli of her surroundings.

As soon as the author felt relatively secure in his control of the situation, the husband was summoned. Fortunately, he was a college graduate with a considerable background in psychology. Rapport with his wife was established for him.

The first measure with him was to inform him extensively concerning the syndrome of Gilles de la Tourette's Disease and to assure him that he would be furnished with references in the literature so that he could understand the peculiarity of his wife's affliction. This was done in his wife's presence in her regressed state, and she was informed of the possibility that sometime in the remote future she might develop such a condition. While she was thinking this over in the trance state, her husband was separately informed of the true state of affairs and of the regressed trance state of his wife as a temporary measure of controlling her problem. In his distress he agreed to let the author attempt experimental therapy, since the author could not inform him of any adequate therapeutic procedure.

The therapy worked out then and instituted was:

1. Informing the patient in the trance state that "in the future" she would be so afflicted.
2. Informing the patient that she was in a somnambulistic regressed trance state and that this was serving to control her problem, which was an actuality in her ordinary waking state.
3. Seeking the patient's cooperation in devising some measure of control of the symptoms.
4. Emphasizing that, since hypnotic regression had effected a temporary relief, hypnotic suggestion could and would undoubtedly be efficacious.
5. Suggesting that the patient be content with minor progress in control and improvement rather than demanding a miraculous cure.
6. Securing her absolute promise to abide by both her condition and the modifications of it that would be suggested.
7. A long discussion concerning the type of motor components that she would willingly permit and the nature of the utterances in regard to both content and volume.
8. The absolute need for her to remain an excellent hypnotic

subject for either the author or any other therapist who might take responsibility for her.

9. The absolute need for her absolute obedience—instant, complete, and without question—upon the slightest request, whether she was awake or in the trance state, and that this obedience would be expected even when she personally objected to instruction.

10. The teaching of the patient of a series of 10 posthypnotic cues by which to develop a trance state and a regression state. (The author did not want to rely upon one or two such cues.)

As this instruction of the patient progressed, it became increasingly difficult to maintain the trance state as well as the state of regression. The patient became increasingly distressed about the author's description of her condition; she obviously did not want to believe his statements, yet the demeanor of her husband, with whom she had been given needed rapport, as well as the emphasis with which she was being given instructions, were most compelling of her belief and acceptance. However, it was apparent that this trance state could not be maintained much longer, and a compromise was offered to the effect that she would arouse from the trance state to remain in the waking state of awareness for whatever time she wished, not to exceed an hour, and that she would then develop a profound somnambulistic regressed trance state. To this she agreed.

She awakened only to burst into a torrent of characteristic utterances accompanied by posturing and gesticulations.

After about 20 minutes of this she managed to express a wish that the author would or could in some way take charge of her situation. This was followed by further uncontrollable behavior and then a brief pause, during which another trance state was induced with explicit and emphatic instructions that henceforth at the first sense of uncontrollable behavior on her part she would immediately regress in age to a period of two years in the past. She accepted this instruction with a facial expression of hope.

After a second brief orientation of her husband concerning her condition, during which the patient listened attentively, attention was given to the task of outlining further the course of therapy for her. This was to include: (1) periodic visits to the author's office; (2) the systematic learning of a pattern of behavior that would meet the compulsions of her illness and yet enable reasonable daily life adjustments. Blind and complete acceptance of these two requirements was demanded and finally agreed to in a most binding fashion.

It was then explained that:

1. She was to continue her symptomatic behavior in a "satisfying"

but "better" manner. That is, since her manifestations would occur in either the presence or absence of others, her symptomatology could be entirely adequate if she alone knew of it. Thus, her utterances need not be so loud, since she could hear even the softest of whispers as well as the loudest of shouts. Additionally, the posturing could also be minimal, since she could be aware of it and any associated thoughts, however minimal the postural movements were. There was added the explanation that her illness, however severe, must necessarily be inconstant in manifestation, since she would have to eat, to drink, and to sleep, and that each of these activities would constitute temporary barriers to symptom manifestation. Hence, thoughtful and careful consideration of these facts would permit realization that there could be other periods of symptom-freedom and hence that extensive therapeutic procedures could be instituted. Much repetition and explanation of these ideas had to be given together with emphatic instruction that all understandings presented were to become an integral part of her waking state regardless of symptom-distress.

2. Systematic instruction was then given and practice insisted upon in uttering in low tones and whispers both her own utterances and some of those the author had voiced. This was demanded most cautiously, with full instruction that a regressed state would develop instantaneously if the author anticipated difficulty for her. This anticipated difficulty, not explained to her, was the possibility of her arousal from the trance and loss of control of the situation. Perhaps unnecessarily, the author did elicit the regressed state several times as a precautionary measure. Also, she was to develop new gesticulations more awkward and less meaningful to the observer than were the "grinds and bumps" which constituted a part of her motor manifestations. Coughing, gasping, choking, yawning, if necessary learning how to belch voluntarily, crossing her legs violently, or whatever else she felt could be bearable were suggested, and she was made to demonstrate the suggested acts.

The patient became most meditative and subdued, and when a regressed state was induced, she was asked to view herself in the future in a thoughtful situation with the author's right hand on her left shoulder and holding her left hand with his left hand. In this way it was possible to pseudo-orient her to the future while in the regressed state with physical contact constituting a part of the conditioning process. Thus, the composure of her regressed state allowed her comfortably to speculate upon her "future needs" as seem indicated by her visual hallucination of herself in suggested special settings, including her actual present condition.

In elaborate detail many ideas about her general and symptomatic behavior were worked out in relation to her home, her family, and her various obligations. Provision was made for her family to leave immediately on a vacation for two weeks with a complete cancellation of all social obligations and all incoming telephone calls. Thus the patient was ensured privacy and opportunity to practice new patterns of behavior.

She made regular visits to the author, but instead of racing the engine, she turned on the car radio to high volume and yielded completely to her vocalizations. Thus, she "got it out of my system" to permit therapeutic interviews with the author. These were barren so far as understandings or information were concerned, but they were most useful in augmenting her ability to modify, control, and direct her symptomatology.

One significant oversight in the proposed therapy was disclosed by the events of one night about a month later. She awakened suddenly and disturbed the whole household by a violent manifestation of her symptoms. When interviewed in both waking and trance states the next day, the explanation was that she had to have "escape valves" as a "safety measure." This led to the provision that weekly, biweekly, or even less frequently she would go into the garage, close it, turn on the car radio full volume, and "let loose with everything."

At first this occurred weekly, but slowly came to be more and more infrequent until the practice was discontinued.

Therapy was continued for two years, first at weekly intervals, then finally at monthly intervals. That the last year of therapy was necessary was questionable in the author's mind. The patient, however, felt that she would feel more comfortable if therapy were continued, even though it was slowly transformed into essentially little more than social visits.

More than five years have elapsed since therapy was discontinued. The patient is free of her symptoms, and has been wholly so since the completion of the first year of therapy. A year ago (1963) she sought an interview with the author on other matters, reminisced with amusement about her previous condition, and declared, "I can say all those things and make all of those movements voluntarily without any distress. Let me show you." She did most comprehensively and then with a laugh remarked, "I am not sure whether some of the things I just said were mine or some of the embellishments with which you horrified me so terribly. Have you or any other psychiatrists any understanding of what an awful mental state descended upon me that time? It makes me shudder to look back upon it, but I remember you telling me that other people got it too. It's really too awful to think about, but I wanted you to be sure I'm over it." (At this writing, she still is.)

Questioning of her during therapy and subsequently of why therapy seemed effective elicited no information. The only conclusion was that it was a blind effort that fortunately succeeded with her.

SECOND PATIENT

A year after therapy with this patient was discontinued, a second, much less severe patient presented himself. His statement was that he was on his way to church one Sunday when, as he caught sight of the church building, he found himself involuntarily bursting into incredible obscenities and profanities with grinding of his teeth and much shaking of his fists. Little description was needed of his symptomatology, since he punctuated the narration of his history with it.

At first only the sight of his own church led to symptom manifestation, then other churches, then the sight of anyone in religious garb. By occupation he was a bartender in an exclusive bar; but as his symptoms continued he discovered that the utterance of a single word of profanity would precipitate an uncontrollable explosion of a minute or two duration from him. At first he avoided going to church, then to streets where there were churches. Finally he had to resign his lucrative position and secure employment in a rough-and-tumble tavern where he soon became favorably known as "The Cussing Bartender" and where his language and behavior attracted a certain clientele, since his episodes were brief though repetitious. In fact, it became a challenge for the tavern's clientele to think up new precipitating phrases which the patient found himself unable to keep from incorporating in his own vocalizations.

His wife resented his reduced income, swore at him in her anger, and became suddenly and painfully aware of her husband's affliction, which he had kept secret from her, enabled to do so by his working hours and careful avoidance of her. She insisted upon psychiatric therapy without delay.

As the patient related his problem, the other patient was called to mind. He differed in that his manifestations seemed to require a "triggering" by sight of something pertaining to religion, religious thinking, or hearing profane and obscene utterances by others.

The patient was then questioned about his willingness to undertake hypnotherapy, and he declared that that was his purpose in seeking the author's assistance.

A satisfactory deep trance was elicited with not too much time or effort being required, and an explanation was given to him in the trance state that before treatment of his problem, there would be undertaken an extensive educational project that would enable more rapid therapy once it was begun. He was reluctant about this since he desired therapy at once, but finally he yielded to the author's persuasions.

Thereupon, a systematic program was instituted to train this patient in selective sensory exclusion of stimuli, visual and auditory, and to establish psychological blocks to render various words "nonsense syllables." This was carefully explained to his wife, ánd her cooperation was won; the patient's own high intelligence and psychological sophistication were of significant value in promoting therapeutic intentions.

Extensive inquiry elicited a satisfactory list of evocative stimuli, and slowly the patient learned a selective blindness that allowed him to see a church as, for example, a "white building," a nun as "a woman dressed in a ridiculous-looking black dress," to listen to oaths and obscenities as "meaningless nonsense syllables," to regard Sunday as his day off duty, and to look upon his wife's church attendance as a special feminine social activity. A thoughtless asking of grace at an evening meal he regarded with confusion and bewilderment, developed a headache, and went to bed without eating. That incident terminated that mealtime practice. Fortunately, there were no children, and the social activities of the man and his wife together were extremely limited.

As for religious thoughts of his own, the patient was extensively instructed in the matter of nonsense syllable experimentation and given to understand that he, too, could devise nonsense syllables. In this way any religious thoughts coming to his mind became transformed into nonsense syllables.

He was seen regularly in the office biweekly for about three months. During this time he was instructed in the trance state to put into force his hypnotically acquired learnings, not constantly, but at first infrequently and then with increasing frequency, so that his symptoms would occur with decreasing frequency. The patient was most cooperative, and by the end of three months he had lost his job as "The Cussing Bartender." However, he secured reemployment on probation in his original position.

After the three months he was seen with decreasing frequency, until he reported not oftener than once a month at the end of two and one-half years of therapy. During the last nine months of therapy much time was given to "There are lost memories coming back to me. I lost them some way, but now they are coming back and I like them." Cautious questioning disclosed that the word *service* had a "special, very special, really wonderful meaning, but just what I don't know. It has something to do with what I want to call 'sacred,' whatever that means." Bit by bit, during the last nine months, he was allowed to recover from his sensory inhibitions and induced aphasia but was cautioned repeatedly in the trance state to do this "comfortably, happily."

A year after discontinuance of therapy he entered the office to request that he be informed why he had ever undertaken psychiatric therapy, why his regular visits were such a blank in his memory, and why his wife would not discuss the matter with him despite the fact that her manner suggested full knowledge on her part.

He consented to go into a trance, and in the trance he was asked the advisability of giving him full conscious information. He assured the author earnestly that all would be well, but he agreed to redevelop a trance state upon the occurrence of any emotional distress.

Aroused, he listened most attentively, demonstrated a slow spontaneous recollection of his original problem, developed a sudden trance in which he explained that his memories horrified him but that he was no longer a victim of that disorder, that he would not be more than distressed by his memories if awakened, that there would be no recurrence. He was awakened, showed reluctance about further discussion, but did assert that he remembered fully and was certain he would not again be so afflicted.

A year later he reported that, shortly after the previous visit, he had begun to go to church without difficulty and that he had had no further symptomatology. He, too, inquired into the author's understandings of his illness and expressed regret that the author knew so little about the condition.

OTHER EXPERIENCE

The author has seen professionally two other cases. One was a 13-year-old boy and the other was a 16-year-old girl. Both had fairly acute onsets but not as sudden as the two patients reported above. In both instances efforts made to treat the patients were utter failures. In all, for each there were no more than four interviews, and no rapport of any sort could be established despite the fact that both patients were of good intelligence. Their parents were demanding, frightened, bewildered, and embarrassed, and even they could not be handled satisfactorily. They wanted immediate results, a prescription preferably, and were not interested in any systematic attempt at therapy. They sought aid elsewhere, completely dissatisfied with the author. The eventual outcome is not known for either of these patients.

SUMMARY

A report is given of the experimental hypnotherapeutic treatment of Gilles de la Tourette's Disease or Syndrome. The experimental therapy consisted of using simple hypnotic trances and hypnotic regression to permit a reeducation of the two patients in a progressively greater control of their condition and with a progressive alteration of symptomatology to render it less severe. Both patients made a recovery in approximately a two-year period. No understanding of the causation of the onset of the condition was discovered in either instance. For further references, see Chapel et al., (1964), and Eisendberg et al., (1959).

11. Hypnotherapy: The Patient's Right to Both Success and Failure

Milton H. Erickson

Many times the author has been asked to publish an account of a failure in hypnotherapy when success was fully anticipated. To date the author has hesitated to do so, since there was no understanding of why the failures occurred (and there have been failures, as one should expect). Why this is so seems best explained in terms of either the therapist's lack of understandings or the patient's own purposes.

The following case history is cited as an excellent example of a failure despite a partial success that still persists but which derived from neither hypnotherapy nor psychotherapy but from an unconventional procedure which changed a serious symptom into a primary nuisance to the patient with its subsequent abolishment. Such could scarcely be considered therapy; it was no more than a symptom removal that enabled him to function adequately within his own restricted limits.

He was an excellent hypnotic subject, but he was passive. He "never got around to it" in carrying out posthypnotic suggestions. Questioning him in the trance state for his history was as futile as in the waking state. He liked to "rest" in the trance state. No measure seemed to stir him into even responsive replies to simple questions. Thus, when asked if he had siblings, he replied "yet." When asked, "How many?" the reply was, "Dottie." In the waking state he gave as his siblings, "Joe."

All he wanted was a symptom correction, nothing more, and while much effort was made by this author and several other psychiatrists, no adequate history was ever obtained from him, although an adequate history was obtained by several psychiatrists from his sister "Dottie."

When first seen by this author, the patient had been shopping around, seeing various psychiatrists, all of whom were requested to undertake the removal of a single symptom and all of whom agreed that he needed intensive psychotherapy for his obviously schizoid condition. Only the author agreed finally to give the therapy requested, believing that it might lead the patient into accepting further treatment. Even so, he continued to shop around to inquire of others if he should have his symptom removed.

Reprinted with permission from *The American Journal of Clinical Hypnosis*, January, 1965, 7, 254-257.

Several told him to go ahead and that he might want to enter therapy. Accordingly, he returned to the author and made his firm restricted demand for the removal of a single annoying symptom, and he was accepted as such a patient.

Neither direct nor indirect hypnotic suggestion was of any avail. The patient remained passive in relation to all hypnotherapy. A nonhypnotic psychotherapeutic approach was equally ineffectual. Thereupon, the author devised the following procedure, which was then presented to him in much the same way as one would present a prescription saying, "Take this to the druggist and get it filled."

This patient's demand of the author was a symptomatic cure of what he called a phobia. Every effort was made to induce the patient to recognize that, though his "phobia" needed correction, he was a decidedly maladjusted person who came from a large family of children, all of whom were, with one exception, neurotic or schizophrenic, and that two of his siblings had committed suicide in state mental hospitals.

The patient, a first-semester college student, declared that, while he had a schizoid personality and that he felt personally inferior, he wanted and would accept therapy for only one thing, his "phobia." This "phobia" was that he could drive a car on only certain streets in Phoenix and Tempe, and that he could reach Tempe (11 miles away) only by following one particular highway. There was one other highway by which he had often tried to leave Phoenix, but he could go no farther than the city limits. If his car passed beyond the city limits sign, he would become dizzy and nauseated; after either vomiting or retching, he would then faint and sometimes remain in that state 10 or 15 minutes.

His brother, his brother-in-law, and various friends had many times gone with him on that highway, but whether he was driving or they were made no difference. If they were driving and kept on going until he recovered from his faint, he would again faint and continue to repeat his fainting if they continued to drive on. The same thing occurred within the city limits of both Tempe and Phoenix, and he often had to park his car on a main street and walk a few blocks to reach certain destinations. On all the main highways except one leading out of Phoenix, he could not even walk beyond the city limits sign without fainting, even though he might be in the company of relatives or friends. For this problem and this problem alone he demanded therapy. Other psychiatrists had refused to accept him on his terms, declaring that they could not help him when he placed restrictions on therapy.

This author told him that he would be accepted as a patient, his terms abided by, but that if he benefited, it was hoped that he would accept further therapy. Since the patient was obdurate and demanding in his attitude, he was given a solemn promise that the author would not make any attempt other than to free him of his car driving problem. Several hours were spent with him in letting him convince himself that the author meant exactly what he said, and in securing from the author an absolute promise that he would do exactly as the patient instructed him.

This promise had been given without any details of procedure being disclosed to the patient. When the promise was finally accepted by the patient, he was handed an envelope bearing in large plain letters, "Anybody curious about me, please read the contents of this envelope." Inside, on the author's letterhead stationery, was the simple statement: "This man is my patient and he is obeying medical orders. If you find that he is unconscious, wait at least 15 minutes. He will then recover and will answer your questions to your satisfaction." There followed my signature.

The patient was then instructed that the next morning at 3:00 A.M., since it was a weekend, he was to take the highway leading to Flagstaff, 150 miles away. Wearing his very best clothes, he was to pin the envelope to the front of his jacket with the notation on the envelope uppermost and to drive to the city limits on that highway. Just before he reached that point, he was to turn off onto the wide shoulder of that highway. (The author was well acquainted with that long, level, wide-shouldered stretch of highway with a sandy, shallow ditch running alongside of the wide shoulders.) As he reached the sign, he was to shift into neutral, turn off the ignition, coast to a stop or brake the car to a stop just beyond the sign, leap out of the car, rush over to the shallow ditch, and lie down on his back, face up, and stay there at least 15 minutes. Then he was to get up, dust the sand from his clothes, get back into the car, start it, shift into first gear, drive one or two car lengths and stop the car, turn off the ignition, put on the brake, and again lie in the ditch as before for another 15 minutes.

This process was to be repeated again and again until he could drive from one telephone pole to the next, and then past the second pole on toward the third, stopping at the first evidence of any symptoms and spending 15 minutes on his back in the ditch each time. It was further explained that traffic on that highway was decidedly slight at that hour in the morning, that if a Highway Patrol car came along the officers would undoubtedly call the author for information, that the only real problem was to be at the city limits at 3:00 A.M.

The patient's reply to all this was, "But that's plain crazy." The author replied, "Agreed, but you want a symptomatic cure, and that is what you are going to get. You made me promise and I made you promise. So, that's it." The patient protested further, "But what if I start to faint when I get up out of the ditch?" "Lie down for another 15 minutes, look at the sky and get mad at me. Then move on in the car to the next spot to lie in the ditch. That's what you want, a symptomatic cure, and you're going to get it."

At about 9:00 P.M. he entered the author's home and stated, "After about the tenth time lying in the ditch I began feeling like a damn fool. I got back in the car and started driving from one telephone pole to the next and then to the curve I could see ahead in the road, and then I got interested in the scenery. I drove to Flagstaff through Oak Creek Canyon and managed the mountain road O.K. I drove around Flagstaff, came back to Phoenix, and I've been driving all over Phoenix and Tempe. I sure as hell was afraid when I started out at 2:30 A.M., and I was scared the first time I laid down in the ditch. Then when I brushed the sand off my clothes I didn't like it. I thought it was a damn fool thing for you to make me promise, and the more I did it, the madder I got, and so I just quit and began enjoying driving."

Thirteen years have elapsed. He graduated creditably from the university in the normal period of time, but he is still very definitely a severe schizoid personality. He has seen a number of psychiatrists but has never remained with any one of them sufficiently long to enter into therapy.

He works irregularly, and although he completed four years of college successfully, he lives at a substandard level. Parental funds keep him from being penniless much of the time, and he has driven his car all over the United States on vacation trips and "job hunting."

When he does work, it is exceedingly well done, and he has been known twice to agree to a year's contract which called for a generous bonus at the expiration of the contract. He broke the contracts a week ahead of time and lost both bonuses. Each position was at a managerial level.

His parents, his normal brother, his neurotic sister, and two normal brothers-in-law have made many ineffectual efforts to get him to stay with some psychiatrist. He is known to have visited at least half a dozen.

His status at the present time is that of one who, in a depressed mood, continued fruitless futile driving about, securing a job, working briefly and then quitting, living at a substandard level and always defeating himself. A typical example of his self-defeating activity was driving 255 miles to see the Grand Canyon, arriving late at night, and then leaving at about 4:00 A.M. the next morning to return to Phoenix without having even looked at the Grand Canyon. His explanation was, "Well, the motel bed wasn't so good."

COMMENT

That the patient wanted and accepted therapy for a troublesome symptom is apparent. That he was definitely an intelligent young man is attested by his good college record and his two managerial positions, each done competently with the exception of breaking the contract at the last week and losing his bonus both times. This, however, did not cause his employers any loss; rather, they profited from his act.

This patient demonstrated a capacity to benefit rather easily and well from the intervention by someone who could create a therapeutic situation but which the patient would accept for one purpose only. The man is not satisfied with his total situation; periodically he seeks but does not accept help from the author and other psychiatrists but that is as far as he will permit matters to go. There seems to be no possible way to motivate him despite his own clear statement, "It looks like I will finally end up in the state mental hospital like my sister, and I sure don't like that idea." He did accept the suggestion that to force mental hospitalization upon himself, he might wander about the streets in a confused way until the police picked him up, but when this occurred (on two occasions) he succeeded in convincing the police that he was just "absent-minded." Thus, twice he competently averted a sanity hearing.

In brief, this man needs help, has a poor prognosis, and, to this author and a number of other psychiatrists, is therapeutically inaccessible, despite the fact that he is a good though completely passive hypnotic subject.

12. Successful Hypnotherapy that Failed

Milton H. Erickson

The following brief case history is reported for the significant values it has in demonstrating the fallibility of success in hypnotherapy.

At a lecture on, and demonstration of, hypnosis before a dental society, the author was asked to "cure" a "gagging" patient. Upon the author's agreement to make such an attempt, the patient, a 45-year-old man, came forward. He gave his own history readily and informatively, and he was aided in this by his family dentist, who was present in the audience and who came forward with his records to offer special items of information. In summary, the history was that, following a toothache and a tooth extraction at the age of 10 years, the patient's mouth had healed satisfactorily. About a month later, when brushing his teeth, the patient noted a slight gagging, but merely wondered at the cause. This slight gagging increased until, at the expiration of another month, the gagging had become so severe that he could not brush his teeth. His family dentist was consulted but could find no cause for this peculiar gagging. The family numbered a psychiatrist and a psychologist among their friends, and both saw the patient separately and together. No explanation of the patient's complaint was found by them despite a searching study. The dentist prescribed mouthwashes and a program of slow, systematic reconditioning of the patient to the use of a toothbrush. This was begun by having the patient close his mouth and touch his lips with the brush, with the intention of slowly introducing the toothbrush into the mouth, and then beginning to initiate the toothbrushing very gently. The psychiatrist and the psychologist worked with the dentist to devise this plan of reconditioning the patient, who was most cooperative.

Unfortunately, the results were worse than the original gagging. The patient shortly began gagging when he merely picked up the toothbrush. Further psychological and psychiatric studies were made with no significant discoveries. The gagging continued to grow worse until eating became a problem. He finally extended the gagging to include the use of a fork or a spoon, and he had to resort to the use of his fingers in eating.

At the age of 22 he fell in love, became engaged to marry, but discovered to his horror that any attempt to kiss mouth-to-mouth resulted

Reprinted with permission from *The American Journal of Clinical Hypnosis*, 1966, 9, 62-65.

in gagging and retching. However, he could give and receive kisses elsewhere than on the mouth.

At the age of 23 he was forced to seek dental care. An examination could be done only under general anesthesia. The dental pathology was so extensive that two dental consultants were called upon for their opinions. All three recommended total extractions of upper and lower teeth. The patient agreed relievedly, since he had had many serious toothaches which he had been forced to endure without dental care except general medication.

General anesthesia was required for the extraction and the preparation of the dentures, and these were fitted in place while the patient was under general anesthesia. To help him become adjusted to the dentures he was heavily drugged first with morphine and then barbiturates.

With the lightening of his narcosis, he began gagging and retching.

After his mouth had healed completely, a new set of dentures was made and fitted in place by means of a general anesthesia. They led only to gagging and retching despite every measure employed to help the patient.

During World War II he managed to enlist for "limited duty" but shortly received a medical discharge because he could not use dentures or eating implements. In civilian life he made an excellent marital, social, and economic adjustment. Repeatedly he was offered promotions that involved meeting people as a salesman if he would wear dentures. Altogether, 10 sets of dentures were made for him with no helpful results. His employer gladly retained him in the lesser occupational position.

In preparation for the dental meeting at which the author was to lecture, his dentist prepared a new set of dentures for him, using, as was customary, general anesthesia. The patient was carrying them in a box in his pocket. He was asked if he wished to be hypnotized and instructed to wear the dentures. He affirmed this to be his desire, but he explained, "First I want you to see this." Thereupon he opened the box, took out the dentures, and slowly moved them toward his mouth. When they were within two inches of his mouth, he began gagging and retching. Moving them away he stated, "That's why I didn't eat breakfast this morning."

With great insistence he was urged to put the dentures in his mouth long enough for the author to see them in place. He agreed to this, but it was noted that he suddenly began perspiring freely. Slowly, with rigid carefulness, he opened his mouth, inserted the dentures, breathing deeply and then holding his breath as his dentist had taught him. He was able to retain the dentures about eight seconds, by which time streams of perspiration were rolling down his face and the front of his shirt was wet with perspiration.

He was asked to put the dentures back in the box, and a simple technique of trance suggestion was employed. The patient developed a somnambulistic trance state within a few minutes. Various phenomena of the somnambulistic trance were demonstrated for the benefit of the audience and to deepen the patient's state of hypnosis. No attempt was made to have him wear the dentures in the hypnotic state. Such an attempt, it was thought, might jeopardize the possibility of success. Hence he was used to demonstrate the phenomena of deep hypnosis as a measure of ensuring extensive learning. Finally, contrary to the author's wishes, he abided by the audience's insistent demand for a test of denture wearing in hypnosis. The patient readily allowed his dentist to insert the dentures. No evidences of discomfort were noted. The patient was then given carefully worded posthypnotic suggestions that he would not notice that he was wearing his dentures when he aroused from the trance state until he was asked to look into a mirror and to smile. He agreed to this readily and aroused upon appropriate suggestions. He had an amnesia for being in the trance and reiterated his statement that he was willing to be hypnotized. He was asked if his dentures were in the box in his pocket. He asserted that they were but that he hoped they would be in his mouth after he had been hypnotized. He was handed a mirror and asked to look at his smile. In a puzzled manner he took the mirror, but as he looked into it, he was obviously most startled. He immediately took the box out of his pocket and found it to be empty. His bewildered behavior was delightful to observe. A member of the audience asked if he would like a steak for luncheon. He stated he would.

The rest of the story is simple. He ate a steak for luncheon in the company of a large group of dentists. He had a second steak for dinner and a third just before midnight, still surrounded by interested dentists. He went home the next morning in the company of his dentist.

All this occurred in the early part of March. Upon arriving at home, his employer gave him a promotion to begin on Monday of the next week. His dentist, whose office was located next to the building where the man was employed, checked daily on the patient's wearing of his dentures. The patient kissed his wife on the mouth for the first time in their 20 years of marriage, and he also kissed his children.

For two months the author received weekly reports from the dentist, whose inquiries had disclosed that the patient was unwilling at first to take his dentures out even to wash them. Then in June letters were received from both the dentist and the patient to the effect that all was well. Another such letter from the dentist was received in July. In August the patient and the dentist went on a fishing trip. All went well. During this fishing trip the patient expressed much appreciation for what had been done for him.

Then on the morning of September 23 the patient awakened, chatted briefly with his wife, and then remarked casually that he was leaving his dentures at home that day. His wife protested, but unemotionally he remarked that it just "seemed to be a good idea." His employer was out of town, and the dentist did not see him that day. In the evening his wife asked him to wear his dentures for dinner. He refused to do so, and she was too bewildered to ask for an explanation.

The patient sat down to dinner, but as the first forkful of food approached his mouth, he gagged. His wife leaped up, secured the dentures, and handed them to him, telling him to put them in his mouth. As he started to do so, he gagged.

He ate the evening meal with his fingers. His wife accompanied him to the dentist the next morning, taking the dentures with her. The dentist induced a deep trance but elicited only the explanation that he did not want to wear the dentures. No additional explanation could be elicited. He manifested no emotional disturbance. His unwillingness to wear his dentures seemed to be no more than a simple statement expressive only of a matter-of-fact attitude.

A long distance telephone call to the author by the dentist led to the advice to refrain from making any issue of the matter. Accordingly, the dentist so instructed the patient's wife, and she accepted the advice.

Two weeks later the patient wrote a simple straightforward account of what had happened, of his intention of not wearing his dentures, of his willingness to be demoted by his employer to his original position, and of his wife's statement that all had gone reasonably well previously and probably would again. He stated further that he knew of no reason for abandoning his dentures, that he regretted disappointing everybody, but that life seemed to be as satisfying one way as another.

A year later the dentist wrote that the patient was contentedly adjusting without his dentures, that the topic of denture-wearing had long been closed, and that the patient and his family were doing well despite the return to the previous lower income.

Another year later the situation was unchanged. The patient, in reply to questions, stated that the only possible explanation that had occurred to him was that the long years without dentures had fully accustomed him to their absence, that he was not sure of this as an adequate explanation, but that he could think of no other explanation. Moreover, he did not mind the requisite adjustment to their absence nor did he feel any loss in not using them nor any desire to return to their use. To a specific question he replied that he now could not understand why he had formerly wanted to wear dentures.

The author has no understanding of the course of events with this patient. Successful therapy was apparently achieved, enjoyed for months by the patient, and then apparently abandoned for no known reason and without regret. The man adjusted well before the extraction of his teeth, and except for his medical discharge from military service, he adjusted well in the edentulous state. He adjusted well during the months of wearing the dentures, and he adjusted well after discarding them. The family dentist and the psychiatrist and the psychologist friends all found nothing of note in their association with the man and his family that would be considered as offering even a semblance of an explanation of the patient's behavior.

13. Visual Hallucination as a Rehearsal for Symptom Resolution

Milton H. Erickson and Ernest L. Rossi

"A doctor and his wife wanted me to cure their 10 year-old son of bed-wetting. It was to be a one-shot effort. I knew the parents well. I had trained the father in hypnosis, and the boy had heard his mother and father speak of me very highly. The boy wanted a dog, but his parents said he could not have one because he wet his bed. I told the parents that the boy could visit me, but they were not to tell the boy that I was supposed to cure his bed-wetting.

TRANCE INDUCTION VIA EXPECTANCY

"The boy came and was intelligent and curious about hypnosis. I told him he could go into a trance and he could have something he wanted very much. He said, 'What?' I repeated that it would be something 'you would want to do very much.' Now when he understood that, he was willing to go into a trance.

"He went into a very nice trance, and I continued, 'Now we will get to find something you would like very much.' His eyes opened, though he remained in trance. 'We will take a walk down the street, maybe we will see something.' I then turned my head to indicate looking into the distance and exclaimed, 'Oh, there is that mother dog; she has got two puppies! [Pause] I think I like the black-and-white one best. Which one do you like best?' The boy looked in the indicated direction and softly said, 'I like the brown-and-white puppy.' I said, 'Would you like to pet it?' The boy reached over the side of his chair and petted the hallucinated puppy. I reached over and petted my puppy and said 'You are going to get a puppy and you can set the date when you are to get the puppy. *I know that! I know you can get a puppy!* Give yourself time, maybe you had better wait for two weeks. And on that day when you come to the breakfast table you will all of a sudden have a bright new idea two weeks from today. You will

---

The first four paragraphs of this paper are an edited version of a taped interview with MHE by the editor who then contributed the analysis that follows.

walk to the table for breakfast, and say to your father and mother, 'Today is the day you are going to bring me a puppy.'

"He did just that, and when they asked him what kind of a puppy, he just said, 'You'll bring the right one, I just know.' I had told his parents it was to be a brown-and-white puppy. But the idea just occurred to him consciously that morning two weeks after his visit with me."

What are the factors involved in this successful hallucinatory experience that lead to a cure of bed-wetting?

1. The parents spoke well of Erickson, so the boy looked up to him.
2. Erickson told the parents not to tell the boy that Erickson was to cure the bed-wetting because that might set up the situation as a challenge, which the boy might feel he had to resist even if he wanted to cooperate on a conscious level.
3. Trance was presented to the boy as an experience where he "could have something he wanted very much." This immediately mobilized his positive expectations and, in particular, probably activated his wish for a dog on either a conscious or unconscious level because, in fact, he did want a dog.
4. These activated associations had an immediate outlet when Erickson mentioned the two puppies.
5. The parents had told him that he could not have a dog until he stopped bed-wetting. Erickson knew this was a frustrating contingency within the boy's mind. It was frustrating because his ego could not control the bed-wetting, and therefore he could not get a dog. Erickson did not have to crudely say or suggest anything further about that painful contingency: *If* you stop bed-wetting, *then* you can have a dog. Erickson simply utilized this already existing contingency and added a few things that would help the boy achieve it:
   a) Erickson gave the boy an intense hallucinatory experience of the dog he wanted. This strengthened the boy's inner image, and his goal became more real by being rehearsed in the trance situation.
   b) Erickson perhaps delivered a strong, secret message to the boy by emphasizing, "I know that! I know you can get a puppy!" The boy knew that Erickson had a lot of prestige with the boy's parents. If Erickson said something, it must carry strong weight with the parents. The boy now had a secret ally in Erickson, so the problem of getting a dog seemed less hopeless.
   c) Erickson gave the boy time: two weeks to learn how to control his bed-wetting with his now vastly strengthened inner resources. Erickson did not have to directly say, "You can have two weeks to learn to control your bed-wetting." Such a crude suggestion was not needed because it was already *implied* when Erickson

said he knew the boy could get a puppy. The parents' contingency plus Erickson's conviction formed a classical logical argument: modus tolons.

Parent's Contingencies   *Symbolic logic*

If you stop bed-wetting,   S
then you can have a dog."   D
or S> D   where > = If . . . then implication

Erickson's Convincing Addition

"I know you can get a puppy."   D

Together these two statements lead to the logical conclusion, S, that bed-wetting will stop. Thus via modus tolons—
  S > D
  D
  ∴ S

6. Erickson utilized another of his favorite hypnotic forms when he made his posthypnotic suggestion contingent on an inevitable piece of future behavior:

Posthypnotic Suggestion	*Commentary*
"When you come to the breakfast table	The time-binding introduction of an implied directive.
you will all of a sudden have a bright new idea two weeks from today.	If it is to be "new," it implies that he will be amnesic for the idea until two weeks pass.
You will walk to the table for breakfast	An inevitable piece of behavior onto which
and say to your father and mother, 'Today is the day you are going to bring me a puppy.'"	this suggestion can be hitchhiked.

The boy's triumphant conviction, "You will bring the right one, I just know," in answer to his parents' question two weeks later about the kind of dog he wanted, is an amusing incidental validation of the connection between Erickson's suggestions and the correct implications the boy drew from them.

III. Utilization Approaches to Hypnotherapy

The papers of this section all demonstrate Erickson's utilization approach to a variety of psychological problems. Utilization theory emphasizes that every individual's particular range of abilities and personality characteristics must be surveyed in order to determine which preferred modes of functioning can be evoked and utilized for therapeutic purposes. Utilization of the patient's own attitudes becomes a basic approach for circumventing what most other therapists term "resistance." The therapeutic process then ideally unfolds as follows: (1) The therapist provides fresh ideas and situations to break through the limiting preconceptions that have blocked the patient's own problem-solving abilities (stages one and two of the microdynamics of trance and suggestion, as outlined in Volume One of this series), thus evoking (2) unconscious processes of search and solution (stages three and four of the microdynamics of trance and suggestion) that lead patients to (3) resolving their own problem in their own way. Following is an edited version of a taped dialogue that occurred in 1973 between Erickson and the editor illustrating this approach.

E: An expert carpenter lost the first three fingers of his right hand. He came out of the hospital and asked me, "What am I going to do to earn a living? How am I going to hold a hammer?" I responded with, "The first task you have is to learn how to shake hands without letting the other fellow know that you've lost three fingers.

He learned how to shake hands without letting the other person discover the missing fingers. He learned how to apply just the right amount of pressure with his thumb, palm, and little finger so the other fellow never realized anything was missing. When he had learned that, his unconscious would automatically know how to hold a hammer. You cannot explain that to anyone.

R: So your hypnotherapy is almost the exact opposite of most conventional hypnotic approaches. Other hypnotherapists believe they have to specify exactly what the patient is supposed to do. But you just open a patient up to knowledge that is within, together with new life experiences, rather than trying to program him with your version of how you believe he ought to behave.

E: Too many hypnotherapists take you out to dinner and then tell you what to order. I take a patient out to a psychotherapeutic dinner and I say, "You give your order." The patient makes his own selection of the food he wants. He is not hindered by my instructions, which would only obstruct and confuse his inner processes.

One of my daughters had a tongue-thrusting problem during swallowing that was interfering with the formation of her teeth. The dentist showed her the more natural way of swallowing and contrasted it with her way. He then told her to go home and practice *both*. And sure enough, after a while my daughter selected, on her own, the natural, correct way to swallow.

R: She was not following any rigid prescription for behavior change given to her by the dentist. He gave her alternatives that enabled her to make her own choice based on her own actual experience.

E: Yes, providing the patient with alternatives sets the stage for inner search and creative problem-solving.

R: You did not tell the carpenter he would have to hold the hammer in exactly such and such a manner, applying pressure here and there in a certain way. He could not learn in such a fashion. The conscious effort to learn *your* way would have interfered with *his own* unconscious manner of learning to deal with his own handicap. You simply gave him a task that would stimulate his inner problem-solving capacities.

E: That's right.

14. Special Techniques of Brief Hypnotherapy

Milton H. Erickson

The development of neurotic symptoms constitutes behavior of a defensive, protective character. Because it is an unconscious process, and thus excluded from conscious understandings, it is blind and groping in nature and does not serve personality purposes usefully. Rather it tends to be handicapping and disabling in its effects. Therapy of such distorted behavior ordinarily presupposes that there must be a correction of the underlying causation. However, such correction, in turn, presupposes not only a fundamental willingness on the part of the patient for adequate therapy but also an actual opportunity and situation conducive to treatment. In the absence of one or both of these requisites, psychotherapeutic goals and methods must be reordered to meet as adequately as possible the total reality situation.

In attempting such modified psychotherapy the difficult problem arises of what can really be done about neurotic symptomatology where the realities of the patient and his life situation constitute a barrier to comprehensive treatment. Efforts at symptom removal by hypnosis, persuasion, reconditioning, etc. are usually futile. Almost invariably there is a return to the symptomatology in either the same form or another guise, with increased resistance to therapy.

Equally futile, under such limiting circumstances, is any effort to center treatment around idealistic concepts of comprehensiveness, or, as is unfortunately too often the case, around the therapist's conception of what is needed, proper, and desirable. Instead, it is imperative that recognition be given to the fact that comprehensive therapy is unacceptable to some patients. Their total pattern of adjustment is based upon the continuance of certain maladjustments which derive from actual frailties. Hence, any correction of those maladjustments would be undesirable if not actually impossible. Similarly, the realities of time and situational restrictions can render comprehensive therapy impossible and hence frustrating, unacceptable, and actually intolerable to the patient.

Therefore, a proper therapeutic goal is one that aids patients to function as adequately and as constructively as possible under those

---

Quoted from the *Journal of Clinical and Experimental Hypnosis*, 1954, 2, 109-129. Copyright by The Society for Clinical and Experimental Hypnosis, 1954.

handicaps, internal and external, that constitute a part of their life situations and needs.

Consequently, the therapeutic task becomes a problem of intentionally utilizing neurotic symptomatology to meet the unique needs of each patient. Such utilization must satisfy the compelling desire for neurotic handicaps, the limitations imposed upon therapy by external forces, and, above all, provide adequately for constructive adjustments aided rather than handicapped by the continuance of neuroticisms.

Such utilization is illustrated in the following case reports by special hypnotherapeutic techniques of symptom substitution, transformation, amelioration, and the induction of corrective emotional response.

SYMPTOM SUBSTITUTION

In the two following case histories neither a willingness for adequate therapy nor a favorable reality situation existed. Hence therapy was based upon a process of *symptom substitution,* a vastly different method from *symptom removal.* There resulted a satisfaction of the patient's needs for defensive neurotic manifestations and an achievement of satisfactory adjustments, aided by continued neurotic behavior.

Patient A

A 59-year-old uneducated manual laborer, who had worked at the same job for 34 years with the expectation of a pension at the end of 35 years, fell and injured himself slightly. He reacted with a hysterical paralysis of the right arm. The company physician agreed to one week's hospitalization. Then, if the patient had not recovered from his "nonsense" at the expiration of that time, he was to be discharged as mentally ill with forfeiture of his pension.

Examination of the man disclosed his arm flexed at the elbow and held rigidly across the chest, with the hand tightly closed. During sleep the arm was relaxed, and the original diagnosis of a hysterical disability was confirmed.

No history other than the above was obtained since the patient was uncommunicative and spent his waking time groaning and complaining about severe pain.

After enlisting the aid of two other physicians, an elaborate physical examination was performed. The findings were discussed with much pessimism and foreboding about his recovery. This was done in low tones, barely but sufficiently audible to the patient. Everybody agreed that it was an "inertia syndrome," but that hypnosis would have to be performed in order to confirm that diagnosis. The prognosis was solemnly discussed and everyone agreed that, if it were the serious condition suspected, its course would be rapid and characteristic. This progression of the disease would be characterized by a relaxation of the shoulder joint, permitting arm movement within the next two days. Unfortunately, this would be accompanied by a "warm, hard feeling" in the right wrist. Then the elbow would lose its stiffness, but this would settle in the wrist. Finally, within the week's time, the fingers would relax and their stiffness would also settle in the wrist. This wrist stiffness would lead to a sense of fatigue in the wrist, but only upon use of the right arm. During rest and idleness there would be no symptomatology. Impressive medical terminology was freely employed during this discussion, but every care was taken to ensure the desired understanding of it by the patient. The patient was approached about hypnosis and readily agreed. He developed a good trance, but retained his symptoms in the trance state.

A physical reexamination was enthusiastically performed, and the same discussion was repeated, this time in a manner expressive of absolute conviction. With definite excitement, one of the physicians discovered signs of relaxation of the shoulder muscles. The others confirmed his discovery. Then "tests" applied disclosed "early changes in the first, fourth, and fifth nerves" of the elbow. All agreed, after solemn debate, that the second and third nerve changes should be slower, and that the general pattern left no doubt whatsoever about the diagnosis of "inertia syndrome," and its eventual and rapid culmination in a permanent wrist impairment. All agreed that there would be free use of the arm and that the wrist fatigue would be apparent but endurable during work. Everyone was pleased that it was a physical problem that could be surmounted and not a mental condition.

The patient's progress was exactly as described to him. Each day the physicians solemnly visited him and expressed their gratification over their diagnostic acumen.

He was discharged at the end of the week with his stiff wrist. He returned to work, completed the year, and was retired on a pension. The wrist had troubled him with its fatigability but had not interfered with his work. Upon retiring all symptomatology vanished.

However farcical the above procedure may seem in itself, it possessed the remarkable and rare virtue of being satisfying to the patient as a person and meeting his symptomatic needs adequately.

Patient B

A factory laborer, following a minor injury at work, developed a hysterical paralysis of the right arm which invalided him. A settlement had been made which would be exhausted in less than another year. At the insistence of the company physician he was sent to the writer for hypnotic therapy. The patient was antagonistic toward treatment, felt that the company was victimizing him, and stated that he would agree to only three sessions.

On taking his history it was learned that, several years previously, he had had removed by hypnotic suggestion a paralysis of the left leg. However, shortly after his "recovery," his left arm became paralyzed. Again hypnotic suggestion had effected a cure, followed shortly by a right leg paralysis. This, too, had been cured by hypnotic suggestion, and now he had a right arm paralysis.

This background suggested both the inadvisability of direct hypnosis and a need by the patient for some neurotic handicap.

Accordingly, the company physician was immediately consulted and therapeutic plans outlined. He agreed to them and promised full cooperation on the part of the company for a work placement for the patient.

A therapeutic approach was made by bringing out medical atlases and discussing endlessly and monotonously, in pseudo-erudite fashion, muscles, nerves, blood vessels, and lymphatic channels. This discussion was increasingly interspersed with trance suggestions until the patient developed a somnambulistic trance state.

The whole discussion was then repeated, and to it was added the reading from textbooks of carefully chosen sentences describing the fleeting, evanescent, and changing symptoms of multiple sclerosis and other conditions, interspersed with illustrative, fabricated case histories. The possibility of a comparable changing symptomatology for him and its possible and probable establishment in a permanent fashion was insidiously and repetitiously hinted.

The next two sessions were of a comparable character, except for the fact that numerous pseudo-tests were made of the nerves in his arms. These tests were interpreted conclusively to signify that a certain final, permanent disability would be an inevitable development. This would be the loss of the functioning of his right little finger but with full use otherwise of the whole arm.

The third session was completed by a review of the pseudo-test findings and a consultation of the medical atlases, with numerous references to textbooks. All this led to the inevitable conclusion that within another month there would be a numbness and stiffness of his little finger, which would always be slightly unpleasant but which would not interfere with his employment.

Approximately a month later the patient volunteered to relinquish half of the remaining weekly disability for a lump sum settlement and reinstatement at work. This was granted, and he applied the money to the mortgage on his home. The company physician secured a placement where a disabled right little finger did not constitute a problem.

Three years later the man was still steadily and productively employed. However, he had informed the company physician that the writer was mistaken in one regard. This was that his finger was not constantly crippled but that the condition waxed and waned from time to time, never really causing difficulty but merely making itself apparent.

Comment

Little discussion of these two case histories is necessary. Apparently both patients desperately needed a neurotic disability in order to face their life situations. No possibility existed for the correction of causative underlying maladjustments. Therefore, as therapy, there was substituted for the existing neurotic disability another, comparable in kind, non-incapacitating in character, and symptomatically satisfying to them as constructively functioning personalities. As a result both received that aid and impetus that permitted them to make a good reality adjustment.

Although more in the way of understanding the total problem could be desired, the essential fact remains that the patients' needs were met sufficiently well to afford them the achievement of a satisfying, constructive personal success.

SYMPTOM TRANSFORMATION

In the next two case histories the therapeutically restricting factors were the limitations imposed by time and situational realities. Accordingly, therapy was based upon a technique of *symptom transformation*. While seemingly similar to symptom substitution, it differs significantly in that there is a utilization of neurotic behavior by a transformation of the personality purposes served without an attack upon the symptomatology itself.

In understanding this technique it may be well to keep in mind the patter of the magician, which is not intended to inform but to distract so that his purposes may be accomplished.

Patient C

During the psychiatric examination, a selectee, otherwise normal in his adjustment, disclosed a history of persistent enuresis since the age of puberty. Though much distressed by this, he had otherwise made a good social, personal, and economic adjustment. However, because of his enuresis, he had never dared to be away from home overnight, although he had often wished to visit his grandparents and other relatives who lived at a considerable distance. Particularly did he wish to visit them because of impending military service. He was much distressed to learn that enuresis would exclude him from service, and he asked urgently if something could be done to cure him. He explained that he had taken barrels of medicine, had been cystoscoped, and numerous other procedures had been employed upon him—all to no avail.

He was told that he could probably get some effective aid if he were willing to be hypnotized. To this he agreed readily, and he developed a profound trance quickly. In this trance state he was assured most emphatically that his bed-wetting was psychological in origin and that he would have no real difficulty of any sort in overcoming it if he obeyed instructions completely.

In the form of posthypnotic suggestions he was told that, upon returning home, he was to go to the neighboring city and engage a hotel room. He was to have his meals sent up to him, and he was to remain continuously in that room until three nights had elapsed.* Upon entering the room he was to make himself comfortable, and he was to begin to think about how frightened and distressed he would be when the maid, as his mother always did, discovered a wet bed the next morning. He was to go over and over these thoughts, speculating unhappily upon his inevitable humiliated, anxious, and fearful reactions. Suddenly the idea would cross his mind about what an amazing but bitter joke it would be on him if, after all this agonized thinking, the maid were surprised by a dry bed.

This idea would make no sense to him, and he would become so confused and bewildered by it that he would be unable to straighten out his mind. Instead, the idea would run through his mind constantly, and soon he would find himself miserably, helplessly, and confusedly speculating about his shame, anxiety, and embarrassment when the maid discovered the dry bed instead of the wet bed he had planned. This thinking would so trouble him that finally, in desperation, he would become so sleepy that he would welcome going to bed, because, try as he might, he would not be able to think clearly.

Then the next morning his first reaction would be one of abject fear of remaining in the room while the maid discovered the dry bed. He would search in his mind frantically for some excuse to leave, would fail, and have to stare wretchedly out of the window so that she would not see his distress.

The next day, beginning in the afternoon, the same bewildered,

---

*The rationale of three nights was simply this: If the plan were effective, the first night would be one of doubt and uncertainty, the second would be one of certainty, and the third would bridge a transition from bed-wetting anxiety to another anxiety situation.

confused thinking would recur with the same results, and the third day would be another repetition of the same.

He was told further that, upon checking out of the hotel after the third night, he would find himself greatly torn by a conflict about visiting his grandparents. The problem of whether he should visit the maternal or the paternal set of grandparents first would be an agonizing, obsessional thought. This he would finally resolve by making the visit to the first set one day shorter than that to the second. Once arrived at his destination, he would be most comfortable and would look forward happily to visiting all of his relatives. Nevertheless, he would be obsessed with doubts about which to visit next, but always he would enjoy a stay of several days.

All of these suggestions were repetitiously reiterated in an effort to ensure the implantation of these pseudo-problems and to effect a redirection of his enuretic fears and anxieties and a transformation of them into anxieties about visits with relatives, and not anxiety about a wet bed for his closest relative, his mother.

Finally he was dismissed after approximately two hours' work with a posthypnotic suggestion for a comprehensive amnesia. Upon awakening he was told briefly that he would be recalled in about three months and that he would undoubtedly be accepted for military service then.

About 10 weeks later he was seen again by the writer as the consultant for the local draft board. He reported in detail his "amazing experience" at the hotel with no apparent conscious awareness of what had occasioned it. He explained that he "almost went crazy in that hotel trying to wet that bed, but I couldn't do it. I even drank water to be sure, but it didn't work. Then I got so scared I pulled out and started to visit all my relatives. That made me feel all right, except for being scared to death about which one to see first, and now I'm here."

He was reminded of his original complaints. With startled surprise he replied, "I haven't done that since I went crazy in the hotel. What happened?"

Reply was made simply that what had happened was that he had stopped wetting the bed and now could enjoy a dry bed.

Two weeks later he was seen again at the induction center, at which time he was readily accepted for service. His apparent only anxiety was his concern about his mother's adjustment to his military service.

Patient D

A selectee, greatly interested in entering military service, disclosed upon psychiatric examination a rather serious, closely circumscribed neurosis which embarrassed him tremendously. His difficulty lay in the fact that he was unable to urinate unless he did so by applying an 8- or 10-

inch wooden or iron pipe to the head of the penis, thus urinating through the tube.

Since, in all other regards, he seemed to be reasonably well adjusted and had a good work and social history, the conclusion was reached that the man might be amenable to brief hypnotherapy.

His history disclosed that as a small boy he had urinated through a knothole in a wooden fence bordering a golf course. He was apprehended from in front and behind and was severely punished, embarrassed, and humiliated. His reaction had been one of a repetition compulsion, which he had solved by securing a number of metal or wooden tubes. These he had carried with him constantly. He gave his story frankly and fully, though much embarrassed by it.

A deep trance was readily induced, and the history already given was confirmed. His attitude toward military service was found to be good, and he was actually willing to enter military service with his handicap, provided it occasioned him no significant embarrassment.

A long, detailed explanation in the form of posthypnotic suggestions was given to him about how this could be done. He was urged to secure a length of bamboo 12 inches long,* to mark it on the outside in quarter inches, to use that in urinating. This he was to hold with his thumb and forefinger, alternately with the right and left hand as convenient, and to flex the other three fingers around the shaft of the penis. Additionally, he was instructed to try with his thumb and forefinger to sense the passage of urine through the bamboo. No actual mention was made of feeling the passage of urine through the urethra with the other fingers. He was also told that in a day or two, or a week or two, he might consider how long the bamboo needed to be and whether or not he could saw off ¼, ½, or even 1 inch, but that he need not feel compelled to do so. Rather he should let any reduction in the length of the bamboo come about easily and comfortably, and he should be interested only in wondering on what day of the week he might reduce the length of bamboo. Also, he was told to be most certain to have the three fingers grasping the shaft of the penis so that he could notice better the flow of urine through the bamboo. As for military service, he would be rejected at the present, but arrangements would be made to have him called up in three months' time for a special psychiatric examination. At that time he would undoubtedly be accepted.

---

*A tube definitely longer than those he had been using was suggested. His acceptance of the longer tube, constituted a reality acknowledgment that the writer could do something about the tube—namely, make it longer. Equally significant is the unrecognized implication that the writer could make it shorter. Additionally, the tube was neither wood nor iron, it was bamboo. Thus, in essence, three transformation processes—longer, shorter, and material—had been initiated.

The interview was closed with two final, posthypnotic suggestions. The first was directed to a total amnesia for the entire trance experience. The other was concerned with the securing and preparation of the bamboo with no conscious understanding of the purpose.

About three months later his local draft board sent him for a special psychiatric examination to the writer, the consulting psychiatrist for that draft board. The young man was surprised and delighted. He explained that he had obeyed instructions, that he had been greatly astonished and bewildered to find himself buying the bamboo and then much embarrassed by the sudden rush of memories. At first distressed by his violation of the amnesia instructions, he soon began to develop a tremendous sense of hope and belief that he would solve his problem. He practiced urinating with the bamboo tube for about a week, then reached the conclusion that he could saw off about ½ inch, and was much puzzled when he actually sawed off a full inch. This pleased him greatly, and he wondered when he would saw off some more, and he realized suddenly that it would occur on a Thursday. (Why Thursday could not be explained.) On that occasion he sawed off 2 inches, and a few days later another inch. At the end of the month he had a ¼ inch ring of bamboo left. While using it one day, he realized that the flexion of the three fingers around the shaft of the penis gave him a natural tube. Therefore, he discarded the remains of the original bamboo and took great delight in urinating freely and comfortably. He did so with both the right and left hand and even experimented by extending the little finger; then he realized that he could urinate freely without resort to any special measure. He was then taken to the lavatory and asked to demonstrate. He immediately raised the question, "Where are you going to stand? Behind me?" Thereupon he laughed and said, "This is not a board fence. That belongs in my past history. You can stand where you want. It makes no difference to me."

A week later he was called up for induction. He was amused by his past difficulties and wondered why he had not had "enough brains" to figure out his particular problem by himself. He was assured that people usually do not know how to handle such simple things, that they have difficulty because of trying too hard.

The total duration of the therapeutic trance, somnambulistic in character, was less than an hour.

The entire procedure and its outcome demonstrate the ease and effectiveness with which symptomatology can be utilized to secure a transformation of a neurotic problem. The incapacitating wooden or metal tube was transformed into bamboo, then into the cylinder formed by the middle, third, and little finger, and then into the tube constituted by the phallus.

Comment

In both of these patients anxiety, precipitated by unhappy reactions of other people, existed in relation to a natural function. Therapy was accomplished by systematically utilizing this anxiety by a process of redirecting and transforming it. By thoroughly confusing and distracting Patient C, his anxiety about a wet bed was transformed into anxiety about a dry bed. Then his anxiety about his wet bed–home relationships was transformed into anxiety about relatives. The final transformation became that of his mother's anxiety about his military service.

For Patient D the transformation of anxiety progressed from: kind of tube; to sensing the passage of urine; to the shortening of the tube; to the question of the day for shortening the tube; and finally, into the unimportant question of where the writer would stand.

Thus, for both patients, the utilization of anxiety by a continuance and a transformation of it provided for a therapeutic resolution into a normal emotion permitting a normal adjustment, known to have continued for nine months while in service. Contact was then lost.

SYMPTOM AMELIORATION

Not infrequently in neurotic difficulties there is a surrender of the personality to an overwhelming symptom-complex formation, which may actually be out of proportion to the maladjustment problem. In such instances therapy is difficult, since the involvement of patients in their symptomatology precludes accessibility. In such cases a technique of *symptom amelioration* may be of value. In the two following cases an overwhelming, all-absorbing symptom-complex existed; therapy had to be based upon an apparently complete acceptance of the symptoms, and it was achieved by ameliorating the symptoms.

Patient E

A 17-year-old, feebleminded boy made poor adjustment when sent to a training school for delinquents. Within a month he had developed a rapidly alternating flexion and extension of the right arm in the horizontal plane at the cardiac level. When he was seen some six weeks later in the hospital, a diagnosis had been made of a hysterical reaction, probably on the basis of masturbation fears and his maladjustment in the training school. Physical examination disclosed essentially a glove anesthesia extending up to the elbow of the right arm and the rapid (135 times a minute) flexion and extension of that arm. Both the anesthesia and the muscular activity disappeared upon physiological sleep and reappeared upon awakening.

Because of his low intelligence, I.Q. 65, efforts at psychotherapy proved futile, and hypnotherapy was suggested.

Accordingly, hypnosis was employed in daily sessions for three weeks before a sustained trance could be obtained. Although he went into a trance readily, he would immediately drift into physiological sleep and would have to be awakened and a new trance induced. Finally, by the measure of hypnotizing him in the standing position and walking him back and forth, a prolonged trance could be secured. The trance state, however, had no effect upon his symptoms.

Efforts made to reduce the frequency of his arm movements failed. His only response was, "Can't stop. Can't stop." Similarly, efforts to discuss his problem or to elicit information failed. His communications were in essence, "My arm, my arm, I can't stop it."

After daily sessions for a week, during which time an intern ostentatiously made repeated counts each day of the movements per minute, a new technique was devised. This was simply a measure of suggesting that the rate would be increased from 135 to 145 per minute and that this increased rate would persist until seen again. The next day the suggestion was offered that it would decrease to the usual 135 until seen again. Again it was increased to 145 and again decreased to 135. After several such repetitions, with the count checked repeatedly by the intern and found to be approximately correct, further progress was made by suggesting alternating increments and decrements—respectively, 5 and 10 points—of the rate of the arm movement. This was continued day after day until a rate of 10 per minute was reached. Then the technique was reversed to increase the rate to 50 movements per minute. Again it was reduced to a rate of 10 per minute. Suggestion was offered that this rate would continue for a few days, then drop to 5 per minute, and then "increase" to 20 or 30 or more a day. A few days later the rate shifted from 5 per minute to scattered, isolated movements per day. The patient himself kept count of these, the daily total ranging around 25. Next the suggestion was given that this count would diminish day by day until it was around 5, and then it would "increase to as high as 25 times a week." The patient responded as suggested, and then he was asked to "guess on what day" there would be no uncontrolled movements.

Shortly he "guessed" the day when no movements would occur and demonstrated the correctness of his conjecture.

Further "guessing" on the patient's part led within a few days to his demonstration that he was free of his disability and was continuing so.

During the process of diminishing the arm movement symptom, there was noted a parallel behavior of the glove anesthesia. It waxed and waned in direct relation to the arm activity. It vanished along with that symptom.

A month later he was returned to the training school and intentionally assigned to the task of kneading bread dough by hand in the institutional bakery. A year later he was still adjusting satisfactorily.

Patient F

A mental hospital employee was referred to the writer because of sudden acute blindness which had developed on his way to work that morning. He was led into the office in a most frightened state of mind. Hesitantly and fearfully he told of having eaten his breakfast that morning, laughing and joking with his wife, and of suddenly becoming extremely disturbed by some risque story his wife related. He had angrily left the house and decided to walk to work instead of taking the bus as was his usual custom. As he rounded a certain street corner, he suddenly became blind. He had developed a wild panic, and a friend passing along the highway in a car had picked him up and brought him to the hospital. The ophthalmologist had examined him immediately and then referred him to the writer. The man was much too frightened to give an adequate story. He did state that he and his wife had been quarreling a great deal recently and that she had been drinking at home; he had found hidden bottles of liquor. She had vigorously denied drinking.

When asked what he was thinking about as he left the house, he explained that he was much absorbed in his anger at his wife, feeling that she should not be telling off-color stories, and that he had a vague feeling of apprehension, believing that he might be heading for the divorce court.

He was asked to trace his steps mentally from his home up to the point of the sudden onset of his blindness. He blocked mentally on this. He was asked to describe that particular street corner, and his reply was that, although he had walked around it many, many times, he could not remember anything about it, that his mind was a total blank.

Since the street corner involved was well known to the writer, various leading questions were asked without eliciting any material from him. He was then asked to describe exactly how the blindness had developed. He stated that there had occurred a sudden flash of intense redness, as if he were staring directly into a hot, red sun. This redness persisted and, instead of seeing darkness or blackness, he was seeing nothing but a brilliant, blinding, saturated red color. He was oppressed by a horrible feeling that, for all the rest of his life, he would never be able to see anything but an intense, glaring red. With this communication the patient became so hysterically excited that it was necessary to sedate him and put him to bed.

After the patient had been put to bed, his wife was summoned to the hospital. With much difficulty, and after many protestations of unfailing love for her husband, she finally confirmed her husband's story of her alcoholism. She refused to relate the story that had precipitated the quarrel, merely stating that it had been a risque story about a man and a redheaded girl which had really meant nothing.

She was told where her husband had developed his sudden blindness and asked what she knew about the street corner. After much hedging she recalled that there was a service station on the opposite side of the street. This she and her husband often patronized in buying gas for their car. After still further insistent questioning, she recalled a service station attendant there who had brilliant red hair. Then finally, after many reassurances, she confessed to an affair with the attendant, commonly known as "Red." On several occasions he had made unduly familiar remarks to her in her husband's presence, which had been intensely resented. After much serious thinking she declared her intention to break off the affair, if the writer would cure her husband of his blindness, and demanded professional secrecy for her confidences. Her husband's unconscious awareness was pointed out to her, and she was told that any further betrayal would rest entirely upon her own actions.

When the patient was seen the next day, he was still unable to give any additional information. Efforts were made to assure him of the temporary nature of his blindness. This reassurance he was most unwilling to accept, and he demanded arrangements to be made to send him to a school for the blind. With difficulty he was persuaded to accept therapy on a trial basis, but on the condition that nothing be done about his vision. When he finally consented, the suggestion of hypnosis was offered as an appropriate, effective therapy for his purposes. He immediately asked if he would know what happened if he were in a trance. Such knowledge, he was told, could remain only in his unconscious, if he so wished, and thus would not occasion him trouble in the waking state.

A deep trance was readily induced, but the patient refused at first to open his eyes or test his vision in any way. However, further explanation of the unconscious mind and of amnesia and posthypnotic suggestions induced him to recover his vision in the trance state. He was shown the writer's bookplate and instructed to memorize it thoroughly. This done, he was to awaken, again blind, and with no conscious knowledge of having seen the bookplate. Nevertheless, he would, upon a posthypnotic cue, describe it adequately to his own bewilderment. As soon as he understood, he was awakened and a desultory conversation was begun. This he interrupted upon the posthypnotic signal to give a full description of the bookplate. He was tremendously puzzled by this, since he knew he had never seen it. Confirmation of his description by others served to give him a great but mystified confidence in the therapeutic situation.

Upon rehypnosis he expressed complete satisfaction with what had been done and a full willingness to cooperate in every way. Asked if this meant he would confide fully in the writer, he hesitated, then determinedly declared that it did.

Special inquiry among his fellow workers on the previous day had disclosed him to have a special interest in a redhaired female employee.

By gentle degrees the question of this interest was raised. After some hesitation he finally gave a full account. Asked what his wife would think of it, he defensively asserted that she was no better than he, and he asked that the matter be kept in confidence.

Immediately, the questioning was shifted to a description of the street corner. He described it slowly and carefully but left mention of the gas station to the last. In a fragmentary fashion he described this, finally mentioning his suspicions about his wife and the redhaired attendant.

He was asked if his suspicions began at the time of his own interest in the redhaired girl, and what did he think he wanted to do about the entire situation.

Thoughtfully, he declared that, whatever had happened, they were both equally guilty, especially since neither had endeavored to establish a community of interests.

Inquiry was then made about his wishes concerning his vision. He expressed fear of recovering it immediately. He asked if the "horrible, bright redness" could be made less glaring, with now and then brief flashes of vision which would become progressively more frequent and more prolonged until finally there was a full restoration. He was assured that everything would occur as he wished, and a whole series of appropriate suggestions was given.

He was sent home on sick leave, but returned daily for hypnosis, accompanied by his wife. These interviews were limited to a reinforcement of the therapeutic suggestions of slow, progressive visual improvement. About a week later he reported that his vision was sufficiently improved to permit a return to work.

About six months later he returned to state that he and his wife had reached an amicable agreement for a divorce. She was leaving for her home state and he had no immediate plans for the future. His interest in the redhaired girl had vanished. He continued at his work uneventfully for another two years and then sought employment elsewhere.

Comment

The procedure with these two patients was essentially the same. The underlying causation was not therapeutically considered. Patient E's intellectual limitations precluded this, and Patient F had demonstrated the violence of his unwillingness to face his problem. Hence for both an amelioration of the overwhelming symptom formation was effected. By a process of alternating increments and decrements a control of E's symptom complex was effected.

For Patient F the reduction of the blinding redness, permission to remain blind and yet to have progressively more frequent and clearer flashes of vision was a parallel procedure.

As a consequence of the amelioration of their symptoms both patients were enabled to make their own personal adjustments.

CORRECTIVE EMOTIONAL RESPONSE

The following case histories concern intensely emotional problems. Therapy was achieved in one case by a deliberate correction of immediate emotional responses without rejecting them and the utilization of time to palliate and to force a correction of the problem by the intensity of the emotional reaction to its definition.

For the second patient the procedure was the deliberate development, at a near-conscious level, of an immediately stronger emotion in a situation compelling an emotional response corrective, in turn, upon the actual problem.

Patient G

An attractive social service student at the hospital entered the writer's office one evening without an appointment. She was clad in scanty shorts and a halter and she sprawled out in the armchair, declaring, "I want something." Reply was made, "Obviously so, or you would not be in a psychiatrist's office." Coquettishly she expressed doubt about wanting psychotherapy and was informed that an actual desire was necessary for therapeutic results.

After some silent thinking she declared that she needed and wanted psychotherapy, that she would state her problem, and then the writer could decide if he were willing to have her as a patient. She expressed the belief, however, that upon hearing her problem, she would probably be ejected from the office.

Thereupon she plunged into her story: "I have a prostitution complex— for the past three years—I want to go to bed with every man I see—most of them are willing—it doesn't make any difference what they are or who they are, drunk or sober, old or young, dirty or clean, any race, anything that can look like a man. I take them singly, in groups, any time, any place. I'm disgusting, filthy, horrible. But I've got to keep on doing it and I want to stop. Can you help me or should I go?"

She was asked if she could control her activities until the next session. Her reply was, "If you'll take me as a patient, I won't do anything tonight. But I will have to give you a new promise in the morning and another at night and keep that up every day until I'm over it."

She was told that she could have the next three days to test her sincerity, and for those three days she reported twice daily at the office to renew her promises. This promise renewal became a routine for her.

During a three-hour session on the fourth day, the patient devoted herself to an intense, verbal self-flagellation by recounting in full detail first one and then another of her experiences. With extreme difficulty she was induced to give such facts as her full name, birthdate, home address, etc. Only by constant interruption of her accounts was it possible to secure the following limited additional history:

Her mother was a "shallow-minded social climber, a complete snob, who is peaches and cream to those she thinks useful and a back-biting cat to everybody else. She rules my father and me by shrill shrieking. I hate her."

Her father was a "big businessman, a nice guy with plenty of money, means well, I love him, but he's nothing but a dirty, stinking grease-spot under my mother's thumb. I'd like to make a man out of him so he'd slap her down."

Both parents taught her to "hate sex, it's nasty they say, and they haven't ever to my knowledge slept in the same bedroom. I'm the only child. I hate sex, and it should be beautiful."

With that she launched into a continuance of her verbal self-flagellation for the rest of the session.

The next three-hour session was equally futile. She devoted herself, despite numerous attempts at interruption, to a bitter, morbid, repetitious account of her experiences.

At the following session, as she entered the office, she was told emphatically, "Sit down, shut up, and don't you dare to open your mouth!"

Peremptorily she was told that the writer would thenceforth take charge of all interviews, that no more time would be wasted, that the course of therapy would be dictated completely by the writer, and that she was to express her agreement by nodding her head and keeping her mouth shut. This she did.

Thereupon, with little effort, a deep, somnambulistic trance was induced, and she was told that thenceforth she would have an amnesia for trance experiences unless otherwise indicated by the writer.

Despite the trance state, however, she was found to be no more accessible than in the waking state—with one exception. She did not speak unless so instructed, but when she did talk, it was exclusively on the subject of her affairs. No more history could be obtained.

Efforts to circumvent her compulsive narration by disorientation, crystal-gazing, automatic writing, and depersonalization resulted only in more specific, detailed accounts.

At the next session, in a deep, somnambulistic trance, she was instructed emphatically:

> We both want to know why you are so promiscuous. We both want to know the cause of your behavior. *We both know that that knowledge is in your unconscious mind.*
>
> For the next two hours you will sit quietly here, thinking of nothing, doing nothing, just knowing that your unconscious is going to tell you and me the reason for your behavior.
>
> *It will tell the reason clearly, understandably, but neither you nor I will understand until the right time comes, and not until then.*
>
> You don't know how your unconscious will tell. I won't know what it tells until after you do, but I will have the reason, and at the right time, in the right way, you will know and I will know. Then you will be all right.

At the end of two hours she was told that the time had come for her unconscious to tell the reason. Before she had time to get frightened, she was handed a typewritten sheet of discarded manuscript. (See Appendix for discussion of this kind of technique.) She was then told:

> Look at this—it's a typewritten page—words, syllables, letters. Don't read it—just look at it. The reason is there—all the letters of the alphabet are there, and they spell the reason. You can't see it. In a minute I'm going to lock that sheet up in my desk with the reason unread. When the times comes, you can read it, but not until then.
>
> Now put the sheet face up on the desk, take this pencil, and in a random fashion, in a scrambled fashion, *underline those letters, syllables, words that tell the reason—quickly."*

In a puzzled manner she rapidly made nine scattered underlinings, while the writer made a numerical notation on another sheet, of the relative positions of the underlinings.

Immediately the sheet was taken from her and locked up face down in a desk drawer.

Then she was told, "Only one thing remains to be done. That is to decide the time when the reason is to be fully known. Come back and tell me tomorrow. Now wake up."

Upon awakening, she was given an appointment for the next day and dismissed. She took her departure without giving her usual promise.

The next morning she again failed to appear to give her promise. However, she kept her late-afternoon appointment, explaining, "I almost didn't come because I have only two silly words to say. I don't even know if I'll keep any more appointments with you. Well, anyway, I'll say the two words—I'll feel better—'Three weeks.'"

The reply was made, "According to the calendar, that would be four o'clock, August the 15th." She answered, "I don't know."

Thereupon, using a posthypnotic cue, a deep trance was induced. She was asked if she had anything to say. She nodded her head. Told to say it, she uttered, "Three weeks, August 15th, four o'clock."

She was awakened and asked when she wanted another appointment. Her reply was that she would like to discuss her plans for the coming year and a possible thesis she might write.

For the next three weeks she was irregularly seen for discussion of her scholastic plans and extracurricular reading. There was no discussion of her problem nor were there any more promises.

During that three weeks she attended a party where a personable young man, newly arrived at the hospital and an advisee of the writer, attempted to seduce her. She laughed at him and gave him the choice of informing the writer of his misbehavior or having her relate it, and she succeeded in so intimidating him that he confessed.

At four P.M., August 15th, she entered the office, remarking, "It's four o'clock, August the 15th. I don't know why I'm here, but I had a strong feeling that I had to come. I wanted to and I didn't want to. There is something awfully scary about coming. I wish I didn't have to."

She was answered by, "You first came to me for therapy. Apparently you drifted away. Maybe so, maybe not. Our sessions were usually three hours long. I used hypnosis. Shall I hypnotize you, or can you finish therapy in the waking state? Just remember both your conscious and your unconscious mind are present. If you want to go to sleep, you can. But at all events, sit down in that chair, be quiet, and at the end of an hour, you name a time by saying, 'I'll be ready at . . . . . . ' and give a specific time."

Uncomprehendingly she sat down and waited awake. At five o'clock she remarked, "I'll be ready at six-thirty, " and continued to wait quietly in a puzzled fashion.

At six-thirty the desk drawer was unlocked and the sheet of paper handed to her.

She turned it over and around in a puzzled fashion, scrutinized the underlinings, suddenly paled, became rigid, gave voice to an inarticulate cry, and burst into choking, shuddering sobs, gasping repeatedly, "That's what I tried to do."

Finally, in better control of herself, she said, "The reason is here—read it."

The underlined material read:

---

i wa nt to f uc K f author*

*The actual numerical order of the underlining was:

1. to
2. I
3. nt
4. wa
5. uc
6. f
7. K
8. f
9. author, with a line joining 8 and 9.

She explained, "It was any man, every man, all the men in the world. That would include father. That would make him a man, not a grease spot under my mother's thumb. Now I know what I have been trying to do, and I don't have to any more. How horrible!"

She reacted by further intense sobbing but finally declared, "That's all in the past now. What can I do?"

The suggestion was offered that she undergo a complete physical examination to check the possibility of veneral disease. To this she agreed.

She completed her next year's training successfully and was not heard from until several years later. Then it was learned from a colleague that she was most happily married and is the mother of three children. Subsequent personal inquiry confirmed the happiness of her marriage.

COMMENT

The entire management of this case was essentially that of a strong dictatorial father with a "bad" child. Her initial emotional attacks upon the writer were immediately corrected by a careful choice of words but without a nullification of her emotions.

Her contempt for her father was corrected by the acceptance of her identification of the writer as a father-surrogate and the utilization of absolute dictatorial authority over her and essentially forcibly continuing it.

The tremendously strong and compelling emotions deriving from her problem were corrected by the emotions of the waiting period, which culminated in the distressing, painful emotionality of the final session.

Patient H

A young man, normally weighing 170 pounds, married a voluptuously beautiful girl, and his friends made many ribald jests about his impending loss of weight.

About nine months later he sought psychiatric advice from the writer because of two problems. One was that he no longer could tolerate his fellow workers jesting about his weight loss of over 40 pounds. More hesitantly he added that the real problem was something else entirely. In fact, it was the failure to consummate the marriage.

He explained that his wife promised each night to permit consummation, but at his first move she would develop a severe panic and would fearfully and piteously persuade him to wait until the morrow. Each night he would sleep restlessly, feeling intensely desirous and hopelessly frustrated. Recently, he had become greatly frightened by his failure to have an erection despite his increased sexual hunger.

He asked if there could be any help for either himself or his wife. He was reassured, and appointment was made for his wife. He was asked to tell his wife the reason for the consultation and to ask her to be prepared to discuss her sexual development since puberty.

They arrived promptly for an evening appointment, and he was dismissed from the room. She told her story freely, though with much embarrassment. She explained her behavior as the result of an uncontrollable, overpowering terror which she vaguely related to moral and religious teachings. Concerning her sexual history, she exhibited a notebook in which the date and hour of onset of every menstrual period had been recorded neatly.

Examination of this amazing record disclosed that for 10 years she had menstruated every 33 days, and that the onset was almost invariably around 10 or 11 A.M. There were a few periods not on the scheduled date. None of these was early. Instead, they were occasional delayed periods, recorded by actual date and with the scheduled date marked by an explanatory note such as, "Been sick in bed with bad cold." It was noted that her next period was not due for 17 days.

When asked if she wanted help in her marital problem, she first declared that she did. Immediately, however, she became tremendously frightened; sobbingly, and with much trembling she begged the writer to let her "wait until tomorrow."

She was finally quieted by the repeated assurance that she would have to make her own decision.

As the next measure she was given a long, vague, general discourse upon marital relations, interspersed more and more frequently with suggestions of fatigue, disinterestedness, and sleepiness until a fairly good trance state had been induced.

Then, accompanied by emphatic commands to ensure continuance of the trance, a whole series of suggestions was given insistently and with increasing intensity. These were to the effect that she might, even probably would, surprise herself by losing forever her fear by suddenly, unexpectedly, keeping her promise of tomorrow sooner than she thought. Also, all the way home she would be completely absorbed with a satisfying but meaningless thought that she would make things happen too fast for even a thought of fear.

Her husband was seen separately and assured of a successful outcome for the night.

The next morning he reported ruefully that, halfway home, 17 days too early, her menstrual period began. He was relieved and comforted by the specious statement that this signified the intensity of her desire and her absolute intention to consummate the marriage. He was given another appointment for her when her period was over.

She was seen again on a Saturday evening. Again a trance was induced. This time the explanation was given her that a consummation must occur, and that the writer felt that it should occur within the next 10 days. Furthermore, she herself should decide when. She was told that it could be on that Saturday night or Sunday, *although the writer preferred Friday night;* or it could be on Monday or Tuesday night, *although Friday was the preferred night;* then again, it could be Thursday night, *but the writer definitely preferred Friday.* This listing of all the days of the week with emphasis about the writer's preference for Friday was systematically repeated until she began to show marked annoyance.

She was awakened and the same statements were made. Her facial expression was one of intense dislike at each mention of the writer's preference.

The husband was seen separately and told to make no advances, to be passive in his behavior, but to hold himself in readiness to respond, and that a successful outcome was certain.

The following Friday he reported, "She told me to tell you what happened last night. It happened so quick I never had a chance. She practically raped me. And she woke me up before midnight to do it again. Then this morning she was laughing, and when I asked her why, she told me to tell you that it wasn't Friday. I told her it was Friday and she just laughed and said you would understand that it wasn't Friday." No explanation was given to him.

The subsequent outcome was a continued, happy marital adjustment, the purchase of a home, and the birth of three wanted children at two-year intervals.

Comment

The psychosomatic response of a 17-day early menstrual period in a woman so sexually rigid is a remarkable illustration of the intensity and effectiveness with which the body can provide defenses for psychological reasons.

The rationale of the 10-day period, the naming of the days of the week, and the emphasis upon the writer's preference may be recognized easily. Ten days was a sufficiently long period in which to make her decision and this length of time was, in effect, reduced to seven days by naming them. The emphasis upon the writer's preference posed a most compelling, unpleasant, emotional problem. Since all the days of the week had been named, the passage of each day brought her closer and closer to the unacceptable day of the writer's preference. Hence, on Thursday, only that day and Friday remained. Saturday, Sunday, Monday, Tuesday, and Wednesday had all been rejected. There, consummation had to occur either on Thursday as her choice or on Friday as the writer's choice.

The procedure employed in the first interview was obviously wrong, but fortunately it was beautifully utilized by the patient to continue her neurotic behavior and to punish and to frustrate the writer for his incompetence.

The second interview was more fortunate. A dilemma she could not recognize of two alternatives was created for her—the day of her choice or of the writer's preference. The repeated emphasis upon the latter had evoked a strong, emotional response, corrective in effect upon her emotional problems. The immediate need to punish the writer and to frustrate his preference transcended her other emotional problem. The consummation effected, she could then taunt the writer with the declaration that last night was not Friday, happily secure that he would understand.

In brief, the resolution of this emotional problem, substantiated by the therapeutic results, was integral to, and contingent upon, an emotional response of corrective effect.

GENERAL COMMENTS

Essentially the purpose of psychotherapy should be the helping of the patient in that fashion most adequate, available, and acceptable. In rendering the patient aid, there should be full respect for and utilization of whatever the patient presents. Emphasis should be placed more upon what the patient does in the present and will do in the future than upon a mere understanding of why some long-past event occurred. The sine qua non of psychotherapy should be the present and the future adjustment of the patient, with only that amount of attention to the past necessary to prevent a continuance or a recurrence of past maladjustments.

Why Patient H refused to permit a consummation of the marriage is of interest only to others, not to her—she is too happy with her children, her marriage, and her home to give even a passing, backward glance at the possible causation of her behavior. To assume that that original malad-justment must necessarily come forth again in some disturbing form is essentially to assume that good learnings have neither intrinsic weight nor enduring qualities but that the only persisting forces in life are the errors.

As an analogy, whatever may be the psychogenic causation and motivation of arithmetical errors in grade school, an ignorance thereof does not necessarily preclude mathematical proficiency in college. And if mathematical ineptitude does persist, who shall say that a potential concert violinist must properly understand the basic reasons for his difficulties in the extrapolation of logarithms before entering upon a musical career?

In other words, in this writer's opinion, as illustrated by the above case histories, the purposes and procedures of psychotherapy should involve the acceptance of what the patient represents and presents. These should be utilized in such a fashion that the patient is given an impetus and a momentum, making the present and the future become absorbing, constructive, and satisfying.

As for the patient's past, it is essential that the therapist understand it as fully as possible but without demanding or compelling the patient to achieve the same degree of special erudition. It is out of the therapist's understandings of the patient's past that better and more adequate ways are derived to help the patient to live in the future. In this way the patient does not become isolated as a neurosis of long duration to be dissected bit by bit, but can be recognized as a living, sentient human being with a present and a future as well as a past.

APPENDIX

There are many variations of the technique used in the case of Patient G, and in the writer's experience they are all often useful, especially in expediting therapy. They are employed by impressing most carefully and emphatically upon a patient the idea that the unconscious mind can and will communicate highly important, even inaccessible, information central to a problem but not necessarily in an immediately recognizable form. Then, as a result of some concrete or tangible performance, the patient develops a profound feeling that the repressive barriers have been broken, that the resistances have been overcome, that the communication is actually understandable, and that its meaning can no longer be kept at a symbolic level.

Essentially, the procedure is a direct clinical utilization of projective test methodology, with the patient's performance committing him decisively to a direct, relatively immediate understanding.

1. The "random" selection from a shelf of a book or books, and thereby unwittingly designating a meaningful title.
2. The checking of dates on a calendar—in one instance a highly important, "forgotten" street address; in another, the age at which a strongly repressed traumatic experience occurred.
3. The spontaneous offer to "count the people in that cartoon" with an oversight of one of the children in it—secret doubts about the paternity of one of her own children.
4. The writing of a series of casual sentences with a misspelled word, a misplaced word, or varied spacing of words in one or more sentences.
5. The writing of a "silly" question—seeking instruction preparatory for marriage to George, she wrote, "Will I marry Harold?" who was known to her only as a casual acquaintance of a friend. She actually married a man named Harry.
6. Scrawling at random on paper, shading a line here and there, and subsequently "finding the lines that make a picture."
7. Drawing a series of related or unrelated pictures, smudging or crossing out one or more partially or completely—the people on the street, with the old lady thoroughly smudged and his recognition of his mother-hostility.
8. The writing of a deliberately false, descriptive account of some casual event—15 people at that party had untidy, straight black hair and unduly long noses.
9. Writing a list of casual words and "underlining one or more which would be or should be difficult or impossible to talk about"—the list was one of various items observed while walking down the street with the one word *flowers* repetitiously included but not underlined—his repressed fears of being a latent "pansy."
10. Tearing out an uninteresting advertisement from some magazine and bringing it to the next session—a picture of doughnuts and

his sudden realization of the extent of his loss of interest in his wife.

11. Picking up and handing over something, just anything: in one instance a pencil stub—phallic inferiority; in another, a burned match—fear of beginning impotence.

12. Glancing briefly at each page in a newspaper. When this has been done, the additional instruction of, "Give a page number quickly"—the alimony story and secret fears about the marital situation.

13. "When you get up and move your chair to the other side of that table, your unconscious mind will then release a lot of important information. Perhaps it will take your unconscious even longer than five or ten minutes to do it, or perhaps it will not be until the next session"—ten years ago giving mother one-half hour early her four-hour dose of tonic and mother's cardiac death five minutes later.

14. Writing to a dutifully loved father a letter filled with unreasonable complaints and hostility and handing it over to be read—an immediate, severe, psychogenic asthmatic attack.

15. Pediatric Hypnotherapy

Milton H. Erickson

As an introduction to what constitutes "Pediatric Hypnotherapy," the question may well be asked, What is the difference between hypnotherapy on the small-sized child, on the medium-sized child, on the large-sized child, and on that older, taller child we encounter so frequently in our offices? Therapy of any kind properly parallels the physical examination in adaptation to the patient as a reality object possessed of needs requiring recognition and definition. And any therapy used should always be in accordance with the needs of the patient, whatever they may be, and not based in any way upon arbitrary classifications.

Psychologically oriented forms of therapy properly employed need always be in relationship to the patient's capacity to receive and to understand. Pediatric hypnotherapy is no more than hypnotherapy directed to the child with full cognizance of the fact that children are small, young people. As such, they view the world and its events in a different way than does the adult, and their experiential understandings are limited and quite different from those of the adult. Therefore, not the therapy but only the manner of administering it differs.

In this connection, and of the utmost importance in the use of hypnosis, is the fact that there governs children, as growing, developing organisms, an ever-present motivation to seek for more and better understandings of all that is about them. This is one of the things that adults so often lose, and which facilitates so greatly the use of hypnosis with all patients. Children have a driving need to learn and to discover, and every stimulus constitutes, for them, a possible opportunity to respond in some new way. Since the hypnotic trance may be defined, for purposes of conceptualization, as a state of increased awareness and responsiveness to ideas, hypnosis offers to the child a new and ready area of exploration. The limited experiential background of the child, the hunger for new experiences, and the openness to new learnings render the children good hypnotic subjects. They are willing to receive ideas, they enjoy responding to them—there is only the need of presenting those ideas in a manner comprehensible to them. This, as in all other forms of psychotherapy for all types of patients, is a crucial consideration.

Reprinted with permission from *The American Journal of Clinical Hypnosis,* July, 1958, *1,* 25-29.

But such presentation needs to be in accord with the dignity of the patient's experiential background and life experience—there should be no talking down to, or over the head of, the patient. There needs to be the simple presentation of an earnest, sincere idea by one person to another for the purpose of achieving a common understanding and a common goal and purpose. The mother croons a lullaby to her nursing infant, not to give it an understanding of the words but to convey a pleasing sense of sound and rhythm in association with pleasing physical sensations for both of them and for the achievement of a common goal and purpose. The child that is cuddled properly, handled in an adequate way, placed at the breast in the right way with the proper "hypnotic touch" is not so likely to develop colic. By "hypnotic touch" is meant no more than the type of touch that serves to stimulate in the child an expectation of something pleasurable, and that is continuously stimulating to the child in a pleasing way.

It is the continuity of the experience that is of importance—it is not just a single touch or pat or caress, but a continuity of stimulation that allows the child, however short its span of attention, to give a continued response to the stimulus. So it is in hypnosis, whether with adults or children, but especially is it so with children. There is a need for a continuum of response-eliciting stimuli directed toward a common purpose.

The child at the breast needs the lullaby continued and the nipple between its lips, even after it has satisfied its hunger and is falling asleep. It needs those continuing stimuli until the physiological processes of sleep and digestion serve to replace them. Similarly in child hypnosis there is a need for a continuity of stimulation, either from without or from within, or a combination of both. Hypnosis, whether for adults or children, should derive from a willing utilization of the simple, good, and pleasing stimuli that serve in everyday life to elicit normal behavior pleasing to all concerned.

Another consideration in using hypnosis therapeutically with children is the general character of the approach to the child. No matter what the age of the child may be, there should never be any threat to the child as a functioning unit of society. Adult physical strength, intellectual strength, force of authority, and weight of prestige are all so immeasurably greater to children than their own attributes that any undue use constitutes a threat to their adequacy as individuals. And since hypnosis is dependent upon a cooperation in a common purpose, a feeling of goodness and adequacy is desirable for both participants. That sense of goodness and adequacy is not to be based upon a sense of superiority of one's own attributes, but upon a respect for the self as an individual dealing rightfully with another individual, with each contributing a full share to a joint activity of significance to both. There is a need, because of the child's lack of experiential background and understanding, to work primarily with, and not on, the child. The adult can better comprehend passive participation.

Nor can there be a linguistic condescension to the child. Comprehension of language always precedes verbal facility. There should not be a talking down to the child, but rather a utilization of language, concepts, ideas, and word pictures meaningful to children in terms of their own learnings. To speak in "baby talk" is usually an insult and a mockery, since any intelligent child knows that the adult possesses vocal facility. One does not imitate the accent of an adult, but one can use a word or phrase respectfully abstracted from the speech of the other. Thus one can speak of "dem bums", but cannot rightfully say "Toity-foist Street." So it is with infantile and childish vocalization.

Similarly, respect must be given to the child's ideational comprehension with no effort to derogate or minimize the child's capacity to understand. It is better to expect too great a comprehension than to offend by implying a deficiency. For example, the surgeon who told four-year old Kristi, "Now that didn't hurt at all, did it?" was told with bitter, scornful contempt, "You're poopid! It did, too, hurt, but *I* didn't mind it." She wanted understanding and recognition, not a falsification, however well-intended, of a reality comprehensible to her. For one to tell a child, "Now this won't hurt one bit" is courting disaster. Children have their own ideas and need to have them respected, but they are readily open to any modification of those ideas intelligently presented to them. Thus, to tell the child, "Now this *could* hurt a lot, but I think that maybe you can stop a lot of the hurt, or maybe all of it," constitutes an intelligent appraisal of reality for the child and offers an acceptable idea of a reasonable and possible responsive participation of an inviting character.

Children must be respected as thinking, feeling creatures, possessed of the capacity to formulate ideas and understandings and able to integrate them into their own total of experiential comprehension, but they must do this in accord with the actual functioning processes they themselves possess. No adult can do this for them, and any approach to the child must be made with awareness of this fact.

To illustrate how one approaches a child and utilizes hypnotic techniques, the following personal example may be cited:

Three-year-old Robert fell down the back stairs, split his lip, and knocked an upper tooth back into the maxilla. He was bleeding profusely and screaming loudly with both pain and fright. His mother and I went to his aid. A single glance at him lying on the ground, screaming, his mouth bleeding profusely and blood spattered on the pavement, confirmed the existence of an emergency requiring prompt and adequate measures.

No effort was made to pick him up. Instead, as he paused for breath for fresh screaming, he was told quickly, simply, sympathetically, and emphatically, "That hurts awful, Robert. That hurts terrible."

Right then, without any doubt in his mind, my son knew that I knew what I was talking about. He could agree with me and he knew that I was agreeing completely with him. Therefore he could listen respectfully to me, because I had demonstrated that I understood the situation fully. *In pediatric hypnotherapy there is no more important problem than so speaking to the patient that he can agree with you and respect your intelligent grasp of the situation as judged by him in terms of his own understandings.*

Then I told Robert, "And it will keep right on hurting."

In this simple statement I named his own fear, confirmed his own judgment of the situation, and demonstrated my good intelligent grasp of the entire matter and my entire agreement with him, since right then he could foresee only a lifetime of anguish and pain for himself.

The next step for him and for me was to declare, as he took another breath, "And you really wish it would stop hurting." Again, we were in full agreement, and he was ratified and even encouraged in this wish, and it was his wish, deriving entirely from within him and constituting his own urgent need.

With the situation so defined, I could then offer a suggestion with some certainty of its acceptance. This suggestion was, "Maybe it will stop hurting in a little while, in just a minute or two."

This was a suggestion in full accord with his own needs and wishes, and because it was qualified by a "maybe it will," it was not in contradiction to his own understandings of the situation. Thus he could accept the idea and initiate his responses to it.

As he did this, a shift was made to another important matter, important to him as a suffering person, and important in the total psychological significance of the entire occurrence—a shift that in itself was important as a primary measure in changing and altering the situation.

Too often, in hypnotherapy or any utilization of hypnosis, there is a tendency to overemphasize the obvious and to reaffirm unnecessarily already accepted suggestions, instead of creating an expectancy situation, permitting the development of desired responses. Every pugilist knows the disadvantage of overtraining; every salesman knows the folly of overselling. The same human hazards exist in the application of hypnotic techniques.

The next procedure with Robert was a recognition of the meaning of the injury to Robert himself—pain, loss of blood, body damage, a loss of the wholeness of his normal narcissistic self-esteem, of his sense of physical goodness so vital in human living.

Robert knew that he hurt, that he was a damaged person; he could see his blood upon the pavement, taste it in his mouth, and see it on his hands. And yet, like all other human beings, he, too, could desire narcissistic distinction in his misfortune, along with the desire even more for narcissistic comfort. Nobody wants a picayune headache, but since a headache must be endured, let it be so colossal that only the sufferer could endure it. Human pride is so curiously good and comforting! Therefore, Robert's attention was doubly directed to two vital issues of comprehensible importance to him by the simple statements, "That's an awful lot of blood on the pavement. Is it good, red, strong blood? Look carefully, Mother, and see. I think it is, but I want you to be sure."

Thus, there was an open and unafraid recognition in another way of values important to Robert. He needed to know that his misfortune was catastrophic in the eyes of others as well as his own, and he needed tangible proof thereof that he himself could appreciate. Therefore, by declaring it to be "an awful lot of blood," Robert could again recognize the intelligent and competent appraisal of this situation in accord with his own actually unformualted, but nevertheless real, needs.

Then the question about the goodness, redness, and strongness of the blood came into play psychologically in meeting the personality meaningfulness of the accident to Robert. Certainly, in a situation where one feels seriously damaged, there is an overwhelming need for a compensatory feeling of satisfying goodness. Accordingly, his mother and I examined the blood on the pavement, and we both expressed the opinion that it was good, red, strong blood, thereby reassuring him not on an emotionally comforting basis only, but upon the basis of an instructional, to him, examination of reality.

However, we qualified that favorable opinion by stating that it would be better if we were to examine the blood by looking at it against the white background of the bathroom sink. By this time Robert had ceased crying, and his pain and fright were no longer dominant factors. Instead, he was interested and absorbed in the important problem of the quality of his blood.

His mother picked him up and carried him to the bathroom, where water was poured over his face to see if the blood "mixed properly with water" and gave it a "proper pink color." Then the redness was carefully checked and reconfirmed, following which the "pinkness" was reconfirmed by washing him adequately, to Robert's intense satisfaction, since his blood was good, red, and strong and made water rightly pink.

Then came the question of whether or not his mouth was "bleeding right" and "swelling right." Close inspection, to Robert's complete satisfaction and relief, again disclosed that all developments were good and right and indicative of his essential and pleasing soundness in every way.

Next came the question of suturing his lip. Since this could easily evoke a negative response, it was broached in a negative fashion to him, thereby precluding an initial negation by him and at the same time raising a new and important issue. This was done by stating regretfully that, while he would have to have stitches taken in his lip, it was most doubtful if he could have as many stitches as he could count. In fact, it looked as if he could not even have 10 stitches, and he could count to 20. Regret was expressed that he could not have 17 stitches, like Betty Alice, or 12, like Allan, but comfort was offered in the statement that he would have more stitches than Bert, or Lance, or Carol, his siblings. Thus the entire situation became transformed into one in which he could share with his older siblings a common experience with a comforting sense of equality and even superiority.

In this way he was enabled to face the question of surgery without fear or anxiety, but with hope of high accomplishment in cooperation with the surgeon and imbued with the desire to do well the task assigned him— namely, to "be sure to count the stitches." In this manner no reassurances were needed, nor was there any need to offer further suggestions regarding freedom from pain.

Only seven stitches were required, to Robert's disappointment, but the surgeon pointed out that the suture material was of a newer and better kind than any that his siblings had ever had, and that the scar would be an unusual "W" shape, like the the letter of his Daddy's college. Thus the fewness of the stitches was well compensated.

The question may well be asked at what point hypnosis was employed. Actually, hypnosis began with the first statement to him and became apparent when he gave his full and undivided interested and pleased attention to each of the succeeding events that constituted the medical handling of his problem.

At no time was he given a false statement, nor was he forcibly reassured in a manner contradictory to his understandings. A community of understandings was first established with him, and then, one by one, items of vital interest to him in his situation were thoughtfully considered and decided, either to his satisfaction or sufficiently agreeably to merit his acceptance. His role in the entire situation was that of an interested participant, and adequate response was made to each idea suggested.

Another example that may be briefly cited is that of the belligerent two-year-old in her crib, who wished no dealings with anybody and was prepared to fight it out on that line for the rest of her life. She had a favorite toy, a rabbit. As she was approached and her jutting jaw and aggressive manner was noted, the challenge was offered, "I don't think your rabbit knows how to sleep."

"Wabbit tan too," and the battle was on.

"I don't think your rabbit can lie down with its head on the pillow, if you show it how."

"Wabbit tan too! See!"

"And put its legs and arms down nice and straight like yours?"

"Tan too! See!"

"And close its eyes and take a deep breath and go to sleep and stay asleep?"

"Wabbit sweep!" a declaration made with pleased finality, and Kristi and her rabbit continued to sleep in a satisfactory trance state.

The entire technique, in this instance, was nothing more than that of meeting the child at her own level and as an individual, presenting ideas to which she could actively respond and thus participate in achieving a common goal acceptable to her and to her adult collaborator.

This type of technique has been employed many times for the single reason that the primary task in pediatric hypnosis is the meeting of the child's needs of the moment. Those are what the child can comprehend, and once that need has been satisfied, there is the opportunity for the therapist to discharge in turn his own obligations.

To conclude, these two case reports have been presented in considerable detail to illustrate the case of the naturalistic hypnotic approach to children. There is seldom, if ever, a need for a formalized or ritualistic technique. The eidetic imagery of children, readiness, eagerness and actual need for new learnings, their desire to understand and to share in the activities of the world about them, and the opportunities offered by "pretend" and imitation games all serve to enable children to accept and to respond competently and well to hypnotic suggestions.

In brief, a good hypnotic technique is one that offers to the patients, whether child or adult, the opportunity to have their needs of the moment met adequately, the opportunity to respond to stimuli and to ideas, and also the opportunity to experience the satisfactions of new learnings and achievements.

The following two articles are suggested for additional reading:

Solovey de Melechnin, Galina. Concerning some points about the nature of hynposis, *J. Clin. and Exper. Hyp.,* IV, 2, April 1956, pp. 83-88.

————.Conduct problems in children and hypnosis, *Diseases of the Nerv. Syst.,* XVI, 8, August 1955, pp. 3-7.

16. The Utilization of Patient Behavior in the Hypnotherapy of Obesity: Three Case Reports

Milton H. Erickson

Requisite to effective hypnotherapy—and the same holds true for experimental hypnosis—is the adequate communication of ideas and understandings to the hypnotized person. Since the object of hypnotherapy is not the intellectual clarification of understandings but the attainment by the patient of personal goals, this cannot be achieved by a simple reliance upon the inherent values of the ideas and understandings to be presented. Rather, communications need to be presented in terms of the patient's personal and subjective needs, learnings, and experiences, whether reasonable or unreasonable, recognized or unrecognized, so that there can be an acceptance and a response and a feeling of personal fulfillment.

To illustrate this need to center the therapeutic use of hypnosis about the individual personality needs and attitudes of the patient, three instances of obesity previously unsuccessfully treated by other procedures will be cited.

CASE 1

A physician's wife in her late forties entered the office and explained that she wished a single interview during which hypnosis was to be employed to correct her obesity. She added that her normal weight was 120 pounds, but that her present weight was 240, and that for many years she had weighed over 200 pounds despite repeated futile attempts to reduce under medical supervision. She stated that in recent years she had been slowly gaining to her present weight, and that she was distressed about her future because, "I enjoy eating—I could spend all the time in the world just eating." Additional history was secured, but the only thing of particular note was her somewhat anxious, unnecessarily repeated

Reprinted with permission from *The American Journal of Clinical Hypnosis*, 1960, 3, 112–116.

assertions that she enjoyed eating and liked to while away time by eating for purely gustatory pleasure.

Since she was insistent upon a single interview and hypnosis, an effort was made to meet her wishes. She was found to be an unusually responsive subject, developing a profound trance almost immediately. In this trance state an understanding of time distortion as a subjective experience, particularly time expansion, was systematically taught to her. She was then instructed to have her physician husband prescribe the proper diet for her and to supervise her weight loss. She was henceforth to eat each meal in a state of time distortion, with time so expanded and lengthened that, as she finished each portion of food, her sense of taste and feeling of hunger for that item would both be completely satiated, as if she had been eating for "hours on end with complete satisfaction." All of this instruction was given repetitiously until it seemed certain she understood fully, whereupon she was aroused and dismissed.

The patient, together with her husband, was seen nine months later. Her weight had been 120 lbs. for the past month, and her husband declared that her weight loss had occurred easily and without any medical complication. Both she and her husband spoke at length about their improved personal, social, and recreational activities, and she commented that, even though she ate much less, her eating pleasures had been intensified, that her sense of taste and smell were more discerning, and that a simple sandwich could be experienced with as much subjective pleasure as a two-hour dinner.

CASE 2

A patient weighing 180 pounds explained half-laughingly, half-sobbingly, that her normal weight was about 125 pounds, but that for over 15 years she had weighed 170 or more "most of the time."

During these years she had been under medical supervision many times for weight reduction. She had always cooperated with the physician, adhering to the recommended diets, obeying every instruction, always losing at least the prescribed poundage each week, usually more. Each time she reduced, she established a goal-weight which varied from 120 to 130 lbs. As she approached this predetermined weight, she invariably experienced much disturbing behavior of an obsessive-compulsive character.

When within 5 or 10 pounds of her goal, she would weigh herself repetitiously throughout the day, and the nearer she came, the more frequent became the weighings with increasing anxiety. When the scales showed exactly the chosen weight, and not until then, she would rush precipitously to the kitchen and "gorge frantically," usually regaining at least 10 pounds the first week. Thereupon the reduction program would cease, and there would occur a progressive, systematic restoration of the lost weight accompanied by a feeling of despair mingled with a profound determination to engage upon another weight-reduction program soon after she had completed regaining her lost weight. She had, in the past, reduced to the goal weight as many as three times within a year, but always under the direction of a different physician.

She now sought reduction to 125 pounds, stating frankly and with some amusement, "I suppose I'll do exactly the same with you, even though you are a psychiatrist, as I do with every other doctor. I'll cooperate and I'll lose and then I'll gain it back and then I'll go to someone else and repeat the same old silly behavior." Here she burst briefly into tears. Recovering her poise she continued, "Maybe if you use hypnosis that will help, but I don't think it will even if you do hypnotize me. I'll just do the same darned thing again and again, and I'm so tired of reducing and gaining. It's just a horrible obsession with me. But I don't want any psychiatry used on me."

Further explanation on the patient's part served only to emphasize more clearly what she had already related.

In accord with her wishes hypnosis was attempted, and by the end of the hour a medium trance characterized by a considerable tendency toward spontaneous posttrance amnesia was induced. She was given a second appointment, at which time her history was taken a second time. The details were essentially the same, and she reiterated her firm belief that she would again follow her pattern of losing and gaining weight, and again she sobbed briefly. She also reaffirmed her unwillingness to accept psychiatric help and restricted emphatically any help given her to the problem of her weight. She also declared her intention of terminating her treatment if any attempt were made to deal with her psychiatrically. Repetitiously she promised her full cooperation in all other regards.

A medium trance state was readily induced, and she was asked to reiterate her promise of full cooperation. She was also induced to restate repetitiously that in the past her problems had centered around "gaining, losing, gaining, losing, gaining, gaining, gaining, losing, losing, losing," and to agree that throughout the proposed course of treatment she would keep this sequence of behavior constantly in mind.

As soon as it was felt that she had accepted these peculiarly but carefully worded statements, the assertion was offered that her treatment this time, "will be the same, yet completely different, *all of your behavior will be used,* your cooperation has been promised and will be given, and all of your behavior that you have shown so many times in the past will be used, but this time used to make you happy, used in a different way."

When it was certain that the patient knew what had been said to her, even though she did not understand what was meant or implied, she was reminded of the firmness of her resolve to cooperate completely, even as she had in the past, but this time, she was told, "things" would be "done differently" and therefore successfully and to her entire happiness and satisfaction.

Thereupon, while she was still in a medium trance, it was explained that always in the past she had approached her problem of obesity by setting a goal weight, by losing and gaining weight, by a performance of obsessional weighing, and then setting a second goal of her original overweight. These same items of behavior, it was emphasized, would again be employed but in another fashion and effectively for the medical purposes desired.

The explanation was continued to the effect that instead of letting her terminate her reducing by a process of gaining, the procedure would be reversed. Therefore, she was under obligation, as a part of her cooperation, to proceed at once, and at a reasonable rate, to gain between 15 and 25 pounds. When this gain had been made, she could then begin reducing.

The patient protested vehemently that she did not want to gain but to lose weight, but it was patiently and insistently pointed out that her reducing programs had always included obsessive weighing, losing weight, gaining weight, the setting of goal weights, and full cooperation with the physicians. No more and no less was now asked. Finally the patient agreed to abide by the instructions. She was then aroused, and the instructions were explained again. She protested vigorously but slightly less so than in the trance state, and finally she reluctantly agreed to the proposed program.

Most unwillingly she began to increase her weight. When she had gained 10 pounds she pleaded to be allowed to begin reducing. She was reminded that an increase of 15 to 25 pounds had been prescribed, and this would be insisted upon. As she approached the gain of 15 pounds, she began weighing herself in a repetitive, obsessive manner and demanded an appointment immediately when the scales showed the 15-pound increase. At that appointment it was carefully explained to her in both the trance and the waking states that the prescribed gain had been for a weight *between* 15 and 25 pounds.

Less than a week later, after much obsessive weighing and eating, which was done with great reluctance, she reported for an interview and hesitantly stated that she had gained 20 pounds, and that this figure was exactly between 15 and 25. She pleaded to be allowed to reduce. Consent was given with the admonition that the *loss of weight must not exceed the average of three pounds a week.*

The patient's progress was most satisfactory. She showed none of her previous obsessive weighing as she approached the weight of 125. She had almost at once calculated the date of her goal weight when she had first begun to reduce, but she had been admonished that weight reduction was on a weekly average. Hence, she could only set the week but not the day of achieving the goal weight.

She was seen only at intervals of three to six weeks. She was always adequately praised for her cooperation in both the trance and waking states, and each time the hope was expressed that no intervening problem would develop to alter the expected week of final achievement.

She forgot her appointment for the final week, but made one for the next week. At that time she weighed 123 pounds instead of 125. She explained that she had failed to weigh herself regularly and hence did not know exactly when she had reached 125 pounds. She declared her intention to remain approximately that weight.

In the nine months that have passed since then the patient has succeeded comfortably in this resolve. In addition she has developed recreational and vocational interests, particularly golf and a book review club, and she has for the first time in her life participated in social and community affairs.

CASE 3

A physician's wife in her middle thirties sought aid for her obesity in an amused, half-hearted manner. This had begun in her junior year in high school, at which time she weighed 110 pounds, and each succeeding year of life had been marked by a progressive increase to the current weight of 270 pounds.

During the past 13 years she had sought help from one physician after another, but each time failed to secure results. Her explanation was, "Oh, I always cooperate with the diet they put me on. I always eat that and everything else I can lay my hands on. I always overeat, and I suppose I always will. As a forlorn hope, I'm trying you to see if hypnosis will work. I know it won't, but my husband will feel better if I do try it. But I warn you not to expect too much because if I know me, and I think I do, I'll overeat as usual."

Hypnosis was attempted. She developed a medium to deep trance readily, but it was difficult to maintain that depth of trance. She would repeatedly arouse, laugh, and explain that she was curious why the writer would be willing to waste his time on her in view of her "unfavorable prognosis" of her own behavior. The explanation was offered to her that neither time nor effort would be wasted since it was intended to utilize her own behavior to effect therapeutic results. Her reply was, "But how can there be therapeutic results when you and I both know that I'll eat any diet you recommend and everything else even if I have to make extra shopping trips? I've had too many years of overeating to give it up, and

I'm here only because my husband wants me to come. I've always tried to cooperate, but it's no use. I know the exact caloric value of any serving of food, but all my knowledge does not keep me from overeating. Even my teenage daughter's embarrassment about my obesity doesn't keep me from overeating. But I'll play along with you, at least for a while, but nothing will work."

Again she was assured that her own behavior would be employed to produce effective results, and she was asked to redevelop a trance state so that hypnosis could be employed. She declared that she would only awaken herself from the trance state if this were done. Even as she completed her statement, she developed a medium to deep trance but almost immediately aroused herself by laughing.

She was then asked to develop and to maintain a light trance and to listen carefully to what was said to her, to understand completely what was said, to go into a deeper trance whenever she wished, or to lighten her trance if she felt so impelled, but at all events to listen to the entire explanation about to be offered her without interrupting it by arousing from the trance. She agreed to cooperate on this basis.

Slowly, systematically, she was instructed:

1. Your weight is 270 lbs.
2. You know the caloric values of any food serving.
3. You always have and always will overeat.
4. Your own behavior has always defeated you in the past.
5. Your own behavior will be used this time to effect therapeutic results. This you do not understand.
6. You will cooperate as you always do, and you will also overeat. (The patient first shook her head vigorously at this, then sighed and slowly nodded her head affirmatively.)

When it was felt that she understood these instructions adequately, she was given the further instructions:

1. You now weigh 270 pounds, not 150 or 140, but 270 pounds. You not only will overeat but you need to eat excessively in order to support that poundage.
2. Now bear this in mind and cooperate fully: During this week overeat, *doing so carefully and willingly,* and overeat enough to support 260 pounds. That is all you need to do, overeat sufficiently to support 260 pounds. Now I am going to arouse you and dismiss you with no further discussion or even comments. You are to return at this same hour one week from today.

She was seen again a week later. Her opening remark was, "Well, for the first time in my life I enjoyed overeating, and I checked on my husband's office scales today, because I don't trust our bathroom scales. I weighed 260 pounds too, a few ounces less in fact, but I call it 260 pounds."

A trance was induced again, light in character, and she was again similarly instructed, but this time to overeat sufficiently to support 255 pounds and to report in another week's time. On that occasion a new goal was established at 250 pounds.

On the next visit she hesitantly explained that she and her husband were going on their annual two weeks' visit at her parental home, and that "I always gain on my mother's cooking, and I hesitate to go this year, but I see no way out of it."

In the trance state she was asked what weight she ought to overeat sufficiently to support on this two-week holiday. She answered, "Well, we'll really be gone 16 days, so I think I ought to eat enough to weigh a good fat 238."

She was emphatically told that she was *to overeat sufficiently to support 238 pounds and also sufficiently to gain 3, 4, or even 5 pounds.*

She returned from the trip jubilant, weighing 242 pounds, and stated happily, "I did just as you said. I gained four pounds. This is a silly game we are playing, but I don't care. It works. I like to overeat and I'm so grateful that I don't overeat as much as I used to."

A variation was introduced into the procedure by insisting that she maintain her weight unchanged on two occasions for a two-week period. Both times she reacted with impatience, declaring "That's too long a time to overeat that much."

In six months' time she has reached the weight of 190 lbs., is enthusiastic about continuing, and is in the process of window-shopping for "something that will look good on a chubby 130 or 140."

SUMMARY

The medical problem for each of these patients was the same, a matter of weight reduction, and each had failed in numerous previous attempts. By employing hypnosis a communication of special ideas and understandings ordinarily not possible of presentation was achieved in relation to personality needs and subjective attitudes toward weight reduction. Each was enabled to undertake the problem of weight loss in accord with long-established patterns of behavior but utilized in a new fashion. Thus, one patient's pleasure in eating was intensified at the expense of quantity, a change of sequence of behavioral reactions led to success for the second, and a certain willfulness of desire to defeat the self was employed to frustrate the self doubly and thus to achieve the desired goal.

17. Hypnosis and Examination Panics

Milton H. Erickson

Over a period of years I have been consulted by many physicians, lawyers, Ph.D. candidates, college students, and high school students who were concerned about the "examination jitters." The vast majority were those who panicked either during the examination or immediately before it, and either failed miserably or made regrettably poor grades. Among the physicians and lawyers have been some persons who have failed the state board or bar examination as many as five times in succession and some who have failed the national specialty certification examinations twice. One particular physician had, following high school days, invariably failed every final examination, but because of his otherwise remarkably excellent record, he had always been given special extra examinations. He always passed these extra examinations with high grades, but only with extreme effort and extended time limits.

The procedure employed with these various applicants for help was essentially constant in character. First a trance was induced that might range in depth from light to somnambulistic. The subjects were then told, in essence:

> You wish to have help in passing your examination. You have sought hypnosis and you have developed the trance state that I know to be sufficient to meet your needs. You will continue in that trance state until I tell you otherwise.
>
> Now, here is the help you wish. Listen carefully and understandingly. You may not want to agree with me, but you must remember that your own ideas have led only to failures. Hence, though what I say may not seem exactly right, abide by it fully. In so doing you will achieve your goal of passing the examination. That is your goal and you are to achieve it, and I shall give you the instructions by which to do it. I cannot give you the information that you have acquired in past study, and I want you to have it available for the examination in the way I specify.
>
> First of all you are to pass this examination, not trying in the

Reprinted with permission from *The American Journal of Clinical Hypnosis,* 1965, 7, 356–358.

unsuccessful ways you have in the past but in the way I shall now define. You want to pass this examination. I want you to pass it. But listen closely: *You are to pass it with the lowest passing grade— not an A or a B. I know you would like a high grade, but you need a passing grade—that's all, and that is what you are to get. To this you must agree absolutely, and you do, do you not?* [An affirmation was always given.]

Next, after leaving this office I want you to feel carefree, at ease, even forgetful of the fact that you are to write an examination. But no matter how forgetful of that fact you become, you will remember to appear on time at the place of examination. At first you may not even remember why you are there, but it will dawn on your mind in time, and comfortably so.

Upon taking your place, you are to read through all the questions. Not one of them will make sense, but read them all. [The purpose of this was to give the subject an unwitting appraisal of the number of questions and the amount of time each would require.]

Then get ready to write, and read the first question again. It will seem to make a little sense and a little information will trickle into your conscious mind. By the time you have written it down, there will be another trickle keeping you writing until suddenly the trickle dries up. Then move on to the next question, and the same thing will happen. When the time is up, you will have answered all of the questions comfortably, easily, just recording the trickle of information that develops for each question.

When finished, turn in your examination paper and leave feeling comfortable, at ease, at peace with yourself.

THE RESULTS

The results have been uniformly good. This was true even for a law student who telephoned long distance to explain that he had repeatedly failed his bar examination, that he was to be reexamined the next day, that he had been hypnotized previously with no satisfactory results, that he had just been referred to the author, and that he wanted immediate last-minute help.

Subsequently he telephoned to report that he had been disappointed in the trance induced over the telephone, that nevertheless he had slept well that night, had reported in a carefree mood for the examination, had written it with no subsequent memory of what the questions were, and had remained mentally comfortable until he was notified several weeks later that he had passed the examination. He then developed a feeling of almost painful urgency to telephone the news to the author. As he offered this information over the telephone, he lost his feeling of urgency and was again mentally at peace.

The above account, with minor variations, is not at all unusual. However, of particular significance has been the effect of insisting upon a low grade, literally the "lowest passing grade." A considerable number of these students have insistently queried the author for his reasons, pointing out that instead of low passing grades, they had received the highest possible grade they felt they were capable of earning. Indeed, A's were common, B's less so, and C's only occasional. There was no instance of a grade of D being received even though, for some of the students, their daily class work was sufficiently good that a final examination grade of D would have led to a passing grade of C. The plausible explanation offered to them has been:

> When you strive for an A, you become tense, overeager, uncertain, and doubtful, and hence you cannot function at your best. When you, obedient to the instructions I gave you, were writing to secure only a C or a D, you were comfortably confident and certain that you could do this with ease. Therefore, you wrote in a state of mental ease and confidence, free of doubt and uncertainty, and you weren't concerned about holding yourself down to a D performance or struggling with doubtful hope for an A. Hence, you were in that mental and emotional frame of thought and feeling that would ensure your optimum performance.

Long experience in psychotherapy has disclosed the wisdom of avoiding perfectionistic drives and wishes on the part of patients and of motivating them for the comfortable achievement of lesser goals. This then ensures not only the lesser goal but makes more possible the easy output of effort that can lead to a greater goal. Of even more importance is that the greater accomplishment then becomes more satisfyingly the patient's own rather than a matter of obedience to the therapist.

This method of handling examination panics has been employed with nearly 100 persons. Physicians, lawyers, candidates for a doctoral degree in medicine, psychology, religion, and education have predominated. The next larger group consisted of college seniors majoring in various fields, but especially in psychology. College juniors and sophomores were fewer in number than were college freshmen, and high school juniors and seniors made up the rest of the students so treated, except for a considerable number of job applicants undergoing a written examination for a promotion. Only one dentist has been handled in this regard.

There have been a few failures, all of whom returned to explain that they, not the author, were at fault, that they had found themselves mistrusting the help offered, and did not use it, with a consequent failure. Now they desired another "treatment" so that henceforth there would be no failures. This was done only upon their agreement to report future results, which they did with pleasure. All of these first-time failures occurred with subjects who developed only light trances and who could not seem to learn deep trances. The deeper the trance, the better pleased was the examinee with the examination results.

It must be recognized, however, that all of these applicants for assistance were highly motivated, which undoubtedly contributed to the success. Also, in the author's opinion some really did not need help.

Subsequently, the physicians and the lawyers in particular sent their wives to the author for training in hypnosis for childbirth.

18. Experiential Knowledge of Hypnotic Phenomena Employed for Hypnotherapy

Milton H. Erickson

INTRODUCTION

In the use of hypnosis for the therapeutic handling of psychogenic problems, there is often too ready a dependence upon hypnosis itself and the immediate use of some well-known structured form of hypnotic approach. For example, the author has seen many instances where hypnotherapy was attempted by a routine use of regression by various therapists with disappointing results, and sometimes with an antagonizing of the patient toward hypnosis. Although hypnotic regression, dissociation, abreaction, and revivification may be useful in general, each patient's problem needs individual scrutiny and the structuring of the therapeutic approach to meet the individuality of the problem.

To illustrate this need, the following account is given in detail to portray the character of a problem that had to be met, the purposes that had to be served, the procedures that had to be considered and utilized in therapy, and the methods that had to be employed in devising a successful therapeutic handling of the problem.

The question of therapeutic procedure will be discussed first to present certain vital aspects of the therapeutic situation as a background for a general understanding of the total problem.

One of the considerations was that therapy would have to be successful on the first completed effort. If there were a failure, there could be no opportunity for any second effort by a revision of therapeutic measures or any measure of "second guessing." One and only one opportunity existed for a successful outcome. Both the patient and the author were aware of this fact, a matter so much in evidence that no mention of it was needed.

The problem was one of long duration and it had many times been confirmed and accepted by respected authoritative persons. Additionally, the patient had been aided and abetted in circumventing his problem most successfully many times. He was now confronted inescapably with the

Reprinted with permission from *The American Journal of Clinical Hypnosis*, April, 1966, 8, 299–309.

need to confront his problem in a situation vital to his whole future with no possibility of any circumvention as had always been done successfully in the past.

He approached the author with a request for help by means of hypnosis but with no adequate understanding that hypnosis could help him only by making more available to him his own potentials for self-help. Nor was he in any frame of mind to be given such understanding. He "knew" beyond all doubt that he was helpless, and he simply surrendered himself to the author with complete dependence upon what the author could do. Hence. any therapeutic procedure would have to be patterned to permit an inclusion of this mistaken understanding by the patient but doing so without invalidating therapy.

The idea of circumvention had become a fixed idea, it was always by the same method, and it had always proved to be the "right and only" method. Now he was barred from circumvention, *hence he had to depend entirely upon the author.*

Since this was the patient's fixed belief, hypnotherapy would have to include circumvention which would not be so recognized by him at the time, since in his own mind he was rigidly convinced that circumvention was impossible. Therefore the structuring of the therapeutic procedure would have to be around something in which the patient fully believed but also fully believed to be impossible of utilization.

The patient himself unwittingly gave the author a rather full statement of how this circumvention could be achieved but which the author did not recognize at the time. Nor did the author recognize, at least consciously and probably not unconsciously, the meaningfulness of the patient's informative statement until after structuring and restructuring the complete plan, and to the author's chagrin he realized he had not listened sufficiently carefully to the patient's own significant statement so vital to the final plan of therapeutic procedure.

Finally, in developing any therapeutic plan that must succeed upon the first effort, the author realized that he would have to do much speculative work and would have to follow the trail of many of his own thoughts on the matter that would turn out to be useless. In this presentation the useless work done will not be reported. The fruitful work only will be reported—and in brief form since the kind, not the extent of the work, is all that is important.

THE PROBLEM

A patient, a professional man seeking certification in a medical specialty, sought the author's aid. His story was that since high school days oral examinations had been nightmarish ordeals. Invariably he developed a multitude of psychosomatic symptoms ranging from mild to severely disabling. He had always been an excellent student, and none of his teachers and instructors, upon seeing the state of his physical collapse when attempting to meet the needs of an oral examination, had ever doubted the genuineness of his reactions.

With a feeling of shame and humiliation when confronted with the possibility of an oral examination, he usually secured a physician's statement affirming his inability to comply and recommending, as a medical necessity, that he be given a written examination. Such medical statements usually stated that there would be no objection to making the written examination much more rigorous and searching than the oral examination would ordinarily be. Invariably he received an excellent grade, since he was a most brilliant and dedicated student.

This special disability had haunted him throughout high school, college and medical school. On several occasions only his earnestness, brilliance, unassuming and modest behavior, and the actual breadth of his knowledge induced some of his instructors to make special allowance for his handicap, or to "humor" him, since a few resented the situation.

State board examinations were trying ordeals for him when both written and oral examinations were required. Only the unusual excellence of the written part of the examination and the documentation of his past experiences induced the two state boards of medical examiners which required an oral examination to accord him special consideration. The reason for examinations by several state boards was his desire to inform himself about the practice of medicine in various parts of the country.

In the actual practice of medicine this patient was well respected and his competence was readily recognized. He experienced no personal problems, and his home and marital adjustments were excellent. He had consulted several psychotherapists, all of whom had regarded his problem as a circumscribed manifestation that did not warrant therapy.

He finally decided to secure certification in a certain specialty. The examining board was considerate about substituting an additional written examination for the customary oral examination part. He received his certification without difficulty. Some years later he decided upon additional certification in an allied field and undertook extensive training for that purpose.

He applied for admission to the examination conducted by the specialty board in that field. He received a letter of acceptance accompanied by a letter from the president of the board of examiners and signed by him. This letter stated that all examinees, in accord with a newly established policy of examination, were required without exception to take an oral examination lasting a minimum of four hours. This would be conducted by the president of the board and two other examiners. The patient recognized the president's name at once as that of a classmate he had had in high school, college, and medical school. That man was fully aware of the patient's oral examination problem; moreover, he had carried throughout the years an unreasoning, intense, and bitter hatred for the patient. With the passage of years occasional encounters at medical meetings had disclosed no abatement of that man's hatred, for which the patient knew no basis and for which no provocation was needed to elicit some unpleasant manifestation.

The patient consulted a colleague who also intended to take the examination at the same time. This colleague had received a letter of acceptance containing the same information, but it was signed by the secretary of the board. He wrote to two other friends with whom he had taken specific postgraduate courses and who were also taking the examination. Their letters were similar in content to his but were signed by the board secretary.

The patient then said simply, "There you have it. The term of office for that man is four years. I need to be certified this year. I know for an absolute certainty that I cannot measure up to an oral examination. I have no doubts about knowing my stuff. I could pass any written examination with flying colors. But I also know with absolute certainty that I cannot take an oral examination, much less one conducted by a man who hates me bitterly for no reason that I know of and who knows my weakness. I regard my situation as hopeless unless hypnosis can do something for me. That is why I have come to you, and I place myself unreservedly in your hands. I am your patient if you will accept me. If you do, you will have my full cooperation in anything that you wish to do or anything that you may wish me to do." This placing of all responsibility upon the author was immediately apparent, as well as his fixed limited understanding of his situation.

INITIAL PROCEDURES AND APPRAISAL OF PROBLEM

He was assured that he was accepted as a patient and he was asked to give in full detail every item of symptomatology he had ever developed in connection with oral examinations. He was asked to execute this task as a simple recounting rather than as a vivification of his symptoms as he recited them.

The patient thoughtfully, slowly, and in a most orderly and systematic fashion detailed his symptoms fully. They were many and included intense fear, uncontrollable tremors, excessive perspiration, nausea and vomiting, palpitation, bladder and bowel incontinence, severe vertigo, and a final

physical collapse resembling shock. He added, with a reflective smile, that
there seemed to be no direct correlation between the severity of his
symptoms and the importance or unimportance of the examination. The
only requisite was that the oral examination must be definitely recognized
as being an examination. A recitation offered no difficulty. He explained
further that even in taking examinations for an automobile driver's
license, he was forced to the measure of taking a pen and a pad of paper
with him. When asked a question, he would simply write the answer on
the paper pad and then "read it aloud." This behavior had occasioned
some lifted eyebrows, but it was a measure by which he "could avoid the
oral examination situation." Even such questions as his age and the
number of years he had been driving an automobile had first to be written
and then "read" to the examining clerk.

The patient was then told that he would not be given any therapeutic or
otherwise helpful hypnotic suggestions until he had been hypnotized a
sufficient number of times to give him an adequate experiential background for therapy. To accomplish this he might be used as an experimental subject in a current project. To this he readily agreed.

He proved to be an excellent somnambulistic subject, but several hours
were spent merely eliciting the various hypnotic phenomena repeatedly.
He was then used as an experimental subject in special work in which the
author was interested with intentional additions for him requiring wide
use of deep trance phenomena. The reason for such use of him in this
experimental work was to secure some measure of his competence for
prolonged hypnotic work of any type.

In the meantime the problem of how to help him was being given
consideration.

His initial account and all subsequent inquiries indicated that his
problem was of a limited, circumscribed character. After much thought it
was reasoned that therapy would need to be similarly circumscribed. That
the patient would have to take additional oral examinations other than the
one impending was considered to be most unlikely. Hence, there would
be no need to devise a therapeutic design to meet future contingencies.

Another consideration was that any measure that met the patient's
needs would also have to include elements that were definitely not
therapeutic but might even serve to enhance his own pattern of circumscribed neurotic structure by a utilization of it. This would be occasioned
by the fact that a vital part of the situation to be met was of an unalterable
character—namely, the man who hated him and who would be examining
him. Any therapeutic or helpful plan would have to include this fact and
be structured accordingly. Furthermore, there could be no clouding or
falsification of this significant aspect of the situation to be met.

The patient, in the time spent with him, had shown himself to be of good strong character, readily able to face all ordinary challenges of life. His war record had been excellent in combat service. Apparently his Achilles heel was only the matter of oral examinations, compounded in this instance by an examiner's intense hatred.

That a simple direct or even indirect therapeutic approach be made was ruled out by several important factors. Foremost was the fact that he came for help in relationship to a specific impending examination, not for therapy. Also, there were his fixed and rigid "certainties" about his condition. These could not be immediately changed; help by the author as the patient understood matters was only to permit success in the examination. Other psychotherapists had assured him he did not need therapy. Also, the usual therapeutic methodologies would take too much time, much more time than was available for him. Then, too, ordinary psychotherapy by whatever school of thought could quite conceivably fail.

Therefore, some plan of procedure had to be devised whereby the patient's needs as he understood them had to be met. It could not include direct or even indirect suggestion, since such suggestions would be in contradiction to the patient's fixed understandings. To attempt some direct procedure such as regression—direct, or indirect by dissociation— offered no promise of success. Nor could there be risked a failure of any sort with hypnosis, since failure would lessen greatly or actually destroy his remaining hope of achieving success.

Since the patient was so rigidly convinced that he had no means whatsoever of his own with which to meet his problem, it was finally decided to devise a "therapeutic" (as he would or might construe whatever the author did) procedure that would give to him various new ways and means of dealing successfully with the impending examination. That it would actually be therapeutic in the usual sense of the word was not of importance. What was important was that the patient would be given entirely new ways of reacting and responding of a sort that would preclude the development of his long-established pattern of behavior. Further thought suggested that the rigid, limited, circumscribed character of his problem be employed to structure the final procedure. To do so might enable him to enter the examination room with his medical knowledge readily available, this to be presented adequately as needed by wholly new and different methods of reacting and responding. All of this would be so structured that it could be achieved within a highly restricted circumscribed frame of reference.

Having reached these conclusions, a systematic plan of therapeutic work was devised. Previous hypnotic work which served primarily to enable the patient to develop a trance satisfactorily was repeated in large part and fitted into the following plan described in detail.

THE THERAPEUTIC PROCEDURE

A deep somnambulistic hypnotic trance was induced on repeated occasions in the patient, and each time he was asked to experience fully, in a fashion entirely unrelated to his problem, all of the various phenomena of the deep trance. Some of this work fitted into a current experimental project, but the patient had no knowledge of what the experimental work was. Most of the work done with him was merely to ensure adequate experiential learning by the patient. Thus, he learned to develop positive and negative visual and auditory hallucinations, superficial and deep anesthesia, regression, revivification, dissociation, selective amnesia, partial or total amnesia, hypermnesia, posthypnotic suggestion, depersonalization, automatism, and time distortion. The patient was given to understand that many of these learnings would be of no service to him, and he was allowed to think that the author was meeting the needs of personal experimental work. In no way was he allowed to realize that this additional work might serve a definite purpose for him—namely, that of preventing him from attaching any of his anxiety and fears to any of those learnings or from distorting those learnings in any way by an overeagerness to benefit from them. Also, the knowledge that the author was already engaged in an hypnotic experiment of which he knew nothing furthered this needed distraction of the patient from the author's work with him. It may be added that if the author had not already been engaged in some experimental work, he would have immediately devised some that would have required the recording of data, this fact of recording being unobtrusively disclosed to the patient without revealing the data. This measure is often most effective in circumventing the hindrance caused by too intense an interest by the patient in his own therapy.

When the author was fully satisfied that the patient was adequately trained, the plan of therapy that had been devised was put into action. This plan was based upon (1) the ability to hallucinate visually, (2) the ability to dissociate from the self and to dissociate the self from objects, (3) the ability to maintain a coherent train of thought while verbally expressing another or while attending auditorially to the utterances of another person, (4) the ability to execute posthypnotic suggestions, (5) the ability to develop amnesia, (6) the ability to behave like an automaton, (7) the ability to distort and to transform realities, and (8) the ability to present an appearance of alert, attentive consciousness, however deep a trance state might develop. Since all instructions given to the patient were permissive in character, the patient was entirely at liberty to utilize these various learnings as best befitted him in the impending situation.

THE RESULTS

In essence, the patient utilized all of the instructions given to him, not always in the order or manner intended by the author but rather in accord with his own understandings of what he was to do. What actually happened is best related in the patient's own words.

"As soon as I got back home, I realized I had to see you again. So I called for an appointment. I had a feeling it was urgent and that you also wanted to see me right away. I literally didn't remember anything until my wife met me at the airport. I read the good news on her face and then I remembered that I had telephoned the good news to both of you. I was in a complete mental daze while going there. I knew I was completely clear-headed and at ease during the examination. I knew I didn't miss a single question. I remembered that they told me my diploma would arrive in about three weeks. Then I telephoned you and my wife. But I forgot all this. Then I must have come home in a daze. I don't remember even checking out of my hotel or catching my plane. I knew where I was. I was just without any memories of what had occurred while I was away from home when my wife met me at the airport. When she said how glad she was I had passed, I could remember notifying her and you. That's all, though. So I told her that I had to go to the office right away on something urgent, and as soon as I got there, I telephoned you and called a cab. Will you put me in a trance and help me to remember?"

The author replied, "The important thing is that you passed your examination. It really is not necessary to induce a trance for a systematic orderly account of what happened. *You can remember now while completely alert and wakeful.*"

In an astonished tone of voice the patient began, "That's right. I was in a daze all the way there. I acted like a robot. I said and did all the right things. I had my notice with me telling me where and at what hour to report. I was there about 20 minutes early. Sat like a robot. Walked in the examination room when the girl called me. My 'friend' showed all his teeth in his smile. They needed cleaning. He said, 'Glad to see you, Jack. Sorry we can't make any special arrangements for you.' But all the time he was speaking, I was looking at his face. It looked as young as when we were in high school. Then I saw it getting older and older, changing like the face of Dorian Grey in the movie. But I just said, 'It's all O.K. with me. I'm ready to go anytime.' Then he said, 'Just take a seat in that chair there.' I looked at it and wondered what a nice chair like that was doing there, but I sat down facing the three of them.

"Then he fired the first question. I heard every word of it, but I kept watching the way his mouth moved. It looked so interesting in such a peculiar way. Then when I told him the answer I knew he wanted but didn't think I knew, you should have seen the look on his face. I knew that he knew my answer was right. But he looked as if he just couldn't believe something about me. I couldn't figure out what it was. Then he asked me a great long question. I tipped my head a bit to hear him better and looked past him, and he disappeared. Just his voice was there. Heard every word but as I heard the words, pages from textbooks appeared before my eyes. I could see the page numbers, and certain paragraphs were in large print. I looked at them carefully while I listened to the words, and when the words stopped, I just summarized what was in those paragraphs. I thought I gave a pretty good summary, but just then my 'friend' came back looking mad. Before I could figure out why, he picked up a sheet of paper and began reading a page-long typewritten question. As he began reading to me, a large sheet of white paper appeared before me, and every word he read showed up in big black print, and I kept reading right along with him about a word or two behind him. When he finished, I just looked that sheet of paper over carefully a few seconds and explained that there were three different possible interpretations. So I told him what they were. You should have seen the agony on his face. That man was in pain." Here the patient interrupted himself to say, "Now I know what really happened. I was in some kind of hypnotic state, and you must have taught me how to use it in the examination situation. It's obvious that I was hallucinating and that I was behaving automatically some of the time. There's probably some things I did that I don't know the technical terms for."

He was assured that his interpretation was entirely correct, but that the author wanted him to continue with his account.

The patient resumed, "Well, then the next man introduced himself and I realized that my 'friend' hadn't done the proper thing. This man looked like an awful nice fellow, and he spoke as if he really needed some help on a problem that was troubling him, so I told him exactly what he needed to know."

Here the patient interrupted himself again, "That's exactly what happened with each of the other two examiners. They each looked like a person you would like to know, and when either of them asked me a question, they looked like they needed help, and so I listened carefully and then I told them what they needed to know. Oh, yes, at the end of an hour and a half they nodded to each other and then to my 'friend.' He looked madder than ever. Then those two stood up and both shook hands with me and congratulated me. Then my 'friend' stepped over and shook my hand and congratulated me and I wondered why, and why he didn't get a rug for his baldness and have the hair on his ears clipped. That was it."

To this the author replied, "Not entirely. Tell me a bit more about what you did in relation to your so-called friend."

"In complete detail? I remember everything and can do it, or will a summary be sufficient?"

He was told that a summary would be satisfactory.

"Well, there was that question where I could see myself standing behind him looking over his shoulder and reading what he was reading and then reading the answer. Then once he seemed to be trying to sing a silly song, so I recited some medical prose. Then he seemed to be beating time while I was talking to him, and I would purposely rephrase what I was saying to get him off beat.

"Oh, yes! There are two especially interesting things, one that puzzled me and both that I enjoyed. Well, several that I enjoyed. The puzzler was where 'friend Henry' looked to be about a block away so I could barely see him. Couldn't recognize him, but I could hear his voice right in front of me. I tried to figure out whether he had moved away from me or if I had moved away from him, but how could his voice be right in front of me? So I replied to him and never did figure that one out till now. But the best ones were when Henry asked about some specific condition or some syndrome and I actually felt myself in white uniform on the ward examining a patient. Each time the patient was Henry and he was in terrible condition—looked awful—and I explained the condition very carefully so that the interns with me could understand fully. I was just one of the fellows taking postgraduate work making rounds with the interns and really enjoying myself.

"In fact, not once did I know what I was there in that examination room for. I just was interested in how I saw things, and I did and said all the right things. Did you teach me how to do all those things in those hypnotic sessions I had with you? And did you make me have amnesia so I just wouldn't worry and fret and get into a horrible stew?"

He was told that such was the case and that he had been taught various other things, all for the purpose of permitting an adequate examination performance with no neurotic distress. He was also told that he was at liberty to ask more questions of the author and also free to remember or to forget his examination experience. However, it was stressed that he retain any measure of learning that might be useful to him and that he could feel comfortably certain that he need never use his hypnotic learnings except appropriately and in times of special need.

The patient has been seen repeatedly many times since then in a casual way. He has referred patients to the author, and he would, if asked, do hypnotic work with the author. He is not interested in employing hypnosis himself, but he has stated that his approach to patients and their problems has been changed for the better. This he explained as, "Perhaps I am unconsciously using hypnotic techniques."

DISCUSSION

It is at once apparent that an unrecognizable (to him) circumvention of the examination situation had been effected. There had been also a bizarre distortion of it, fully as bizarre as his own neurotic behavior that disabled him. This distortion of the examination situation had been amusing, puzzling, even bewildering, but in no way distressful, nor did it interfere with the examination procedure. Posthypnotic suggestion had served to enable him to present an appearance of ordinary wakefulness, alertness, and responsiveness. Well-learned forms of the various types of hypnotic behavior were posthypnotically employed by him in his own private personal manner of meeting the requirements of the examination.

Paradoxically, such an elaborate procedure was not evolved for the patient's sake. A general explanation can be found in the question, "Why do neurotic and psychotic patients so frequently develop such elaborate psychological structures to give expression to their illness?" Undoubtedly because the expression they do give is so inadequate. As for the patient, why did he have such elaborate and so many and such intense symptoms? Nausea and vomiting alone were sufficient. Certainly bladder and bowel incontinence were more than adequate to prevent an oral examination. Then why were there all the other symptoms? Did they serve some other purposes or relate to unrecognized significances? As in the case with other patients, the author simply does not know. Nor does he know of anybody who has ever really understood the variety and purposes of any one patient's multiple symptoms despite the tendency of many psychiatrists to hypothecate, to their own satisfaction, towering structures of explanation often as elaborate and bizarre as the patient's symptomatology.

As for the therapy evolved for this patient, it was he who developed it, not the author. The patient was taught simply how to experience various hypnotic phenomena. Thus he learned how to develop a negative hallucination for the author, for a part of the author such as his hand, his head, or his torso. He was taught to alter visual stimuli by experiencing them as coming from near at hand or from a remote distance. He was taught to hallucinate printed pages and printed words and various other objects, as well as movements by the author or by objects in the office. He learned to change and to distort visual stimuli. He could see the author smiling and experience it as frowning, and vice versa. He learned to see tears streaming down the face in a picture on the author's desk, he saw that face burst into a smile, and then he saw that face in the picture talking and he hallucinated the apparently spoken words. He saw a black-and-white picture in bright colors. He experienced visually a small oblong ashtray as square, as a circle, as tall, as flat, as transparent, as opaque, as of many different colors, as twisted into various shapes, as floating in midair, as moving back and forth or up and down rapidly, slowly, in various rhythms. In each of these teachings care was taken to make sure he understood the nature or kind of experience he was to learn; but, unless absolutely necessary, never the degree or extent of the suggested experience. Thus it was he who decided that a negative hallucination for a part of the author's body should be of the hand, the foot, the head, or the torso. The shapes in the twisting of the ashtray were determined entirely by him, and no effort was made to inquire what those shapes were. The words hallucinated as spoken by the face in the picture remained unknown to the author. The *kind* of task was the author's responsibility in this hypnotic teaching of the subject. The *content* was the patient's. *All of the teachings that he had been given or that would be given to him by the author,* he was told, *he was to use profitably and well in any needful situation.*

In relation to the auditory field one precaution was emphasized—namely, that he would hear clearly and easily every verbal stimulus and that he would listen most understandingly to all utterances. If he wished, he might have the speaker standing up, sitting down, or leaning on a chair, but always he was to hear clearly and understand thoroughly.

Each of the various hypnotic phenomena was developed in this same detailed fashion until the author was convinced of the patient's competence. Great care was taken to ensure his appearance as a person alert, attentive, interested, understanding, responsive, and fully wide awake regardless of what hypnotic phenomena he was experiencing.

Posthypnotic suggestion and amnesia, while taught with the same meticulous care, were used directly by the author to ensure certain things. These were that the patient make the trip to the city where the examination was held with a generalized amnesia, but with a responsive alertness to meet every expected or unexpected development concerning the trip itself. Thus he made the trip and appeared in proper time for the examination but with an amnesia for, and a total unconcern about, the purpose of the trip. In his own words, "I just went comfortably. I read a novel that I had long wanted to read and I took it with me." His telephone calls to the author and to his wife were both the outcome of posthypnotic suggestion. He was told that he might forget telephoning his wife, but that he could "read" that fact upon seeing her and that this might make him realize the importance of promptly seeing the author, who knew the hour of his return flight. The amnesia on the way there was to prevent any building up of tension, and on the way back it served to let him rest without sensing unduly his fatigue or building up an elated tension over his probable success.

The final interview with the author was to give the patient a full recollection of all that occurred, all or any part of which he was at liberty to remember or to forget. Since then he has forgotten much that occurred, but of noteworthy significance is the fact that he can speak of his past oral examination experiences casually and that he took his next examination for a renewal of his driver's license quite unconcernedly. As for his "friend Henry," the patient now speaks of him as a rather absurdly emotional man.

BACKGROUND OF EXPERIMENTATION

Since 1935 the author has many times induced hypnotic trances in normal college students to discover if they could take an examination successfully in a college course while in a posthypnotic trance state. The results were always equal to, or better than, what might have been expected in relation to their class grades. Unless special understandings had been given to the students, they always developed persistent spontaneous amnesia for having taken the examination, which had to be removed by the author. In some instances this amnesia was allowed to persist for as long a period as a year.

These experiences led the author to induce in professional persons the development of posthypnotic trance states during which they might give to students or colleagues (even psychiatrists) a prepared or impromptu lecture, present patients at a staff conference, discharge a day's duties on the ward, or spend a social evening or day with friends without the trance state being detected. They always succeeded, and similarly developed spontaneous amnesia which had to be removed by the author.

A third-year resident in psychiatry, who was an experimental subject of the author's but who was unaware of this special work, asked to be taught autohypnosis. Without inducing a hypnotic trance, the author casually and conversationally outlined various methods of autohypnosis, intending to give more adequate instruction later. About a month afterward, before any further instruction had been given, the author received a telephone call from the resident, who declared, "I must see you. It's four o'clock in the afternoon, and there's something I do not understand. May I come to your office?"

Upon arriving at the office, the resident stated very simply, "This morning I dressed to go to town [Detroit] for some shopping with a friend. I looked at the clock on the dresser and it was a few minutes of eight. I saw that I had just time to meet Dr. ——, have breakfast, and then catch the bus to town. I took a second look at the clock, and it read four o'clock. Then I noticed that the sun was shining through the west window, and then I turned and looked at the rest of the room. There was my bed all made up, with a lot of packages on it. I looked at some of the wrappings.

They were from stores in Detroit. I opened a couple of them. They were things I had promised myself to buy months ago, but had completely forgotten about. That's when I knew I ought to see you, and here I am. Put me in a trance and see if my unconscious knows anything at all about this, because I don't."

The author gave a cue used in experiments with this subject, and a somnambulistic trance ensued. The subject, with open eyes, smiled and waited expectantly. The author then asked, "Do you know what happened?" The reply was, "I do now, but I don't when I'm awake." The author asked, "What do you want me to do?" "Ask me about everything, then wake me up and tell me." The author answered, "Would it be all right if I just awakened you and let you remember everything sequentially?" "I think that would be better, so wake me up so I can start."

The subject aroused from the trance state, appeared astonished, and said, "I'm sure you must know everything, but I'm just beginning to remember. Today I was off duty, and I had arranged to go to Detroit by bus with Dr. ——, who was also off duty, after we had breakfast together. But just after I looked at the clock I went into an autohypnotic trance. I had been thinking about autohypnosis since the day you discussed it with me. I had been impressed by your statements that, in developing autohypnosis, you cannot tell your unconscious mind all the things it should do and how it should do them, because that would be making it a conscious task. And it's also a useless task because your unconscious mind already knows what you know a lot better than you do. So I knew that I would have to go into autohypnosis unexpectedly. Now I have just remembered that this morning my unconscious mind simply took over, and there I was in an autohypnotic trance. Now I'll tell you what happened, because I am remembering things one by one just as they happened."

Then there followed a long, sequential detailed narrative of the day's events, with interspersed comments. The account included conversations with Dr. —— (also a psychiatrist) and with other friends, an accidental meeting with two former high-school classmates who had not been seen for more than eight years, eating lunch with Dr. —— and the two friends at a favorite restaurant, shopping in various stores, purchasing four items long wished for but always previously forgotten, returning on the bus with Dr. ——, putting the packages on the bed, and then turning to look at the clock as a self-determined cue for awaking.

This account was then related by both the resident and the author to various members of the hospital psychiatric staff. A few of them indignantly declared, with all the weight of their lack of knowledge, that a person in a hypnotic trance would necessarily act "like a zombi." This was disputed with equal indignation by Dr. ——.

A few weeks later, at a staff conference, the same resident presented several patients, discussed the clinical records, and answered questions adequately, even those asked by some unexpected visitors at the staff conference. The fact that the resident was in an autohypnotic trance throughout the conference was recognized only by the author, although it was strongly suspected by another staff member (not Dr. ——). He later demanded confirmation of his suspicions from the author. This being given, he emphatically discredited to his colleagues the "zombi" misunderstandings which had been previously expressed. To substantiate his statements, he called upon the resident, who was found to have a total and seemingly unbreakable amnesia for that particular staff conference, even when confronted by the typewritten record.

The fact was then established that behavior in an autohypnotic state may be difficult to differentiate from ordinary waking behavior. The author was then called upon to "restore" the resident's "loss of memory." A few cues given to the resident served to effect a recovery of the amnestic material along with a full awareness of the previous conscious unawareness. The resident then disclosed that such an occurrence had been secretly intended but for a much later staff conference.

19. The Burden of Responsibility in Effective Psychotherapy

Milton H. Erickson

The following case material is presented because it offers so concisely and clearly a modus operandi in hypnotherapy with a type of patients who have had long experience in failing to derive desired benefits from extensive, traditionally oriented therapy. The three persons reported upon are typical of dozens of others that this author has seen over the years, and the results obtained have been remarkably good despite the fact that the patients were seen on only one occasion for an hour or two.

In each instance hypnosis was used for the specific purpose of placing the burden of responsibility for therapeutic results upon the patient himself after he himself had reached a definite conclusion that therapy would not help and that a last resort would be a hypnotic "miracle." In this author's understanding of psychotherapy, if a patient wants to believe in a "hypnotic miracle" so strongly that he will undertake the responsibility of making a recovery by virtue of his own actual behavior and continue that recovery, he is at liberty to do so under whatever guise he chooses, but neither the author nor the reader is obliged to regard the success of the therapy as a hypnotic miracle. The hypnosis was used solely as a modality by means of which to secure their cooperation in accepting the therapy they wanted. In other words, they were induced by hypnosis to acknowledge and act upon their own personal responsibility for successfully accepting the previously futilely sought and offered but actually rejected therapy.

CASES 1 AND 2

A telephone call was received in the office from a man who stated that he wanted an appointment. He refused to give any reason except that it was for a proper medical reason he preferred to explain in person.

At the interview the man stated that he was suffering from Buerger's

Reprinted with permission from *The American Journal of Clinical Hypnosis*, January, 1964, *6*, 269–271.

disease, that he was a diabetic, and that he had cardiac disease and high blood pressure—"Too much for a man with a family the size of mine and only 50 years old." He went on, "That isn't all. I've been psychoanalyzed for eight months for five hours a week. During that time my insulin dosage has had to be increased, I've gained 40 pounds, my blood pressure has gone up 35 points, and from 1½ packs of cigarettes I have gone up to 4½ packs a day. I am still the psychoanalyst's patient, I have an appointment with him for Monday, but he is paid up to date. He says he is slowly uncovering the psychodynamics of my self-destructive behavior. I myself think that I'm digging my grave with power tools."

Then with utter gravity he asked, "Would it be unethical for you, knowing that I am another physician's patient, to give me the benefit of two hours of hypnotherapy this afternoon? My analyst disapproves of hypnosis, but he certainly hasn't done me any good."

The simple reply was made that, from my point of view, the question of professional ethics did not enter into the situation at all, that every patient, including mine, has the right to seek from any duly trained and licensed physician whatever proper help he desires, that medical ethics should properly be centered about the patient's welfare rather than a physician's desire to keep a patient.

He was then told to close his eyes and repeat his story from beginning to end, to do this slowly, carefully, to drop out the question of ethics and in its place to specify what he wanted from the author. This he was to do slowly, thoughtfully, appraisingly, and as he did so, the mere sound of his own voice would serve to induce in him a satisfactory trance in which he could continue to talk to the author, listen to the author, answer questions, *do anything asked of him by the author and that he would find himself under a most powerful compulsion to do exactly that which was indicated.*

The man was taken aback at these unexpected instructions, but leaned back in his chair, closed his eyes, and slowly began his recitation with pertinent additions. Shortly his voice began to trail off, indicating that he was developing a trance, and he had to be told several times to speak more loudly and clearly.

No mention was made of the question of ethics, but with a wealth of detail *he outlined the therapy which he thought to be indicated.* He was asked to repeat this several times, and each time he did so more positively, emphatically, and inclusively.

After four such repetitions the author pointed out that he, as a physician, had offered no advice or therapeutic or corrective suggestions, that every item in that regard had come from the patient himself, *and that he would find himself under the powerful compulsion arising from within him to do everything that he thought was indicated.* To this was added that he could remember any selected parts of his trance state, but regardless of what he remembered or did not remember *he would be under a most powerful compulsion to do all that he himself thought to be indicated.*

He was aroused, a casual conversation initiated, and he left.

A year later, in excellent physical shape, he brought in an old childhood friend of his and stated very briefly, "I eat right, I sleep good, my weight is normal, my habits regular, my diabetes is under good control, my Buerger's disease has not progressed, my blood pressure is normal, I never went back to my analyst, my business is better than ever, I'm a new man and my whole family thanks you. Now this man is my boyhood pal, he's got emphysema, a very bad heart, look at his swollen ankles, and he smokes like a chimney. He's been under a doctor's care for years." (This man was smoking one cigarette and had another out of the package ready to light.)

"Treat him the way you did me, because I told him you talked to me in a way that just takes complete hold of you."

He left the office with the new patient remaining.

Essentially the same procedure was carried out, checking against the first patient's file as this was done, and almost precisely the same words were used that were applicable.

At the close of the interview the man left, leaving his cigarettes behind him.

Six months later a long distance call was received from the first patient, stating, "Well, the news is bad but you should feel good. Joe died last night in his sleep from a coronary attack. After he left your office, he never smoked another cigarette, his emphysema was much better, and he enjoyed life instead of worrying all the time about running out of cigarettes and about the cigarettes making his condition worse."

CASE 3

A telephone call was received early in the morning. A man's voice said, "I've just realized that my condition is an emergency. How soon can I come in?" He was told that a cancellation had just been received and he could be seen in one hour's time. At the specified time a 32-year-old man walked in, smoking a cigarette, and stated hastily, "I'm a chronic smoker. I need help. I've been in psychotherapy twice a week for two years. I want to quit smoking. I can't. Look! I've got six packs in my pockets right now so I can't run out of them. My analyst says I am making progress, but I was only carrying two packs a day when I first went to him. Then slowly I increased my reserve and emergency supplies until it is up to six packs a day. I'm afraid to leave home without at least six packs in my pocket. I read about you. I want you to hypnotize me out of smoking."

He was assured that *this could not be done,* but that the author would like to have him retell his story slowly, carefully, with his eyes closed, and to give it in good detail, letting his unconscious mind (he was a college graduate) take over all dominance, and that, as he related his story, he was to specify in full and comprehensive detail exactly what it was he wished in relation to cigarettes, but that during his narrative he would find himself going unaccountably into a deep and deeper trance without any interruption of his story.

The procedure and results were almost exactly comparable to the two preceding cases.

Two years later another telephone call was received from the same man asking for a half-hour appointment at noon and volunteering to pay an hour's fee. He again declared it to be an emergency.

Exactly at noon he came striding into the office and remarked. "You won't recognize me. You only saw me for an hour two years ago. I am Mr. X, and I had had two years of analysis for excessive smoking with only an increase in my smoking. I can't remember what went on when I saw you, but I do know that I haven't smoked a cigarette since then. It's embarrassing, too, because I can't even light one for my girl. I've tried many times, but I can't.

"But I went back to that analyst, and he took all the credit for my stopping smoking. I didn't tell him about you. I thought I needed to see him about what he called a character defect in me. Here I am with a college education, and the longest I've worked at a job has been three months. I can always get a job, but I'm 34 now, and four years of psychoanalysis has wound up with my last job lasting only five weeks. But I'm 34 now, and I've got the promise of another job with a future to it. Now I want you to do something about whatever is wrong with me because I've quit the analyst. I've had better jobs than the one coming up, but there is nothing to hold me to it. It will be the same old story. Now, hypnotize me and do what I should have had you do two years ago, whatever that was."

His former case record was looked up to refresh the author's memory. As precisely as possible the technique of the previous occasion was followed, and he was again dismissed.

Two years later he was still at the "new job" but had been promoted to a managerial position which he has held for over a year. A chance meeting with him disclosed this fact and also that he is married and a father and that his wife voluntarily gave up smoking.

SUMMARY

Three of a long series of similar cases are reported here to illustrate the use of hypnosis as a technique of deliberately shifting from the therapist to the patient the entire burden of both defining the psychotherapy desired and the responsibility for accepting it. Often this is the most difficult part of psychotherapy. In all the patients this author has handled successfully in this manner, all had a history of a steady, persistent search for therapy, but a failure to take the responsibility of accepting it. Additionally, all such patients with whom the author has had a known success were of a superior intelligence level.

In traditional ritualistic and conventional psychotherapies much, often futile, effort is made to induce patients to assume adequately the responsibility for their own behavior and for future effort. This is done without regard for the patients' consciously thinking and firmly believing as an absolute truth the futility of any effort on their own part.

But utilizing hypnosis as a technique of deliberately and intentionally shifting to the patients their own burden of responsibility for therapeutic results and having them emphatically and repetitiously affirm and confirm in their own thought formulations and their own expressed verbalizations of their own desires, needs and intentions at the level of their own unconscious mentation, forces the therapeutic goals to become the patient's own goals, not those *merely offered* by the therapist he is visiting.

That this procedure always is successful is not true. There are many patients who want therapy but do not accept it until adequately motivated. There are other patients whose goal is no more than the continuous seeking of therapy but not the accepting of it. With this type of patient hypnotherapy fails as completely as do other forms of therapy.

20. The Use of Symptoms as an Integral Part of Hypnotherapy

Milton H. Erickson

In dealing with any type of patient clinically there is a most important consideration that should be kept constantly in mind. This is that the patient's needs as a human personality should be an ever-present question for the therapist to ensure recognition at each manifestation. Merely to make a correct diagnosis of the illness and to know the correct method of treatment is not enough. Fully as important is that the patient be receptive of the therapy and cooperative in regard to it. Without the patient's full cooperativeness therapeutic results are delayed, distorted, limited, or even prevented. Too often the therapist regards patients as necessarily logical, understanding, in full possession of their faculties—in brief, as reasonable and informed human beings. Yet it is a matter of common knowledge often overlooked, disregarded, or rejected that patients can be silly, forgetful, absurd, unreasonable, illogical, incapable of acting with common sense, and very often governed and directed in their behavior by emotions and by unknown, unrecognizable, and perhaps undiscoverable unconscious needs and forces which are far from reasonable, logical, or sensible. To attempt therapy upon a patient only apparently sensible, reasonable, and intelligent when that patient may actually be governed by unconscious forces and emotions neither overtly shown nor even known, to overlook the unconscious mind for possible significant information, can lead easily to failure or to unsatisfactory results. Nor should seemingly intelligent, rational, and cooperative behavior ever be allowed to mislead the therapist into an oversight of the fact that the patient is still human and hence easily the victim of fears and foibles, of all those unknown experiential learnings that have been relegated to his unconscious mind and that he may never become aware of or ever show just what the self may be like under the outward placid surface. Nor should therapists have so little regard for their patients that they fail to make allowance for human weaknesses and irrationality. Too often it is not the strengths of the person that are vital in the therapeutic situation. Rather, the dominant forces that control the entire situation may derive from weaknesses, illogical behavior, unreasonableness, and obviously false and misleading attitudes of various sorts.

Reprinted with permission from *The American Journal of Clinical Hypnosis,* July, 1965, *8,* 57–65.

Therapists wishing to help their patients should never scorn, condemn, or reject any part of a patient's conduct simply because it is obstructive, unreasonable, or even irrational. The patient's behavior is a part of the problem brought into the office; it constitutes the personal environment within which the therapy must take effect; it may constitute the dominant force in the total patient-doctor relationship. Since whatever patients bring into the office is in some way both a part of them and a part of their problem, the patient should be viewed with a sympathetic eye appraising the totality which confronts the therapist. In so doing therapists should not limit themselves to an appraisal of what is good and reasonable as offering possible foundations for therapeutic procedures. Sometimes—in fact, many more times than is realized—therapy can be firmly established on a sound basis only by the utilization of silly, absurd, irrational, and contradictory manifestations. One's professional dignity is not involved, but one's professional competence is.

To illustrate from clinical experience, case history material will be cited, some from a nonhypnotic therapeutic situation, some from situations involving the use of hypnosis.

CASE REPORT 1

George had been a patient in a mental hospital for five years. His identity had never been established. He was simply a stranger around the age of 25 who had been picked up by the police for irrational behavior and committed to the state mental hospital. During those five years he had said, "My name is George," "Good morning," and "Good night," but these were his only rational utterances. He uttered otherwise a continuous word-salad completely meaningless as far as could be determined. It was made up of sounds, syllables, words, and incomplete phrases. For the first three years he sat on a bench at the front door of the ward and eagerly leaped up and poured forth his word-salad most urgently to everyone who entered the ward. Otherwise, he merely sat quietly, mumbling his word-salad to himself. Innumerable patient efforts had been made by psychiatrists, psychologists, nurses, social service workers, other personnel, and even fellow patients to secure intelligible remarks from him, all in vain. George talked only one way, the word-salad way. After approximately three years he continued to greet persons who entered the ward with an outburst of meaningless words, but in between times he sat silently on the bench, appearing mildly depressed but somewhat angrily uttering a few minutes of word-salad when approached and questioned.

The author joined the hospital staff in the sixth year of George's stay. The available information about his ward behavior was secured. It was learned also that patients or ward personnel could sit on the bench beside him without eliciting his word-salad so long as they did not speak to him. With this total of information a therapeutic plan was devised. A secretary recorded in shorthand the word-salads with which he so urgently greeted those who entered the ward. These transcribed recordings were studied, but no meaning could be discovered. These word-salads were carefully paraphrased, using words that were least likely to be found in George's productions, and an extensive study was made of these until the author could improvise a word-salad similar in pattern to George's, but utilizing a different vocabulary.

Then all entrances to the ward were made through a side door some distance down the corridor from George. The author then began the practice of sitting silently on the bench beside George daily for increasing lengths of time until the span of an hour was reached. Then, at the next sitting, the author, addressing the empty air, identified himself verbally. George made no response.

The next day the identification was addressed directly to George. He spat out an angry stretch of word-salad to which the author replied, in tones of courtesy and responsiveness, with an equal amount of his own carefully contrived word-salad. George appeared puzzled and, when the author finished, George uttered another contribution with an inquiring intonation. As if replying the author verbalized still further word-salad.

After a half-dozen interchanges, George lapsed into silence, and the author promptly went about other matters.

The next morning appropriate greetings were exchanged employing proper names by both. Then George launched into a long word-salad speech to which the author courteously replied in kind. There followed then brief interchanges of long and short utterances of word-salad until George fell silent and the author went to other duties.

This continued for some time. Then Goerge, after returning the morning greeting, made meaningless utterances without pause for four hours. It taxed the author greatly to miss lunch and to make a full reply in kind. George listened attentively and made a two-hour reply, to which a weary two -hour response was made. (George was noted to watch the clock throughout the day.)

The next morning George returned the usual greeting properly but added about two sentences of nonsense. The author replied with a similar length of nonsense. George replied, "Talk sense, Doctor." "Certainly, I'll be glad to. What is your last name?" "O'Donovan, and it's about time somebody who knows how to talk asked. Over five years in this lousy joint" . . . (to which was added a sentence or two of word-salad). The author replied, "I'm glad to get your name, George. Five years is too long a time" . . . (and about two sentences of word-salad were added).

The rest of the account is as might be expected. A complete history sprinkled with bits of word-salad was obtained by inquiries judiciously salted with word-salad. His clinical course—never completely free of word-salad, which was eventually reduced to occasional unintelligible mumbles—was excellent. Within a year he had left the hospital, was gainfully employed, and at increasingly longer intervals returned to the hospital to report his continued and improving adjustment. Nevertheless, he invariably initiated his report or terminated it with a bit of word-salad, always expecting the same from the author. Yet he could, as he frequently did on these visits, comment wryly, "Nothing like a little nonsense in life, is there, Doctor?" to which he obviously expected and received a sensible expression of agreement to which was added a brief utterance of nonsense. After he had been out of the hospital continuously for three years of fully satisfactory adjustment, contact was lost with him except for a cheerful postcard from another city. This bore a brief but satisfactory summary of his adjustments in a distant city. It was signed properly, but following his name was a jumble of syllables. There was no return address. He was ending the relationship on his terms of adequate understanding.

During the course of his psychotherapy he was found hypnotizable, developing a medium to deep trance in about 15 minutes. However, his trance behavior was entirely comparable to his waking behavior, and it offered no therapeutic advantages, although repeated tests were made. Every therapeutic interview was characterized by the judicious use of an appropriate amount of word-salad.

The above case represents a rather extreme example of meeting a patient at the level of his decidedly serious problem. The author was at first rather censoriously criticized by others, but when it became apparent that inexplicable imperative needs of the patient were being met, there was no further adverse comment.

The next report is decidedly different. Although no psychosis was involved, there existed such an irrational rigidity of emotional conviction that the patient appeared to be inaccessible.

CASE REPORT 2

A man in his early forties approached a dentist friend of the author, explaining his situation at great length, perspiring freely as he did so and manifesting much fear and trepidation. His account was that he had recently read a news story about the use of hypnosis in dentistry. This reminded him of his college days, when he had many times acted as a hypnotic subject for experimental purposes in the psychology laboratory. In these experiences he easily and invariably achieved the somnambulistic state with profound amnesias still persisting for his trance experiences as such, but with a still present fair memory of the experimental accounts subsequently shown to him.

For some reason not recalled by him but referred to as "some horribly painful experience connected with dentistry in some way" he had not visited a dentist for over 20 years despite the fact that he was well aware that he was seriously in need of dental care. His direct explanation was, "I just can't bring myself to see a dentist. Dentistry is a painful thing. It has to be painful. There are no ifs, ands, or buts about it. Dentistry has to be connected with pain. Even with an anesthetic there is pain after it wears off. No matter what you do in dentistry, there is some place that becomes terribly sensitive." There was more of this almost irrational obsessional thinking, but the foregoing is an adequate example.

The news story about hypnodontia made him hopeful that in some way his terror of dentistry could be overcome. Hence he made telephone calls about hypnodontia until he located the author's friend.

That dentist agreed to see him and in a preliminary session gave the patient a careful explanation of hypnoanesthesia. The man developed an excellent somnambulistic trance and easily developed glove anesthesia and then a profound anesthesia of the fingers as tested by overflexing forcibly the terminal phalanx. The dentist then attempted to produce mandibular anesthesia. This failed completely, arousing the dentist's intense interest in the problem apparently confronting him. An entire evening was spent the next day by the dentist endeavoring by one technique or another to produce dental anesthesia. The patient could develop surgical anesthesia anywhere except in relation to his mouth. Instead of anesthesia a seeming hyperesthesia developed.

Another dentist well-experienced in hypnosis was called in to work with the patient hypnotically. The two dentists spent an intensive afternoon and evening with a profoundly somnambulistic hypnotic subject who was surgically anesthetic and able to withstand any painful stimulus they were willing to administer to his body. The patient had his eyes open throughout the trance, and he was most interested in his hypnoanesthesia.

However, a touch on the patient's lip, chin, or the angle of his jaw would result in a flood of perspiration, a flushing of the skin, and complaints that the slightest touch seemed to be extremely painful, and the patient would break down hypnotically established neck and body rigidity in order to wince and to withdraw from such touches.

Other dentists were questioned for suggestions and advice to no avail, and the patient was finally sent to the author together with a typed account of the findings of the two dentists and with a typed example of the patient's verbalizations about dental pain.

The interview with the patient and the induction of a deep trance permitted an easy confirmation of the report by the dentists.

Scrutiny of the typed account of his obsessivelike utterances about pain and dentistry, and close listening when he verbalized afresh his convictions about dentistry and pain, suggested a possible likely course of action. Since the dentists had expressed their interest in any experimental work the author might do, the patient was dismissed with an instruction to make an appointment with the first dentist. When the appointment was made, the dentist telephoned his friend and the author.

At the proper time the patient appeared and at the author's request took a seat in the dental chair with his face flushed and perspiring and in a general state of utter fear. In spite of that he developed a deep somnambulistic trance in rapport with the two dentists as well as the author.

The intended approach to dental anesthesia and its rationale had been previously discussed with the dentists, and it was agreed the entire procedure should be done with no preliminary preparation of the patient.

When all was in readiness, the patient, still in a deep somnambulistic trance, tremulous, and with his face flushed and perspiring, was asked to listen closely to a reading of a typed account of his statements about dentistry and pain, which included the statements quoted above. He listened with utter intensity, and as the last statement was read, he was told seriously and impressively, "You are entirely right, absolutely right, and you summarize it most adequately in one of your statements. Let me read it again, 'No matter what you do in dentistry there is always some place that becomes terribly sensitive.' You are completely correct. As you sit there in the dental chair, the dentist will be to your right. Hence, you may now, at once, safely extend your left hand and arm, there to let it stay suspended as if frozen rigidly in place. And you may turn your face and see it there, and as you do so you will note that your left hand, so completely out of reach of everything, safe from any touch, from the slightest breath of air, is becoming so terribly, so awfully, so horribly hypersensitive, so unbelievably hypersensitive that in another minute all of the sensitivity of your entire body will drain into that hand. And since the dentist in working with you will not touch your hand where all the hypersensitivity is, he can easily do all the dental work you need. Now make an unforgettable mental note of just where that hypersensitive left hand is, and turn your head and let the dentist go to work."

The patient turned his head, fearfully voiced a plea that the dentist be careful of his left hand, and, comforted by the dentist's reassurance, opened his mouth in complete readiness.

The facial flush and the perspiration had vanished. It was noted that his left hand was flushed and perspiring. The dentist then took charge completely and, by means of posthypnotic suggestions, convinced the patient that each time he sat in the dental chair, he would develop left-handed hyperesthesia so that his dental work could be done. At no time was any oral anesthesia ever suggested.

The rationale of this approach is rather clear and simple. The patient was rigidly fixated on the idea that a painful hypersensitivity must inevitably accompany dentistry. Attempts at oral anesthesia fixated his attention on oral sensations. Acceptance of his neurotic belief and employing it to create hypnotically an area of extreme hypersensitivity met his need to be able to experience pain without having to do so. Thus all pain expectation was centered in his hand, resulting in an anesthesia of the rest of his body, including his mouth.

On the occasion of the termination of the last dental visit, the dentist tested the patient for pain sensitivity elsewhere in his body and found that a general surgical anesthesia existed.

This second case represents the hypnotic utilization, with an augmentation of it, of the actual barrier to the patient's capacity to develop the needful manifestation that he wished. It is true that the logic of the entire procedure is decidedly specious, but it must be borne in mind that the patient's total attitudinal set was equally specious. Cold hard logic, presentation of scientific facts, any sensible reasonable approach would have been useless. Utilizing the patient's own neurotic irrationality to affirm and confirm a simple extension of his neurotic fixation relieved him of all unrecognized unconscious needs to defend his neuroticism against all assaults. A systematic analysis of exactly what kind of thinking the patient brought into the office led readily to the solution of his problem. This same sort of situation existed in the third case to be cited immediately.

CASE REPORT 3

A thrice-divorced young woman sought psychiatric help "for just one problem, that's all, and I will tell you the problem right away, but I don't want any treatment for anything else. That you must promise me."

The gist of her story was that at age 18 she had impulsively married a handsome and, as she discovered later, dissolute man of 25 very much against parental wishes. The wedding night she discovered that he was a secret alcoholic, and the attempted consummation of the marriage in his state of intoxication was a hideous travesty to her. He blamed her entirely, berated her unmercifully, described her rudely as "having a refrigerated derrière," left her alone, and spent the night with a prostitute. Nevertheless, she continued to live with him hopefully despite his continued use of the description that he had bestowed on her the first night. After some months of wretched effort to prove to him that she was a woman of normal sexuality, she secured a divorce, secretly fearing that he was correct in his appraisal of her lack of sexuality.

A year later, in an overcompensatory effort to avoid the kind of trouble she had encountered in her first marriage, she married a highly effeminate man whose latent homosexuality disclosed itself on their wedding night by his horrified aversion to her body. His reason for marrying her, since she did have some wealth in her own name, was to secure "proper social standing in the community." He was completely outraged and incensed by her "indecent haste" to consummate the marriage and administered a rather rigidly prim reprimand. He spent the night, as she learned later, with a male friend who helped him bemoan his unfortunate plight. Her reaction was one of complete self-blame, no understanding of her husband's actual sexuality, and she succeeded in convincing herself that he had applied the same derogatory description of her as had her first husband. The marriage continued for nearly a year, chiefly by virtue of the fact that he spent most of his nights at his mother's apartment. An actual attempt at consummation after about four months proved to be only a revolting experience for him and a conviction, because of her entire lack of response to him, that she was absolutely lacking in sexual feelings.

After they finally got a divorce, she secured employment and gave up any hope of a normal life. After about two years, while living a very sheltered, retiring life, she met by chance a man five years her senior who was successfully engaged in an exciting, but to soberer minds, a somewhat questionable, promotional activity in real estate. His charm, his easily likeable personality, his knowledge of the world, his attentiveness and courtesy led her to make a third venture into matrimony.

They were married in the morning and then went to an expensive suite in a hotel in a nearby town, where he spent the day with her presenting innumerable plausible reasons in an effort to persuade her to turn over to him all of her property for him "to develop," thus to secure larger returns.

As he presented his arguments with increasing persuasiveness but with no display of emotional interest in her, a recollection of the beginnings of her first marriage raised sickening doubts in her mind. Her husband, becoming impatient with her slowness to accept his arguments, suddenly noted the horrified, doubting expression on her face. Infuriated, he threw her on the bed and had violent intercourse with her while he denounced her for her lack of response, ridiculed her, told her how he had spent the previous night with a responsive prostitute; he finally walked out on her "to find someone who didn't have what my first husband said I had." A divorce was promptly secured by her.

Now she was interested in a young man who met the approval of her lawyer, her banker, her parents, her minister, and her friends. She desperately wanted to marry him, yet was equally desperate in her desire not to cause him any unhappiness. Her purpose in seeking psychiatric aid was to have her "deficiency corrected." With extreme embarrassment, in plain simple Anglo-Saxon so that there could be no possibility of any misunderstanding by the author, she made matters painfully clear. She wanted, no more, no less, the chill she felt continuously, no matter what she wore, no matter how warm the seat she sat on, to be removed from her buttocks. This wretchedly cold feeling had been present, painfully present, since the first evening of her third marriage. The prompt dissolution of that marriage had not lessened the feeling of a subjectively recognizable coldness that had developed following the third husband's devastating criticism of her. This had plagued her continuously, and she found herself to be too embarrassed to seek medical aid. Recently, in night school courses she was taking, she had read about hypnosis, hypnotic phenomena, and hypnotherapy. Seeing the author's name given as a reference, she had come to Arizona for immediate, direct, and specific therapy.

Her desire for therapy was almost irrational in its intensity. She was convinced of the circumscribed character of her problem and could not even listen to any attempted exposition of the general character of her difficulties. She was rigidly certain that once the "coldness" was removed, all would be well. She asserted an absolute willingness to cooperate in any way to achieve her goal of a slightly elevated temperature in place of the gluteal coldness. In the desperateness of her desire for help it was not possible for her to see the humorous effect of her use of vulgar language to ensure the author's exact understanding of her problem in terms of the exact words that had been used to describe it to her originally.

After a laborious three-hour effort to secure her interest in the author's views, it became apparent that therapy would have to be accomplished, if possible at all, in full accord with her persistent demands.

Much speculative thought was given to the content of her limited understandings to devise some kind of therapeutic approach. Since she wanted hypnosis desperately, she became an easy somnambulistic subject, as is sometimes the case with this type of patient. Indeed, she was one of the most receptive and amenable subjects the author has encountered, and she agreed readily to accept and act upon any hypnotic suggestion given her. The specious explanation given her was that, since she wanted her problem corrected by hypnosis, it was requisite that she be thoroughly trained in all hypnotic phenomena so that every possible necessary hypnotic element requisite for her cure would be experientially known to her. Actually, the real purpose was to develop in her a receptiveness, a responsiveness, a feeling of complete acceptance, and a willingness to execute adequately any suggestion offered her.

The next step was to ask her to make a systematic study by filling her bathtub with water of increasingly higher temperature until the water was hot enough to produce goose bumps on her legs, which were the only part of her to be immersed in the bathtub. After much labor she succeeded in achieving this. She was then presented with a laboriously detailed explanation of how an overloading of the thermal receptors by excessive warmth would overflow into the cold receptors of the skin, thereby resulting in gooseflesh. The success of this venture, in the author's opinion, played a large part in the successful therapy. It supplied her with indisputable visual proof that heat can produce the concomitants of coldness and that this could be done in a definitely limited area of the body. From that point on there existed for her no doubts or fears of the author's understandings or competence.

Therapy was then continued by inducing a deep trance and by carefully worded suggestions, making her feel privately—a feeling just to be enjoyed within herself—an exaggerated, utterly intense, and inordinate pride in having the secret knowledge shared only with me that at least a part of her body could experience heat by a subjective cold response. Thus, by repetitious suggestion it was emphatically impressed upon her that this must always and forever be regarded as her own private pleasurable joy. The reason for this secrecy was to intensify her feeling and to preclude any disparagement by anyone in whom she might confide.

Then, bit by bit, suggestions were cautiously given her that, just as her calves had developed cold receptor responses to heat, so could the cold receptors of her thighs, of her buttocks, and her abdomen. Her acceptance of these ideas was ensured by a sudden shift to a discussion of the "thrills and tingles of complete happiness and ecstatic joy that race so delightfully up and down the spine of the little girl who receives the new dolly so desperately wanted and never really expected."

This complex idea was impressed upon her with much repetition and with careful changes in the key words of "thrills" and "tingles" by making the phrase "thrills and chills and tingles" and then in a random fashion omitting one and then another of the three words. Also, since she came from a northern state and had a reasonably happy childhood, the "tingling delights of sledding down hill on a tinglingly cold day," "the rapturous joys of a cold, cold dish of ice cream on a hot summer's day," and similar plays on words associated with pleasures safely remote in her history, were woven into a whole series of suggestions.

This was repeated for a number of sessions, always impressing upon her the need for an unconscious retention of the ideas, the need to incorporate them, and everything else she had been taught in therapy, into the warp and woof of her very existence, and yet to keep the knowledge of all this safely secret forever from her conscious mind, just knowing in some vague and satisfying way that she possessed within her a knowledge and an understanding of a personal value, beauty, and happiness.

Very rapidly there occurred a marked change in her general behavior. The tension, the urgency, the overall anxiety disappeared; she went for long scenic drives, and she began speaking of visiting Phoenix again.

Then one day she entered the office hesitantly, diffidently, blushing deeply and keeping her eyes downcast. After about 15 minutes, almost in the voice of a small child, she asked, "Can I tell you a secret, a very important secret that's all mine, my special secret that belongs all to me?" The reply given her was, "I think that if you think it over very carefully, you will find that you probably can tell your psychiatrist because he will understand."

After another seven minutes she said softly, "I've got to tell it in a special way that I know you will understand. It's what I said when I first came to you, only it's all different now." Then, in completely vulgar terms, with many blushes, she stated in essence, "I like being a frozen-posteriored creature."

To the author that signified that she needed no further therapy, and the years that have passed, her successful fourth marriage, her completion of college during the first years of this marriage, and her subsequent entrance happily into the pleasures of motherhood have all confirmed the success of therapy.

And what was her problem? An impulsive marriage in the best of good faith, but a wretchedly mistaken marriage as she immediately discovered; a second mistaken marriage to correct the trauma of the first, promptly discovered to be another mistake that was slowly corrected only so far as the marital state was concerned, but with only an intensification of her traumas; a third desperate marriage entered in good faith to correct, if possible, the injuries of the past, which only resulted in further injury. Then came the acute realization of her therapeutic needs when a genuinely good marriage presented itself.

And what was her therapy? An unhappy succession of events had progressively emphasized the trauma centering about a vital need in her life, her fulfillment as a woman. These events had degraded her in her own eyes and had led her unconsciously to summarize her total unhappiness in a circumscribed way. Then she sought circumscribed therapy, only circumscribed therapy. This was presented to her in such a fashion that, even as she had circumscribed everything, she was in a position to enlarge properly her whole problem. Her thinking about her problem had been emotionally repressed, largely at an unconscious level. Her therapy permitted her to do the same type of thinking but to include in it not only the events leading to her problem but the emotional values dating all the way back to her childhood. Then, once she had achieved her goals, at the level of unconscious motivation she felt compelled to verbalize her original presenting complaint but with a totally different meaning and perspective. By doing this she freed herself from any dependency upon the therapist and then could go her way, finding her own proper goals in life.

CONCLUDING COMMENT

These three different case histories are presented to illustrate the importance in therapy of doing what appears to be most important to the patient, that which constitutes an expression of the distorted thoughts and emotions of the patient. The therapist's task should not be a proselytizing of the patient with his own beliefs and understandings. No patient can really understand the understandings of his therapist nor does he need them. What is needed is the development of a therapeutic situation permitting the patient to use his own thinking, his own understandings, his own emotions in the way that best fits him in his scheme of life.

Each of the patients reported on has no real understanding of what their therapist thinks, knows, believes, likes, or dislikes. They know primarily that in some peculiar way they began to unsnarl their lives in a fashion as inexplicable as was the fashion in which they had once snarled their thinking and their emotions.

21. Hypnosis in Obstetrics: Utilizing Experiential Learnings

Milton H. Erickson

To present in 20 minutes the subject of hypnosis in obstetrics is a rather difficult task. However, I shall assume that my major obligation is to present to you certain general considerations and then to rely upon your own interests and desires for more detailed information which will lead you into further exploration of this topic.

I shall begin by defining hypnosis, as one needs to understand it in a clinical sense. It is a state of consciousness—not unconsciousness or sleep—a state or consciousness or awareness in which there is a marked receptiveness to ideas and understandings and an increased willingness to respond either positively or negatively to those ideas.

It derives from processes and functionings within the patient. The operator is merely someone who can offer intelligent advice and instruction to the patient and thus elicit from the patient the behavioral responses best fitted to the situation.

Hypnosis is not some mystical procedure, but rather a systematic utilization of experiential learnings—that is, the extensive learnings acquired through the process of living itself. For example, mention may be made of hypnotic anesthesia, or hypnotic amnesia, but these are no more than learnings of everyday living utilized in an orderly, controlled, and directed fashion. For example, nearly everyone has had the experience of losing a painful headache during a suspense movie without medication of any sort. Similarly, everyone has developed an anesthesia for the sensation of shoes on the feet, glasses on the face, and a collar around the neck.

Comparably we all know how effectively the news of the sudden, unexpected death of a loved one can instantly destroy a ravenous appetite or even completely arrest the physiological processes of digestion already under way.

All of us have a tremendous number of these generally unrecognized psychological and somatic learnings and conditionings, and it is the intelligent use of these that constitutes an effectual use of hypnosis.

In obstetrics, as in no other field of medicine, the patient occupies a dominant role for months as an individual undergoing an extensive

Unpublished manuscript, circa 1950s.

progressive alteration, not only somatically but psychologically, in all personal, social, economic and temporal relationships. Hence, there comes into play throughout pregnancy, as well as delivery, a multitude of forces deriving from the personality as a whole and from the special attitudes, beliefs, understandings, learnings, and conditionings acquired during the patient's lifetime.

The history of obstetrics is marked by a continual striving to introduce into the delivery room various procedures intended to facilitate delivery and to render it a pleasing experience both to the patient and to the physician. Medications of many varieties, surgical procedures, and mechanical aids have all been introduced from time to time, with various acclaims, but the obstetrician's search for improved methodologies still continues with an awareness that the search should embrace every avenue of understanding and not be restricted to a further development of just one field of understanding.

It is for this reason that there is a growing interest in the use of hypnosis in obstetrics. The slow progressive development of psychosomatic medicine since the 1920s, and the many experimental and clinical studies demonstrating effectively the extensive interrelationships between the mental functioning of the individual and his physiological processes, have now served to make many people aware that a business worry or a hysterical fear can manifest itself in a stomach ulcer, colitis, chronic backache, or migrainous headaches—just to cite common examples.

Against this general background of the general understandings derived from psychosomatic medicine, hypnosis is gaining increasing acceptance in obstetrics as a significant scientific methodology. And it is gaining that acceptance not because it is a mystical art or a dramatic procedure of thrusting needles through tissues and suggesting, "arms as rigid as iron bars." Instead, it is gaining acceptance because of its valuable ability to enlist as fully as possible the patient's own capabilities and potentialities at both psychological and physiological levels of functioning.

It matters not whether the use of hypnosis in obstetrics is called psychosomatic obstetrics, or systematic education of the mother in childbirth as a normal physiological process, or the *Grantley Dick Read Method of Childbirth Without Fear,* or progressive psychosomatic relaxation, or simply hypnosis in obstetrics. The essential consideration is the enlistment of the expectant mother as an adequately responsive participant in a normal physiological process of great personal and social significance.

Now the questions arise:

1. At what time, or when, does one use hypnosis in obstetrics?
2. Who can be hypnotized?
3. What are the dangers?

4 What type of case warrants its use?
5. How is it done?
6. Where can a knowledge of hypnotic techniques be obtained?
7. What specifically can hypnosis accomplish, both generally and in individual cases?
8. And finally, just what excuse is there for using hypnosis when there are many other methods?

To take up the last question first, whenever there is a wealth of remedies for any one condition, their inadequacy is thereby signified. For example, each week a new tranquilizer comes on the market, guaranteed to cure everything, until replaced by next week's preparation with the same claims.

But more seriously, the real need for introducing hypnosis into the obstetrical field is the opportunity it offers to secure from the patient full, earnest, happy, and confident cooperation with the physician during pregnancy, delivery, and the postpartum period. Anything that can effect good cooperation between patient and physician in achieving an important goal is worthy of consideration.

Perhaps the next question should concern the dangers of hypnosis.

In over 30 years of experimental and clinical work with hypnosis I have not been able to discover any harmful effects, nor have colleagues with extensive experience in the use of hypnosis reported any to me—despite repeated inquiries. I do know that people of little and even no experience with hypnosis will gladly tell all manner of tales about the harmfulness of hypnosis, sometimes even believing the tales themselves. And I do know that stupid or uninformed people sometimes use hypnosis in the wrong way, but any harm that results comes not from the hypnosis, but from the mistaken or misdirected behavior associated with hypnosis.

As for the next question—who can be hypnotized—the answer is simply that any normal person and some abnormal persons can be hypnotized, provided there is adequate motivation. In pregnancy there is usually a great deal of motivation to achieve a delivery and a postpartum recovery of a most pleasing sort, hence the motivation among informed obstetrical patients is high.

As for the question of where one can learn medical hypnosis, I can state emphatically, in agreement with the AMA recommendations, that it can best be learned and should only be learned under medical, or dental, or psychological auspices. There are instructors who are reputable and competent clinicians as well as teachers; they can meet the needs of physicians interested in hypnosis as a professional methodology. Instruction by quacks, stage hypnotists, charlatans who brag about being the world's fastest hypnotists, and the numerous variously named American Institutes of Accredited Hypnotists, are all to be avoided in the same way a physician would avoid taking instruction in physical examination from a chiropractor. Medical teaching properly should always be on a high ethical and professional level, and the stage hypnotist or the charlatan with no degree or with a diploma-mill degree does not qualify.

As for the appropriate time at which to use hypnosis in obstetrics, the answer is that some obstetricians prefer the last trimester, some the first trimester, but actually it should be a matter of clinical choice and judgment. If employed only for the delivery and postpartum period, the third trimester is adequate time.

However, it is only reasonable to employ hypnosis to meet the problems of nausea and vomiting and weight gain during pregnancy, since the patient's full cooperation in all regards is desired, and hypnosis is a method of securing that full cooperation and participation.

As for the type of case warranting the use of hypnosis, the answer is simply any case in which you wish full, free, and easy cooperation to the patient's fullest capacity. Such cases range from the mother who is happily anticipating her child to the anxious, tense, hysterically fearful woman who dreads the entire experience and who consequently needs special care and attention.

As for the final question—what specifically can hypnosis do in general and in the individual case?—the comprehensive reply can be offered that it enables a woman to undergo her pregnancy, her delivery, and the postpartum period in that fashion most nearly in accord with her needs and her psychological and physiological capabilities.

It is not in any way a replacement for other obstetrical procedures, but it is a scientific adjunct that serves greatly to reduce the need for some other medical procedures. For example, while in some cases hypnosis may produce complete anesthesia, in others it serves primarily to reduce extensively the amount of medication or chemoanesthesia required. But primarily hypnosis serves to permit the patient to cooperate much more adequately with her physician and to participate more satisfactorily.

Whether the patient is in a light trance, a medium trance, or a deep trance, the following general effects can be achieved.

1. The patient can be taught physical relaxation, adjustment to progressive changes in physical sensations and alterations, and a feeling of comfort and well-being, so desirable in pregnancy.
2. Weight changes, nausea and vomiting, and fear and anxiety states are much more adequately handled.
3. An attitude of cooperation and understanding can be developed, with greater trust and confidence in the physician and his or her competence.
4. The patient can be taught, in accord with her actual capacities to learn, an anesthesia or an analgesia or an amnesia for the

discomfort of labor, and thus she can enter the delivery room and participate at a full level of awareness, and do so enjoyably, in the actual experience of childbirth.

5. The patient's behavior during the postpartum period can be directed toward the promotion of sleep, physical comfort, freedom from anxiety, and feelings of physical comfort and well-being.

6. The patient's breast behavior and her attitudes and anxieties in this regard can be handled more adequately.

To summarize, obstetrics is a branch of medicine that centers around a patient-physician relationship extending over a period of many months and involving a physiological process of profound psychological significance and paramount in importance to the patient. Hypnosis, facilitating as it does a receptiveness and a responsiveness to ideas, is of value in every aspect wherein instruction, advice, counsel, guidance, direction, reassurance, comfort, and all those manifold values of interpersonal relationships are so significant.

22. A Therapeutic Double Bind Utilizing Resistance

Milton H. Erickson

A 12-year-old boy, 5 feet 10 inches tall and weighing 170 pounds, was brought almost forcibly into the office by his irate and despairing parents. He was described as sullen, rebellious, stubborn, hardheaded, uncooperative, self-willed, lazy, and a chronic bed-wetter. They explained that he had had a wet bed every day of his life and that they had reached the absolute limit of their patience in attempting every known method of curing him other than taking him to a psychiatrist. They now wished to turn the forbidding task over to the writer, and they would be willing to limit their participation to a simple morning inspection of his bed. They were promptly instructed to relegate this task entirely to the household maid.

Systematic questioning disclosed the following information: The father was an inch taller and 10 pounds heavier than his son. The father's interests were restricted to his business and to philosophical reading. The mother was a demanding woman, interested in drama and club work. She was an inch shorter than her son, but equalled his weight. The boy's interests were negligible. He had no interest in athletics nor in such groups as the Boy Scouts, nor did he seem to have any friends. He enjoyed comic books and "eating." He usually spent the weekends "forgetting" to do either his schoolwork or his assigned chores at home. He was not interested in schoolwork, was content with poor grades, and expressed the hope that he would not have to go to high school. He spent his summers swimming—a skill at which he was most proficient.

As the first measure of therapy, the parents were instructed to relinquish completely all interest in the therapy of their son for a period of at least six months—to make no inquiry or show interest in any way. To this they readily agreed.

TRANCE INDUCTION UTILIZING RESISTANCE

The boy was then invited into the office. He expressed an unwillingness for an interview and offered the statement that he was "tired enough to go

Unpublished manuscript, 1952.

to sleep" and that he would rather go home. Reply was made that he could defeat the purpose of the office interview by deliberately going to sleep and not listening to what the writer had to say. He accepted this as a challenge and proved to be an excellent hypnotic subject to the rather simple testing of suggestion—"Just go to sleep, just don't listen to me; you can sleep restfully and comfortably, even if I do talk"—and similar such suggestions until a deep trance was secured.

He was then instructed that he did not need to bother to listen, but that he could understand everything that was said to him; however, he would nonetheless sleep restfully and comfortably. Thus it became possible to meet both his personal needs and those of the therapeutic situation. An explanation was then offered that because of his parents it would be necessary to see him repeatedly, but that the writer would try to make it as infrequent as possible.

Therapy was then begun by stating that his parents had demanded that the writer correct the bed-wetting problem, but that the parents were regarded as somewhat unreasonable in this matter. The conclusions were elaborated in the following fashion, while he continued in a deep trance:

> Your parents want you to have a permanently dry bed right away, and that is simply unreasonable. In the first place, you have been too darned busy to bother to learn to have a dry bed. You have a great big beautiful frame, with great big powerful muscles to handle it. Your chassis is one that took a lot of energy to build and it is almost as big as your father's and you are only 12 years old. It took an awful lot of energy to build a body as big and strong as that one you've got, and you didn't have any energy left over for such unimportant things as a dry bed or mowing grass or being a teacher's pet. But you will soon be full-grown, bigger than your father, and you haven't got far to go to beat him. Then you'll have all that energy and horsepower you have been putting into growing to spread around to the other things you want, like a permanently dry bed. In fact, you are so close to being finished with building that great big powerful body that you've probably already got extra energy to spare.
>
> But let's get it straight. I don't think it's reasonable to expect you to have a permanently dry bed this month—it's only the first part of January. I don't even expect you to have just one dry bed this week. That's too darned soon. It's not reasonable. But what puzzles me is whether you will have a dry bed next week on Wednesday or on Thursday. I don't know and you don't know and we'll have to wait to find out, and that is a long wait because today is only Monday of this week and you really won't know

until Friday of next week whether you will have a dry bed on
Wednesday or Thursday of next week.

The double-bind suggestions were variously worded and repeated in the
above verbose casual manner, thus to ensure the patient's acceptance of
them and to avoid any resistance on his part.

The suggestions were continued: "You can come in next Friday and let
me know whether it was Wednesday or Thursday, and you will just have
to wait and see."

On the specified Friday he entered the office to report happily that he
had had a dry bed on both Wednesday and Thursday.

The discouraging remark was made to him, "Let's be reasonable about
this. You just can't expect to have that happen again too soon. It just isn't
reasonable to expect you to begin to have a permanently dry bed this
month, even if January is a long month."

The patient looked first troubled and then rebellious at these comments, as he settled back resentfully in his chair and looked away from the
writer. Comment was offered that he probably felt tired enough to sleep,
and a new trance was promptly induced by the original technique.

On this occasion posthypnotic suggestions were carefully given to
ensure ready trance development with the minimum of time expenditure.
Also, instruction was given for him to have a general amnesia for all office
events but a ready understanding and recall of everything necessary in the
office. Therapeutic suggestions were continued:

It really was interesting to wait and see whether it was Wednesday
or Thursday, but you were sure surprised when Thursday came
along with another dry bed. A nice surprise, too, but it can't
always happen yet—it's too darned soon.

Of course, I don't know when your next batch of dry beds will
come along, this month or early in February, but it's too soon for
your permanently dry bed in January, and February is a short
month. So, what puzzles me is will your permanently dry bed
begin on St. Patrick's Day or on April 1st, which is April Fool's
Day, or on any day between March 17th and April 1st. But let's
get it straight. Whatever day your permanently dry bed begins is
strictly your business. It is none of my business. That just belongs
to you as your own private business, and even though I would like
to know if it's St. Patrick's Day or April Fool's Day, or any day in
between, it is still strictly none of my business and even though I
want to know, don't tell me. That's something that just belongs to
you.

The above double-bind suggestions were reiterated in various ways to ensure his acceptance of the idea that only the date was in doubt, not the actuality of the permanently dry bed.

Thereafter the patient was seen at irregular intervals. Double-bind suggestions were variously employed to reinforce the general ideas already given and to emphasize the purported rationale of the argument originally presented to the patient. There was no direct seeking of information, nor were direct therapeutic suggestions given. After the first two sessions the interviews tended to be casual, friendly boy-man conversations, rather than doctor-patient interviews. Occasionally a trance state was induced for some "extra sleep just to spread that extra energy around."

The weeks of March and April passed with neither comment nor inquiry, but a carefully worded telephone inquiry of the household maid late in April disclosed that there had been a continuously dry bed for some weeks. Early in May the patient, during a casual conversation, commented that one of his friends was a bed-wetter and that he would like to help this friend, and would the writer be willing to see that boy professionally? This indirect communication was the one and only reference made to the original problem. The patient is still a personal friend, has become a most successful college student, and from time to time refers bed-wetters for therapy.

23. Utilizing the Patient's Own Personality and Ideas: "Doing It His Own Way"

Milton H. Erickson

A newly married 22-year-old man entered the office with the specific request that he be hypnotized and his practice of irresponsible, reckless driving be corrected. He added, however, that he doubted that he could be hypnotized and that he even had doubts about the need to alter his driving. His reason for the latter belief was his long experience in stunt driving, in which he had learned to wreck cars deliberately and to emerge unscathed. The only current justification for changing his driving behavior was the fact that he always took his wife with him, but even so, his car was in good condition, and his confidence in his ability to meet any driving hazard was unlimited. He denied any other reason for his visit and was explicit in his demand that the writer limit himself to the stated purpose.

TRANCE INDUCTION AND POSTHYPNOTIC SUGGESTION

The patient developed a fairly deep trance, affirmed his need to change his driving behavior, explained that he averaged around 90 miles an hour on the straightaway, and often reached speeds of 70 to 90 miles on mountain roads. When he was asked what he wished the writer to do, he explained that the writer could do nothing at all, that he himself would have to quit speeding, and that he would have to do it his own way, and only in his own way. He explained further that nothing that the writer could do or say would help, but that he did want help in some way from the writer.

Accordingly, he was asked how soon he wished to drive sensibly and in accord with the legal limits. His reply was that it was now early April and that by the first of May he should be driving properly. He was then asked to explain what he thought he would have to do. He merely repeated his previous statement that he would have to quit in his own way.

This statement was seized upon and repeated to him in various

---

Unpublished manuscript, 1954.

wordings as a posthypnotic suggestion, but without altering the meaning. This was done repetitiously in a most insistent, compelling manner. This acceptance of a patient's declaration and turning it back upon him in the form of posthypnotic suggestions is often a most effective therapeutic procedure. It gives the patient a feeling of being committed to his own intentions and wishes, and intensifies his ability to act accordingly, without a feeling that he is being forced to accept proferred help. For a patient as independent-minded as this young man, it was of crucial importance to *utilize his own ideas* rather than attempt to impose those of the therapist.

He was awakened with the suggestion that nothing sufficiently important for conscious recollection had been said. Upon awakening he commented that he probably was too difficult to hypnotize, that his own request for help appeared rather useless, and that obviously it was up to him to do it his own way. Regretfully he took his departure.

Two weeks later he appeared at the office to report that he was "still driving like a fool" and taking his wife with him on all his trips. He added that, somehow, he would have to quit in his own way. Again he left reluctantly.

Two weeks later he reported again, this time jubilant, declaring that he had handled things in his own way. His story was that the previous week, on his day off, he had overhauled his car completely with the aid of a friend. When this task was finished, he announced to his wife that he was taking a ride over a certain mountain road she had frequently asked him to travel. However, he refused to take her or his friend. Ten miles down the road he came to a long stretch of reasonably straight road. Immediately he decided to have a final fling at speeding and rejoiced at such an opportunity to do it without making his wife frightened. He reached the speed of 90 miles an hour, but before he came to the end of the open stretch, he discovered that he was losing control of the car. Before he could formulate any ideas, he realized that he would have to abandon the car. He succeeded in leaping out of it, suffering only minor bruises in so doing, just before it hurtled down the mountainside.

The long walk back home was spent in repetitious thinking of, "You've done it your own way." He explained what he had done to his wife, and later purchased another car which he began driving safely and within legal limits. Three months later he dropped into the office casually to comment that he was still driving safely. To this he added it had been rather expensive for him to do it in his own way and that he had merely wasted his time and money seeing the writer, except that possibly the writer had given him some psychological impetus.

IV. Hypnotherapeutic Approaches to Pain

We have seen how Erickson's personal life experience led him to develop the "naturalistic methods" of pain resolution with hypnosis (see "Autohypnotic Experiences of Milton H. Erickson" in Volume One of this series). Pain relief through hypnosis is simply an extension and utilization of many natural life experiences that diminsh or completely obliterate the subjective experience of pain. In many talks and workshops Erickson has expressed this point as follows:

"Pain is a phenomenon with which human beings have frequent, extensive, and greatly diversified experiences, but as a phenomenon in itself pain is little understood by scientists or laymen. We know that it is a subjective experience that need not necessarily be present even though there can be adequate physiological evidence that it should be a most noticeable psychological experience of the moment. Conversely, we know that pain can be most excruciatingly experienced even though there has been no organic, physiological basis, having only a psychological stimulus as its origin.

"To illustrate these various points, the following instances may be cited. The soldier, in the excitement of battle, may discover only later that he has been wounded severely. Upon discovering this fact, he reacts with appropriate pain. Yet that pain can be less than he would have experienced if he were aware that such injury was shortly to be inflicted. We know that pain originating from observable physical injury can be forgotten and even lost by the development of an intense, absorbing interest in something else, by the simple distraction of attention, or by the introduction—either accidentally or intentionally—of an irrelevant, confusing, or even amusing external stimulation.

"An example is the psychologically oriented patient suffering a fresh third degree burn of the right hand who "forgot" or "lost" the intense pain when confronted with the intriguing (to him) problem of devising simple and reliable tests of right- or left-thumbedness. There is also the pain of cancer, which can be excruciatingly severe and unresponsive to powerful analgesic drugs, but completely responsive to a horror picture on the TV.

"Then there is, finally, the example of the patient with severe body burns, who was suffering extensive pain and was about to be transferred out of the general ward because of his continued low moaning. Suddenly, an illiterate 40-year-old man, totally unacquainted with and completely frightened by hospital procedures, began running wildly about the ward in an open-backed hospital gown, trailing an enema bag and pursued by a nurse and an orderly. The patient with the severe burns burst into laughter and laughed, as he explained, until he "hurt all over." Then he asked with surprise what had happened to his burn pains, as the mere recall of that ludicrous sight proved to be analgesic. He was not the only patient on the ward who found that scene and its recollection a satisfying analgesic."

All the papers of this section are essentially explorations of how the hypnotherapist utilizes these naturalistic pathways to facilitate pain relief.

24. An Introduction to the Study and Application of Hypnosis for Pain Control

Milton H. Erickson

INTRODUCTION

Hypnosis is essentially a communication of ideas and understandings to a patient in such a fashion that he will be most receptive to the presented ideas and thereby motivated to explore his own body potentials for the control of his psychological and physiological responses and behavior. The average person is unaware of the extent of his capacities of accomplishment which have been learned through the experiential conditionings of this body behavior through his life experiences. To the average person in his thinking, pain is an immediate subjective experience, all-encompassing of his attention, distressing, and to the best of his belief and understanding, an experience uncontrollable by the person himself. Yet as a result of experiential events of his past life, there has been built up within his body—although all unrecognized—certain psychological, physiological, and neurological learnings, associations, and conditionings that render it possible for pain to be controlled and even abolished. One need only think of extremely crucial situations of tension and anxiety to realize that the severest of pain vanishes when the focussing of the sufferer's awareness is compelled by other stimuli of a more immediate, intense, or life-threatening nature. From common experience one can think of a mother suffering extremely severe pain and all-absorbed in her pain experience. Yet she forgets it without effort or intention when she sees her infant dangerously threatened or seriously hurt. One can think of men seriously wounded in combat who do not discover their injury until later. There are numerous such comparable examples common to medical experience. Such abolition of pain occurs in daily life in situations where pain is taken out of awareness by more compelling stimuli of another character. The simplest example of all is the toothache forgotten on the way to the dentist's office, or the headache lost in the suspenseful drama portrayed at the cinema. By such experiences as these in the course of a

Proceedings of the International Congress for Hypnosis and Psychosomatic Medicine, edited by J. Lassner Springer Verlag, Berlin, Heidelberg, New York. Reprinted with permission of Springer Verlag.

lifetime, be they major or minor, the body learns a wealth of unconscious psychological, emotional, neurological, and physiological associations and conditionings. These unconscious learnings, repeatedly reinforced by additional life experiences, constitute the source of the potentials that can be employed through hypnosis to control pain intentionally without resorting to drugs.

CONSIDERATIONS CONCERNING PAIN

While pain is a subjective experience with certain objective manifestations and accompaniments, it is not necessarily a conscious experience only. It occurs without conscious awareness in states of sleep, in narcosis, and even under certain types of chemoanesthesia as evidenced by objective accompaniments and as has been demonstrated by experimental hypnotic exploration of past experiences of patients. But because pain is primarily a conscious, subjective experience, with all manner of unpleasant, threatening, even vitally dangerous emotional and psychological significances and meanings, an approach to the problem it represents can be made frequently by hypnosis—sometimes easily, sometimes with great difficulty, and the extent of the pain is not necessarily a factor.

In order to make use of hypnosis to deal with pain, one needs to look upon pain in a most analytical fashion. Pain is not a simple, uncomplicated noxious stimulus. It has certain temporal, emotional, psychological, and somatic significance. It is a compelling motivating force in life's experience. It is a basic reason for seeking medical aid.

Pain is a complex, a construct, composed of past remembered pain, of present pain experience, and of anticipated pain of the future. Thus, immediate pain is augmented by past pain and is enhanced by the future possibilities of pain. The immediate stimuli are only a central third of the entire experience. Nothing so much intensifies pain as the fear that it will be present on the morrow. It is likewise increased by the realization that the same or similar pain was experienced in the past, and this and the immediate pain render the future even more threatening. Conversely, the realization that the present pain is a single event which will come definitely to a pleasant ending serves greatly to diminish pain. Because pain is a complex, a construct, it is more readily vulnerable to hypnosis as a modality of dealing successfully with it than it would be were it simply an experience of the present.

Pain as an experience is also rendered more susceptible to hypnosis because it varies in its nature and intensity, and hence, through life experiences, it acquires secondary meanings resulting in varying interpretations of the pain. Thus the patient may regard his pain in temporal terms, such as transient, recurrent, persistent, acute, or chronic. These special qualities each offer varying possibilities of hypnotic approaches.

Pain also has certain emotional attributes. It may be irritating, all-compelling of attention, troublesome, incapacitating, threatening, intractable, or vitally dangerous. Each of these aspects leads to certain psychological frames of mind with varying ideas and associations, each offering special opportunities for hypnotic intervention.

One must also bear in mind certain other very special considerations. Long continued pain in an area of the body may result in a habit of interpreting all sensations in that area as pain in themselves. The original pain may be long since gone, but the recurrence of that pain experience has been conducive to a habit formation that may in turn lead to actual somatic disorders painful in character.

Of a somewhat similar character are iatrogenic disorders and disease arising from a physician's poorly concealed concern and distress over his patient. Iatrogenic illness has a most tremendous significance because in emphasizing that if there can be psychosomatic disease of iatrogenic origin, it should not be overlooked that, conversely, iatrogenic health is fully as possible and of far greater importance to the patient. And since iatrogenic pain can be produced by fear, tensions, and anxiety, so can freedom from it be produced by the iatrogenic health that may be suggested hypnotically.

Pain as a protective somatic mechanism should not be disregarded as such. It motivates the patient to protect the painful areas, to avoid noxious stimuli, and to seek aid. But because of the subjective character of the pain, there develop psychological and emotional reactions to the pain experience that eventually result in psychosomatic disturbances from unduly prolonged protective mechanisms. These psychological and emotional reactions are amenable to modification and treatment through hypnosis in such psychosomatic disturbances.

To understand pain further, one must think of it as a neuro-psycho-physiological complex characterized by various understandings of tremendous significance to the sufferer. One need only to ask the patient to describe his pain to hear it variously described as dull, heavy, dragging, sharp, cutting, twisting, burning, nagging, stabbing, lancinating, biting, cold, hard, grinding, throbbing, gnawing, and a wealth of other such adjectival terms.

These various descriptive interpretations of the pain experience are of marked importance in the hypnotic approach to the patient. The patient who interprets his subjective pain experience in terms of various qualities of differing sensations is thereby offering a multitude of opportunities to the hypnotherapist to deal with the pain. To consider a total approach is possible, but more feasible is the utilization of hypnosis in relation first to minor aspects of the total pain complex and then to increasingly more severely distressing qualities. Thus, minor successes will lay a foundation for major successes in relation to the more distressing attributes of the neuro-psycho-physiological complex of pain, and the understanding and cooperation of the patient for hypnotic intervention are more readily elicited. Additionally, any hypnotic alteration of any single interpretive quality of the pain sensation serves to effect an alteration of the total pain complex.

Another important consideration in the matter of the understanding of the pain complex is the recognition of the experiential significances of various attributes or qualities of subjective sensation, and their differing relationships in such matters as remembered pain, past pain, immediate pain, enduring pain, transient pain, recurrent pain, enduring persistent pain, intractable pain, unbearable pain, threatening pain, etc. In applying these considerations to various of the subjective elements of the pain complex, hypnotic intervention is greatly accelerated. Such analysis offers greater opportunity for hypnotic intervention at a more understanding and comprehensive level. It becomes easier to communicate ideas and understandings through hypnosis and to elicit the receptiveness and responsiveness so vital in securing good response to hypnotic intervention. It is also important to recognize adequately the unrecognized force of the human emotional need to demand the immediate abolition of pain, both by the patient himself and by those in attendance on him. In hypnotic intervention there is a need to be aware of this and not to allow it to dominate a scientific hypnotic approach to the problem of pain.

HYPNOTIC PROCEDURES IN PAIN CONTROL

The hypnotic procedures in handling pain are numerous in character. The first of these, most commonly practiced but frequently not genuinely applicable is the use of *direct hypnotic suggestion for total abolition of pain.* With a certain limited number of patients, this is a most effective procedure. But too often it fails, serving to discourage the patient and to prevent further use of hypnosis in his treatment. Also, its effects, while they may be good, are sometimes too limited in duration, and this may limit the effectiveness of the *permissive indirect hypnotic abolition of pain.* This is often much more effective, and although essentially similar in character to direct suggestion, it is worded and offered in a fashion much more conducive of patient receptiveness and responsiveness.

A third procedure for hypnotic control of pain is the utilization of *amnesia.* In everyday life we see the forgetting of pain whenever more threatening or absorbing experiences secure the attention of the sufferer. An example is the instance already cited of the mother enduring extreme pain, seeing her infant seriously injured, and forgetting her own pain in the anxious fears about her child. Then of quite opposite psychological character is the forgetting of painful arthritis, headache, or toothache while watching an all-absorbing suspenseful drama on a cinema screen.

But amnesia in relationship to pain can be applied hypnotically in a great variety of ways. Thus one may employ partial, selective, or complete amnesias in relationship to selected subjective qualities and attributes of sensation in the pain complex as described by the patient as well as to the total pain experience.

A fourth hypnotic procedure is the employment of *hypnotic analgesia,* which may be partial, complete, or selective. Thus, one may add to the patient's pain experience a certain feeling of numbness without a loss of tactile or pressure sensations. The entire pain experience then becomes modified and different and gives the patient a sense of relief and satisfaction, even if the analgesia is not complete. The sensory modifications introduced into the patient's subjective experience by such sensations as numbness, an increase of warmth and heaviness, relaxation, etc., serve to intensify the hypnotic analgesia to an increasingly more complete degree.

Hypnotic anesthesia is a fifth method in treating pain. This is often difficult and may sometimes be accomplished directly, but is more often best accomplished indirectly by the building of psychological and emotional situations that are contradictory to the experience of the pain and which serve to establish an anesthetic reaction to be continued by posthypnotic suggestion.

A sixth hypnotic procedure useful in handling pain concerns the matter of suggestion to effect the *hypnotic replacement or substitution of sensations.* For example, one cancer patient suffering intolerable, intractable pain responded most remarkably to the suggestion of an intolerable, incredibly annoying itch on the sole of her foot. Her body weakness occasioned by the carcinomatosis and hence inability to scratch the itch rendered this psychogenic pruritis all-absorbing of her attention. Then hypnotically, there were systematically induced feelings of warmth, of coolness, of heaviness and of numbness for various parts of her body where she suffered pain. And the final measure was the suggestion of an endurable but highly unpleasant and annoying minor burning-itching sensation at the site of her mastectomy. This procedure of replacement substitution sufficed for the last six months of the patient's life. The itch of the sole of her foot gradually disappeared, but the annoying burning-itching at the site of her mastectomy persisted.

Hypnotic displacement of pain is a seventh procedure. This is the employment of a suggested displacement of the pain from one area of the body to another. This can be well illustrated by the instance of a man dying from prostatic metastatic carcinomatosis and suffering with intractable pain, particularly abdominal pain, in both the states of drug narcosis and deep hypnosis. He was medically trained and understood the concept of referred and displaced pain. In the hypnotic trance he readily accepted the idea that, while the intractable pain in his abdomen was the pain that would actually destroy him, he could readily understand that equal pain in his left hand could be entirely endurable, since in that location it would not have its threatening significances. He accepted the idea of referral of his abdominal pain to his left hand, and thus remained free of body pain and became accustomed to the severe pain in his left hand, which he protected carefully. This hand pain did not interfere in any way with his full contact with his family during the remaining three months of his life. It was disclosed that the displaced pain to the left hand often gradually diminished, but the pain would become increased upon incautious inquiry.

This possibility of displacement of pain also permits a displacement of various attributes of the pain that cannot otherwise be controlled. By this measure these otherwise uncontrollable attributes become greatly diminished. Thus the total complex of pain becomes greatly modified and made more amenable to hypnotic intervention.

Hypnotic dissociation can be employed for pain control, and the usual, most effective methods are those of *time and body disorientation*. The patient with pain intractable to both drugs and hypnosis can be hypnotically reoriented in time to the earlier stages of his illness, when the pain was of minor consideration. And the disorientation of that time characteristic of the pain can be allowed to remain as a posthypnotic continuation through the waking state. Thus the patient still has his intractable pain, but it has been rendered into a minor consideration, as it had been in its original stages.

One may sometimes successfully reorient the patient with intractable pain to a previous time predating his illness and, by posthypnotic suggestion, effect a restoring of the normal sensations existing before his illness. However, although intractable pain often prevents this as a total result, pleasant feelings predating his illness may be projected into the present to nullify some of the subjective qualities of his pain complex. Sometimes this effects a major reduction in pain.

In the matter of *body disorientation* the patient is hypnotically dissociated and induced to experience himself as apart from his body. Thus one woman with the onset of unendurable pain, in response to posthypnotic suggestions, would develop a trance state and experience herself as being in another room while her suffering body remained in her sickbed. This patient explained to the author when he made a bedside call, "Just before you arrived, I developed another horrible attack of pain. So I went into a trance, got into my wheelchair, came out into the living room to watch a television program, and left my suffering body in the bedroom." And she pleasantly and happily told about the fantasied television program she was watching. Another such patient remarked to her surgeon, "You know very well, Doctor, that I always faint when you start changing my dressings because I can't endure the pain, so if you don't mind, I will go into a hypnotic trance and take my head and feet and go into the solarium and leave my body here for you to work on." The patient further explained, "I took a position in the solarium where I could see him [the surgeon] bending over my body, but I could not see what he was doing. Then I looked out the window, and when I looked back he was gone, so I took my head and feet and went back and joined my body and felt very comfortable." This particular patient had been trained in hypnosis by the author many years previously, had subsequently learned autohypnosis, and thereafter induced her own autohypnotic trance by the phrase, "You know very well, Doctor." This was a phrase that she could employ verbally or mentally at any time and immediately go into a trance for the psychological-emotional experience of being elsewhere, away from her painful body, there to enjoy herself and remain until it was safe to return to her body. In this trance state, which she protected very well from the awareness of others, she would visit with her relatives, but experience them as with her in this new setting while not betraying that personal orientation.

A ninth hypnotic procedure in controlling body pain, which is very similar to replacement or substitution of sensations, is *hypnotic reinterpretation of pain experience.* By this is meant reinterpreting for the patient in hypnosis of a dragging, gnawing, heavy pain as a feeling of weakness, of profound inertia, and then as relaxation with the warmth and comfort that accompanies muscular relaxation. Stabbing, lancinating, and biting pains may sometimes be reinterpreted as sudden startle reactions, disturbing in character but momentary and not painful. Throbbing, nagging, grinding pain has been successfully reinterpreted as the unpleasant but not distressing experience of the rolling sensations of a boat during the storm, or even as the throbbing that one so often experiences from a minor cut on the fingertip and of a no greater distressing character. Full awareness of how the patient experiences pain is requisite for an adequate hypnotic reinterpretation of his pain sensation.

Hypnotic time distortion, first described by Cooper and then later developed by Cooper and Erickson (1959) is often a most useful hypnotic measure in pain control. An excellent example is that of the patient with intractable attacks of lancinating pain which occurred approximately every 20 to 30 minutes, night and day, and which lasted from five to 10 minutes. Between the attacks the patient's frame of mind was essentially one of fearful dread of the next attack. By employing hypnosis and teaching him time distortion, it was possible to employ, as is usually the case in every pain patient, a combination of several of the measures being described here. In the trance state the patient was taught to develop an amnesia for all past attacks of pain. He was then taught time distortion so that he could experience the five- to 10-minute pain episodes in 10 to 20 seconds. He was given posthypnotic suggestions to the effect that each attack would come as a complete surprise to him, that when the attack occurred, he would develop a trance state of 10 to 20 seconds' duration, experience all of the pain attack, and then come out of the trance with no awareness that he had been in a trance or that he had experienced pain. Thus the patient, in talking to his family, would suddenly and obviously go into the trance state with a scream of pain, and perhaps 10 seconds later come out of the trance state, look confused for a moment, and then continue his interrupted sentence.

An eleventh hypnotic procedure is that of offering *hypnotic suggestions effecting a diminution of pain,* but not a removal, when it has become apparent that the patient is not going to be fully responsive. This diminution is usually brought about best by suggesting to the hypnotized patient that his pain is going to diminish imperceptibly hour after hour without his awareness that it is diminished until perhaps several days have passed. He will then become aware of a definite diminution either of all pain or of special pain qualities. By suggesting that the diminution occur imperceptibly the patient cannot refuse the suggestion. His state of emotional hopefulness, despite his emotional despair, leads him to anticipate that in a few days there may be some diminution, particularly that there may be even a marked diminution of certain of the special attributes of his pain experience. This in itself serves as an autosuggestion to the patient. In certain instances, however, he is told that the diminution will be to a very minor degree. One can emphasize this by utilizing the ploy that a one percent diminution of his pain would not be noticeable, nor would a 2 percent, nor a 3 percent, nor a 4 percent, nor a 5 percent diminution, but that such an amount would nevertheless be a diminution. One can continue the ploy by stating that a 5 percent diminution the first day and an additional 2 percent the next day still would not be perceptible. And if on the third day there occurred a 3 percent diminution, this, too, would be imperceptible. But it would total a 10 percent diminution of the original pain. This same series of suggestions can be continued to a reduction of pain to 80 percent of its original intensity, then to 70 percent, 50 percent, 40 percent, and sometimes even down to 10 percent. In this way the patient may be led progressively into an ever greater control of his pain.

However, in all hypnotic procedures for the control of pain one bears in mind the greater feasibility and acceptability to the patient of indirect as compared with direct hypnotic suggestions, and the need to approach the problem by indirect and permissive measures and by the employment of a combination of various of the methodological procedures described above.

SUMMARY

Pain is a subjective experience, and it is perhaps the most significant factor in causing people to seek medical aid. Treatment of pain as usually viewed by both physician and patient is primarily a matter of elimination or abolition of the sensation. Yet pain in itself may be serving certain useful purposes to the individual. It constitutes a warning, a persistent warning of the need for help. It brings about physical restriction of activity, thus frequently benefitting the sufferer. It instigates physiological changes of a healing character in the body. Hence, pain is not just an undesirable sensation to be abolished, but rather an experience to be so handled that the sufferer benefits. This may be done in a variety of ways, but there is a tendency to overlook the wealth of psycho-neuro-physiological significances pain has for the patient. Pain is a complex, a construct composed of a great diversity of subjective interpretative and experiential values for the patient. Pain, during life's experience, serves to establish body leanings, associations, and conditionings that constitute a source of body potentials permitting the use of hypnosis for the study and control of pain. Hypnotic procedures, singly or in combination, for major or minor effects in the control of pain described for their application are: Direct Hypnotic Suggestion for Total Abolition of Pain; Permissive Indirect Hypnotic Abolition of Pain; Amnesia; Hypnotic Analgesia; Hypnotic Anesthesia; Hypnotic Replacement or Substitution of Sensations; Hypnotic Displacement of Pain; Hypnotic Dissociation; Reinterpretation of Pain Experience; Hypnotic Suggestions Effecting a Diminution of Pain.

25. The Therapy of a Psychosomatic Headache

Milton H. Erickson

INTRODUCTION

Too often, trite observations are made to disparage experimental findings. For example, a professor of internal medicine, after reading a psychiatric report upon a single patient, remarked that one case proves nothing. Reply was made that a single instance of an untried medication administered to only one patient with lethal results proved much more than could possibly be desired. The nature and character of a single finding can often be more informative and valuable than a voluminous aggregate of data whose meaning is dependent upon statistical manipulation. This is particularly true in the field of human personality where, although each individual is unique in all of his experiential life, single instances often illustrate clearly and vividly aspects and facets of general configurations, trends, and patterns. Rather than proof of specific ideas, an illustration or portrayal of possibilities is often the proper goal of experimental work.

In a comparable fashion another type of assumption places limitations unwarrantedly upon experimental findings. For example, many psychotherapists regard it as almost axiomatic that therapy is contingent upon making the unconscious conscious. When thought is given to the unmeasurable role that the unconscious plays in the total experiential life of a person from infancy on, whether awake or asleep, there can be little expectation of doing more than making some small parts of it conscious. Furthermore, the unconscious as such, not as transformed into the conscious, constitutes an essential part of psychological functioning. Hence, it seems more reasonable to assume that a legitimate goal in therapy lies in promoting an integrated functioning, both singly and together, and in complementary and supplementary relationships, as occurs daily in well-adjusted living in contrast to the inadequate, disordered, and contradictory manifestations in neurotic behavior.

Quoted from the *Journal of Clinical and Experimental Hypnosis* (October, 1953, *I* (4), 2-6). Copyright by The Society for Clinical and Experimental Hypnosis, 1953.

THE PATIENT

To illustrate the above considerations, the following case history is reported.

A professionally trained female employee of a state hospital was referred to the writer for therapy after extensive medical study. Her complaint was one of severe headaches, for which numerous medical studies had found no physical basis, and severe personality disturbances manifested in quarrelsomeness and uncooperativeness. At the time she was seen, she had been given notice of her discharge to take effect either immediately or, if she sought therapy from the writer, in six weeks' time.

Under these adverse circumstances, the patient sought out the writer, explained the situation bitterly, and declared that she was confronted with "the choice of wiring home for transportation money or being messed around with by a damn hypnotist." (The fact that the writer was wholly innocent of any part of her situation was totally disregarded by her.) She added ungraciously, "So here I am. What do you want? Go ahead."

An effort was made to secure her history, but she was uncommunicative and remained so throughout the course of therapy. The only material obtained was the following fragments:

For the past four years, beginning when she parted ties with her childhood home, she had been suffering from intense, unlocalized headaches. These sometimes occured twice a week and were accompanied by nausea, vomiting, and physical incapacitation from two to four hours' duration. Also they were always associated with intense, inexplicable emotional disturbances characterized by extreme quarrelsomeness, bitterness, and violent verbal attacks on everyone about her. Usually these emotional disturbances presaged the headaches, and upon recovery from that symptom she would remain seclusive, subdued, and somewhat socially adjusted for a day or two until the next attack.

Every attempt to secure more adequate information from her failed. She resented any questions or even casual conversation about herself. Also, she was embittered by the fact that she had been given notice of her impending discharge and only then had been referred for psychotherapy, "as if to make up for firing me."

This behavior of hers had caused her to lose one position after another as well as all of her friends and even the possibility of making new friends. Hence, she felt most lonely and wretched about her situation.

THERAPEUTIC PROCEDURE

She was unfriendly and uncooperative at the first interview and so was told only that hypnosis might possibly be of value but that it would first be necessary to see her during one of her headache seizures.

A few days later word was received that she was confined to bed with a sudden headache. She was found to be pale and drawn in appearance. She flinched whenever she moved her head or body, and was dazed, slow, and unresponsive in her general behavior.

A few hours later she was found recovered from her headache, spasmodic and excitable in her movements. She spoke in a high-pitched tone of voice, scolded and excoriated everybody, and seemed to take a sadistic delight in making cutting, painful remarks. She was most unwilling to discuss her condition, denounced the hypnotist, and demanded to be left alone. The next day her characteristic depressive reaction set in, and she was silent, seclusive, but would occasionally make self-condemnatory remarks.

A few days later, in a pleasant, affable mood, she approached the hypnotist spontaneously for hypnotic therapy. However, she dismissed all attempts at questioning, declaring politely but emphatically that her only problem was her headaches and that all therapy should be directed entirely to that one symptom. If this were done, she explained, her other difficulties would vanish, since they all derived from the headaches and her reactions to them.

Finally it became necessary to accept her on her own terms, with the mental reservation to resort to experimental measures.

Repeated attempts at hypnosis produced only light trances, but these were capitalized upon to secure her cooperation as a demonstration subject for a teaching clinic. By this measure it was possible to induce a profound trance in which she was given adequate training and instruction to permit the induction of profound trances in the future.

During the course of the next four weeks a total of 15 profound trances were induced. These trances were utilized to give repeatedly, emphatically, and insistently the following suggestions, until, more or less under duress, she accepted them and agreed to obey them:

1. Should a headache develop unexpectedly, or should she develop the irritability that experience had taught her presaged a headache, she was to go to bed at once and sleep soundly for at least half an hour. This, she was told repeatedly, would serve to abort either of the manifestations.

2. Following this half-hour of sleep she was then to spend at least an hour, preferably more, in mentally reviling, denouncing, condemning, and criticizing anybody and everybody she wished, giving free rein to her fantasies as she did so. This was to be done at first in obedience to the instructions given her, but sooner or later she was to carry out these instructions solely because of her own sadistic desires.

3. She was further told that, after she had secured adequate emotional satisfaction from these fantasied aggressions, she was to sleep soundly and restfully another half-hour. Then she might awaken and go about her work freely and comfortably with no need to "hate herself." This would be possible, it was explained, because obedience to the foregoing instructions would result in a hypnotic sleep that would persist until she finally awakened to go about her work in a rested, comfortable fashion. Of all this she would know only that she had gone to bed, fallen asleep, and had finally awakened feeling comfortable and rested in every way.

During the first three weeks the subject obeyed these instructions a half-dozen times by excusing herself from her work, returning to her room, and falling asleep. She would remain in this sleep from two to three hours and then rouse up and seem refreshed and comfortable. Several check-ups during periods when she was sleeping disclosed her to be in a trance state, but not in good rapport with the writer.

During the fourth week a new procedure was introduced. This was also in the form of a posthypnotic suggestion to the effect that on a certain day, at a specified hour, she was to develop a severe headache. As this developed, she was to fight against it and to persist in working until she could no longer stand it. Then she was to go hastily to her room and obey the first series of suggestions.

These instructions were carried out fully. At 1 P.M. on that day, three hours after her headache had begun, she returned to work, socially adjusted in a satisfactory fashion. Her only complaint was a comment on her ravenous hunger, since she had missed her lunch. On previous occasions such an event had often been seized upon to justify her irritability. Thus, she had been given experimental proof of the effectiveness of hypnotic suggestion and of the possibility of a good therapeutic response.

About a week later, in another trance state, she was given posthypnotic instructions to develop at a given time the emotional disturbance that often presaged a headache. As this developed, she was to resist it, to control her tongue except for a few disagreeable remarks, and finally to develop an overwhelming desire to return to her room, to which she would finally yield. There she was to follow the routine suggested previously.

All instructions were obeyed, and after nearly three hours of sleep she returned to her work in a pleasant frame of mind.

These two special trance sessions were purposely included in the course of therapeutic or instructive trances as a measure of forcing the subject to act responsively upon the earlier trance instructions. Subsequent trance states in which the suggestions cited above were given were augmented in force by reference to the experiential values of the posthypnotically induced headache and emotional disturbances and the benefits of following instructions.

In addition, every effort was made to impress upon her the future effectiveness of the general procedure and the desirability of yielding at once to the posthypnotic suggestions.

The last trance session was devoted to a general review of the instructions given to her, the posthypnotic disturbances suggested to her, her learned ability to meet the whole general problem, and the future applicability of the procedure in the event of further headaches and emotional disturbances.

Repeatedly during trance sessions efforts were made to learn the content of her thinking during the periods of mental aggression, but she proved uncommunicative. It was, she declared, "too terrible" to relate.

Questioning in the waking state disclosed her to have a complete amnesia for all except the superficial facts that she had been hypnotized repeatedly and that there had been a number of occasions on which she felt a headache developing, and that this had been warded off by a compulsive need to sleep. Every effort to secure additional data from her failed. She did attribute her change in behavior to the hypnosis, but was not curious about what had been done.

THE RESULTS

After leaving the hospital, she was not seen for three months. At the next meeting with her she related that she had only two threatened headaches, but had promptly warded them off with a little sleep, and that they had been the happiest three months of her life.

Immediately she began to thank the writer effusively, declaring that her freedom from headaches was unquestionably the result of his hypnotic work. Efforts to secure her reasons for this conclusion elicited only more expressions of certainty, conviction, and gratitude, but with no evidence of any true understanding or knowledge of what had occurred therapeutically.

She was interrupted in her thanks and the suggestion was given insistently that adequate expression of gratitude could come only from continued satisfactory adjustment in the future. With this remark the interview was closed.

More than 15 years have elapsed, and the therapeutic outcome has been good. She secured a position in another part of the country and has been promoted progressively until she is now a department head. Each Christmas a greeting card expressing briefly her gratitude is received. Occasionally a business letter is received, asking for references concerning somebody the writer knows, or recommending to him somebody needing therapy or a job placement.

One additional fact is that acquaintance has been made with several persons who have worked for her. They have been found to entertain the highest regard, personal liking, and respect for her and to be most enthusiastic about her charming personality.

In response to a specific letter of inquiry she stated that she had on the average three headaches a year, but that these responded readily to brief rest. She expressed the belief that these headaches were "different" from her former headaches, and she attributed them to reading without her glasses.

She is now in her early forties, unmarried, wholly content, absorbed in her work and the creature comforts of her tastefully decorated apartment. She was described by a competent psychiatrist who knew her well, but nothing of the above history, as "one of those delightful people you like to number among your friends. She looks upon men as charming companions but nothing more. She's most enthusiastic about her work and inspires everyone who works under her. After the day is over she likes her home, or the theater, or concerts, or has some of us in for a social evening. She is content and happy. You must have enjoyed knowing her."

COMMENT

A definitive discussion, even of a single aspect of this case history, is impossible since it is restricted entirely to overt symptoms. The only things known are what the therapist tried to do, but not the experiential significances thereof to the patient, and the subsequent, definitely successful therapeutic results.

At most it can be said that an experimental procedure was employed which in some manner permitted the patient's unconscious, distorted and disorganized in its functioning, to achieve a satisfactory role in the total experiential life of the patient, and to do so without becoming a part of the conscious. That such an outcome was possible with one patient suggests strongly that a comparable procedure could be adapted satisfactorily to the therapeutic needs of other patients.

26. Migraine Headache in a Resistant Patient

Milton H. Erickson

An admonition from William Alanson White, M.D., then Superinten-
dent of St. Elizabeth's Hospital, was given to this writer early in his
psychiatric career, and a year or so later he was again given the same
admonition by Adolf Meyer, M.D. Both strongly advised the writer never
to refuse to consult with a patient. A single interview graciously granted
during which the patient's story was listened to attentively, while not
especially remunerative, had often permitted them to encounter many
unusual instances of psychopathology and to achieve, in many cases,
astonishingly effective results. These results had sometimes proved to be
far better than the doctors had considered possible at the time of the
interview, even if long-term therapy could have been instituted. They
likened such instances to the processes of behavior wherein "love at first
sight" has drastically and positively altered the lives of various individuals.
One such historical example was the schoolteacher who thought it wrong
for an adult man making his living as a tailor (Andrew Johnson) to be so
uneducated. The events that unfolded began with teaching and led to
love, marriage, a law degree, a judgeship, and eventually the presidency
of the United States.

Adolf Meyer particularly stressed the utility of hypnosis in eliciting the
potentialities of these transient patients and urged this writer to see such
patients for both the educational values of the experience and the
possibility of effecting unexpected results. Throughout the passing years
the writer has conducted many "one-shot" interviews and sometimes as
much as 20 years later has received an appreciative letter or a personal
visit confirming the therapeutic impact of the brief encounter.

One such case is as follows: In 1936 the author lectured to his first class
of medical students at the Wayne State University College of Medicine.
During one of the last two lectures of the year the subject of hypnosis was
discussed. One of the students hostilely and aggressively interrupted the
lecture to denounce hypnosis as a hoax and challenged the author to
hypnotize him. He proceeded to berate the author; one of his classmates
who was well known to the author rushed up and quietly explained that no
notice should be given to the student's misconduct. He was a known
sufferer of migraine headaches, which developed unexpectedly; the

Unpublished manuscipt, 1936.

headaches were always preceded by an outburst, as had just occurred; this behavior was merely the prodomes of a migraine headache, which would last for one to three days; and finally, such outbursts would occur in the most unexpected of situations—on the street, in the classroom, at parties, football games, etc. After the outburst the student would slowly become flushed of face and neck, followed shortly by projectile vomiting, and culminating in a violent, incapacitating headache of perhaps several days' duration. He had been examined by many competent physicians and had almost been refused admission to the medical school. So far no medication or treatment had been found for his malady. (Several of the rest of the class members confirmed this account of the student's history.)

Within 10 minutes the student apologized for his conduct, declared that he was in the process of developing a migraine headache for which nothing could be done, in that about 15 or 20 minutes he would begin vomiting; after that happened, could he and a friend be excused so that he could be taken home. He also explained that his emotional outburst was a part of the aura. He was still getting angrier within himself, but he wanted to stay at the lecture as long as possible, since past experience had taught him how to judge his condition. Consent was given, but a challenge was issued that he might try hypnosis, since nothing else had worked. He bristled at this suggestion, but suddenly said, "Well, I've got nothing to lose but my breakfast, so go ahead with your silly hypnosis."

He was asked to take a seat in front of the class, facing the author and with his back to the audience. Slowly it was explained that he was to rotate his chair (it was a four-legged chair) bit by bit until he had made a complete turn of 360 degrees. His hostile manner and attitude suggested the inadvisability of attempting any routine traditional technique. Additionally, such a technique as moving his chair in a circle as he sat in it would be utterly incomprehensible to him as well as a difficult task. Yet, by so doing, he would be caught in the situation of actually participating with the author in a joint undertaking. Thus, he would validate by his own actions the idea that he was going into a trance.

As he gradually rotated his chair, the author explained to the class that the subject would do this task slowly, that each little movement would become slower and more difficult, that there was no hurry, no rush, that the subject could take his time and ought to, that each time he moved his chair a little, he would feel increasing fatigue and sleepiness, that the chair would seem to get more and more difficult to move, that his efforts would increasingly become less and less effective, and that shortly his eyes would close, he would take a deep breath, he would give up trying to move the chair, and simply relax by going into a deep trance.

All of the above was said as if it were no more than an explanation to the rest of the class. Thus, the subject would hear these suggestions as an explanation to the class but not as commands personally addressed to him.

He would develop no counterset to the suggestions and would thus tend to respond to them more readily, since he was already cooperating by slowly rotating his chair. Another important factor was the impending threat of a disabling migraine headache and the undoubtedly strong desire to escape from it in some way, even if that "way" appeared silly to him. Indeed, the entire situation favored the development of a trance state—the long history of migraine, the prodromes of hostility, aggressiveness, and belligerency, his own feeling of helplessness, his unwillingness to experience the projectile vomiting, and his dread of the utterly painful incapacitation that awaited him.

By the time he was facing the audience, he had developed a deep trance. He was peremptorily told that the author was now in charge of him and that all instructions were to be carried out. To this he nodded his head affirmatively. He was instructed to awaken, to speak derogatorily about hypnosis and the author, and to declare that such nonsense as hypnosis made him sick to his stomach. He should then *try* to prove that statement by going to the window, opening it, and *trying* to vomit projectilely, *but that he would fail completely.*

He was aroused, appearing surprised to find himself facing his classmates, made several unpleasant remarks as instructed, and then opened a window overlooking a vacant lot. He apparently did his best to vomit but failed, stating, "By this time I should have lost the lining of my stomach, but I'm beginning to feel better. I always vomit when I am about to have a migraine and I sure had all the warning signs this morning. But if I can't vomit, perhaps I won't have it [the migraine]."

This utterance was seized upon by the author to expand the idea that maladies, whether psychogenic or organic, followed definite patterns of some sort, particularly in the field of psychogenic disorders; that a disruption of this pattern could be a most therapeutic measure; and that it often mattered little how small the disruption was, if introduced early enough. After some discussion of this for the class (and as disguised suggestions to him) he was challengingly asked if he thought there was such a thing as hypnosis, and did he dare to volunteer to be a subject.

His reply was most informative: "I just told you it was silly nonsense, but I'm beginning to believe in it and I almost feel that you could hypnotize me. But what I don't understand is that something has happened to my headache. I knew this morning when I woke up that I was going to have one, and when I came into this classroom I was in my usual, helpless, ugly mood. But now I feel fine."

The answer given was, "It's all very simple, and as I explain you will go into a trance, a deep trance, remember everything, and then awaken, knowing that you never need to have another migraine headache. So rouse up!" He awakened from the trance that developed as the above remarks were made and had a total recovery of all events.

27. Hypnosis in Painful Terminal Illness

Milton H. Erickson

The use of psychological measures in the treatment of human illness, whether organic or psychological or a combination of both, is as old as human history. In fact, the psychological aspect of medicine constitutes the art of medicine and transforms the physician from a skillful mechanic or technician into a needed human source of faith, hope, assistance, and, most importantly, of motivation for the patient toward physical and mental health and well-being.

With this integral relationship between psychology and medicine it is not surprising that hypnosis as a psychological measure should be considered, seriously and rightly, in the treatment of painful terminal illness, particularly the last stages of malignant disease. However, as a preliminary statement, it must be emphasized that hypnosis is not an absolute answer and that it cannot replace other medical procedures. Rather, it is no more than one of the adjuvants or synergistic measures that can be employed to meet the patient's needs.

To present this topic to you, it might be well first to define both hypnosis and the rationale of its use. Essentially, hypnosis is a state of intensified attention and receptiveness and an increased responsiveness to an idea or to a set of ideas. There is nothing magical or mystical about it; it is attentiveness to, absorption in, and responsiveness to an idea or a whole group of ideas. We see this sort of thing repeatedly in everyday living where hypnosis is not involved—the automobile driver who forgets everything he should keep in mind because he is fascinated by the white line in the middle of the highway or by the scenery along the roadside, or the man unwisely and so intensely interested in a woman that he literally forgets everything that common sense has taught him.

In medicine as well as in dentistry this normal everyday capacity for intensely directed attention can be employed to concentrate and redirect a patient's attentiveness and responsiveness to selected stimuli. This constitutes the use of hypnosis in painful terminal disease.

Presented before the Eighty-Second Annual Session of the Arkansas Medical Society, May 6, 1958, at Hot Springs, Arkansas, and being published simultaneously by *The Journal of the Arkansas Medical Society*. Reprinted with permission from *The American Journal of Clinical Hypnosis,* January, 1959, *1*, 117-121.

In treating such patients, the question is not one of treating the illness itself, since the patient is both dying and suffering painfully. The primary problem is how to treat the patient so that his human needs may be met as much as possible. Thus, it becomes a complex problem of what the physical body has to have and what the patient as a personality needs, since cultural and individual psychological patterns are of as much and perhaps greater importance than the physiological experience of pain.

Before this audience there is no need to offer suggestions concerning the proper medically oriented procedures to employ in meeting the physical needs of the body. However, a statement should be made about meeting the physical needs of the body: Such treatment is just as important as the treatment of the psychological needs of the patient as a personality and should never be discredited. In fact, it is a prerequisite for any psychological treatment. Therefore, the question becomes, What is the adequate but at the same time the minimal treatment of the body? That it be minimal though adequate is essential, because in painful terminal disease sedatives, analgesics, and narcotics are employed that may deprive the patients of the privilege of knowing that they are alive and of enjoying what pleasures yet remain; also, they deprive relatives of adequate contacts with the patient. Hence, medication should be administered only in those quantities that meet the physical requirements without obstructing or defeating those psychological needs vital to the total life situation and which also require satisfactions even more than the physical.

To illustrate this point and to clarify the foregoing discussion, three case reports will be cited:

REPORT 1

The first patient was a 37-year-old woman of grade-school education, mother of four children, dying of advanced metastatic carcinomatous disease originating in the uterus. For the three weeks preceding hypnosis she had been kept in a narcotic semistupor, since this was the only way to control her pain, to enable her to sleep, and to enable her to eat without extensive nausea and vomiting. The woman understood her condition and resented helplessly her inability to spend the remaining weeks of her life in contact with her family. The family physician finally decided to have hypnosis employed.

The situation was explained to the woman, and narcotics were omitted on the day she was to be hypnotized so that this could be done without excessive drug interference.

Approximately four continuous hours were spent with the woman, systematically teaching her how to go into a trance despite her attacks of pain, how to develop a numbness of her body, how to absorb herself in a state of profound fatigue so that she could have physiological sleep despite pain, and how to enjoy her food without gastric distress. No elaborate explanations were necessary, since her educational limitations and the desperateness of her situation motivated a ready acceptance of suggestions without questioning doubts. Additionally, she was trained hypnotically to respond to her husband, her oldest daughter, and to her family physician, so that hypnosis could be readily reinforced in the event of any new development.

This one time was the only occasion on which the patient was seen by the writer. Her motivation was so great that the one hypnotic training session was sufficient.

The previous medication, it was found, could actually be discontinued, except for one heavy hypodermic administration late Thursday evening. This gave her additional relief, and it allowed her to be in full contact with her family in a rested state on the weekends. Also she shared in the family evening activities during the week.

Six weeks after her first trance, while laughing and talking to her daughter, she suddenly lapsed into a coma and died two days later without recovering consciousness. Those six weeks had been decidedly happy and pain-free for her.

REPORT 2

This 35-year-old woman, the mother of four small children and the wife of a professional man, was seen five weeks before her death from lung cancer. For a month before hypnosis, she had been almost continuously in a narcotic stupor, since the pain she experienced was unbearable to her. She asked that hypnosis be employed and voluntarily went without medication that entire day in her own self-determined effort to ready herself for hypnosis.

She was seen at 6:00 P.M., bathed in perspiration, suffering acutely from constant pain and greatly exhausted. Nevertheless, approximately four hours of continuous effort were required before a light trance could be induced. This light stage of hypnosis was immediately utilized to induce her to permit three things to be accomplished, all of which she had consistently refused to allow in the very intensity of her desire to be hypnotized. The first of these was the hypodermic administration of ⅛ grain of morphine sulfate, a most inadequate dosage for her physical needs, but one considered adequate for the immediate situation. The next was the serving to her of a pint of rich soup, and the third was the successful insistence upon an hour's restful physiological sleep. By 6:00 A.M. the patient, who finally proved to be an excellent somnambulistic subject, had been taught successfully everything considered to be essential to meet the needs of her situation.

The procedure followed was probably unnecessarily comprehensive, but the situation did not warrant any approach less inclusive. The first step was to teach her positive and negative hallucinations in the modalities of vision, hearing, taste, and smell. Then she was taught positive and negative hallucinations in the areas of touch, deep sensation, and kinesthesia, and in relation to this latter type of sensation, she was taught body disorientation and dissociation. When these learnings were sufficiently well acquired, the patient was given suggestions for glove and stocking anesthesias, and these were extended over her entire body. Thereupon it became possible to teach her rapidly combined partial analgesias and anesthesias for both superficial and deep sensations of all types. To this was added a combination of both body disorientation and body dissociation, so that these latter could supplement the former.

The patient was not seen again, either professionally or socially, but her husband telephoned or gave reports in person daily concerning the patient's condition.

She died suddenly five weeks later, in the midst of a happy social conversation with a neighbor and a relative.

During that five-week period she had been instructed to feel free to accept whatever medication she needed. Now and then she would suffer pain, but this was almost always controlled by aspirin. Sometimes a second dose of aspirin with codeine was needed, and on half a dozen occasions ⅛ grain of morphine was needed. Otherwise, except for her gradual progressive physical deterioration, the patient continued decidedly comfortable and cheerfully adjusted to the end.

REPORT 3

The third patient was a professionally trained man of advanced years, who understood fully the nature of his carcinomatous illness. Because of his educational background it was both necessary and advantageous to develop the hypnotic suggestions with care in order to secure both his intellectual and his emotional cooperation. While resigned to his fate, he resented greatly the narcotic stupors he developed when given sufficient medication to control his pain. It was his earnest desire to spend his remaining days in the fullest possible contact with his family, but this he found difficult because of the severely agonizing recurrent pains he suffered. As a solution, he requested hypnosis, and he himself discontinued medication for 12 hours in order to avoid a possible narcotic interference with a trance development.

At the first hypnotic session all suggestions were directed to the induction of a state of profound physical fatigue, of overwhelming sleepiness, and of a need to enter physiological sleep and to rest sufficiently to permit the induction of a hypnotic trance. A light trance was induced that almost immediately lapsed into a physiological sleep of about 30 minutes' duration. He aroused from this definitely rested and most firmly convinced of the efficacy of hypnosis.

A second and, this time, medium trance was then induced. Systematically a series of suggestions was given in which a direct use was made of the patient's actual symptomatology. The rationale for this was to validate the hypnotic suggestions through utilization of the experiential validity of his symptoms.

Thus the patient was told that his body would feel tremendously heavy, that it would feel like a dull, leaden weight, so heavy that it would feel as if sodden with sleep and incapable of sensing anything else except heavy tiredness. These suggestions, repetitiously given and in varying phraseology to ensure comprehensive acceptance, were intended to utilize the patient's feeling of distressing weakness, previously unacceptable to him and to combine it with the complaint of "constant, heavy, dull, throbbing ache." In addition, suggestions were given that, again and again as he experienced the "dull, heavy tiredness" of his body, it would periodically go to sleep, while his mind remained awake. Thus his distressing feeling of weakness and his dull, throbbing ache were utilized to secure a redirection and a reorientation of his attentiveness and responsiveness to his somatic sensations and to secure a new and acceptable perception of them. Also, by suggesting a sleeping of the body and wakefulness of the mind, a state of dissociation was induced. The next step was to reorient and redirect his attentiveness and responsiveness to the sharp, brief, constantly recurring, agonizing pains from which he suffered, usually less than 10 minutes apart. These pains, while brief, less than one minute in duration as timed by a watch, were experienced by the patient subjectively as "endless" and as essentially "continuous" in character.

The procedure followed included several steps.

First of all, he was oriented in relationship to subjective time values by asking him, at the expiration of a sharp pain, to fix his attention rigidly on the movement of the minute hand of a clock and to await the next sharp pain. The slightly more than seven minutes of waiting in anticipatory dread seemed hours long to the patient, and it was with definite relief from his feeling of wretched expectation that he suffered the next sharp pain. Thus anticipation and pain, as separate experiences, were differentiated for him. Also, he acquired in this way an understanding of time distortion (Cooper & Erickson, 1959), particularly that aspect of time distortion related to the lengthening or expansion of subjective time experience.

Next a careful explanation was given to him that freedom from the experience of pain could be accomplished in several ways—by anesthesia and by analgesia, both of which he understood, and by amnesia, which he did not understand. The explanation was offered that in amnesia for pain one could experience pain throughout its duration, but that one would immediately forget it and thus would not look back upon the experience with a feeling of horror and distress, nor look forward to another similar pain experience with anticipatory dread fear. In other words, each recurrent sharp pain could be and would become a totally unexpected and completely transient experience. Because it would be neither anticipated nor remembered, it would seem experientially to have no temporal duration. Hence, it would be experienced only as a momentary flash of sensation of such short duration that there would be no opportunity to recognize its character. In this fashion the patient was taught another aspect of time distortion—namely, a shortening, contraction, or condensation of subjective time. Thus, in addition to the possible hypnotic anesthesia, analgesia, or amnesia for the pains, there was also the hypnotic reduction of their subjective temporal duration which, in itself, would serve to diminish greatly the pain experience for the patient.

When these matters had been made clear to him, he was urged most insistently to employ all of the mechanisms that had been suggested—alteration of body sensations, body disorientation, dissociation, anesthesia, analgesia, amnesia, and subjective time condensation. In this way, it was argued, he could quite conceivably free himself from pain more readily than by employing a single psychological process. In addition, the suggestion was also offered emphatically that he employ subjective time expansion to lengthen experientially all periods of physical comfort, rest, or freedom from pain.

By this variety of differently directed suggestions, repetitiously given and in different phrasings to ensure adequate comprehension and acceptance, the patient's sharp recurring pains were abolished in large part insofar as observation of his objective behavior and his own subjective reports were concerned. However, it was noted that periodically he would lapse into a brief unresponsive stuporlike state of 10 to 50 seconds' duration, an item of behavior suggestive of a massive obsuring reaction to pain. It was noted that these were less frequent and shorter in duration than the original sharp pains had been. It was also observed that the patient appeared to have no realization whatsoever of his periodic lapses of awareness.

No systematic inquiry could be conducted into the actual efficacy of the suggestions. The patient simply reported that hypnosis had freed him almost completely of his pains, that he felt heavy, weak, and dull physically, and that not over twice a day did any pain "break through." His general behavior with his family and friends validated his report.

Some weeks after the beginning of hypnotic therapy the patient lapsed suddenly into coma and died without recovering consciousness.

SUMMARY AND GENERAL COMMENTS

A presentation has been offered of the utilization of hypnosis in terminal painful disease. Three case reports, not entirely typical, have been presented in order to illustrate more adequately the actual possibilities of therapeutic benefits.

An effort has been made to describe the therapeutic methodologies employed, but this effort is not fully possible. Hypnotherapeutic benefits, especially in such cases as reported here, are markedly contingent upon a varied and repetitious presentation of ideas and understandings to ensure an adequate acceptance and responsiveness by the patient. Also, the very nature of the situation precludes a determination of what elements in the therapeutic procedure are effective in the individual case.

These three case reports indicate definitely that hypnosis can be of value in treating painful terminal illness. However, it is not to be regarded as an absolute answer to all the medical problems involved. Rather it is one of the possible approaches in the handling of the patient's problems that possesses special and highly significant values at both psychological and physiological levels.

While hypnosis can sometimes be used alone as a means of pain control in carcinomatous disease, more often it is properly used as an adjuvant. In that capacity it can serve to diminish significantly the actual drug dosage and to effect a much greater relief both mentally and physically. In all probability the more comprehensive psychologically the hypnotic approach, the greater is the possibility of therapeutic results.

28. The Interspersal Hypnotic Technique for Symptom Correction and Pain Control

Milton H. Erickson

Innumerable times this author has been asked to commit to print in detail the hypnotic technique he has employed to alleviate intolerable pain or to correct various other problems. The verbal replies made to these many requests have never seemed to be adequate since they were invariably prefaced by the earnest assertion that the technique in itself serves no other purpose than that of securing and fixating the attention of patients, creating then a receptive and responsive mental state, and thereby enabling them to benefit from unrealized or only partially realized potentials for behavior of various types. With this achieved by the hypnotic technique, there is then the opportunity to proffer suggestions and instructions serving to aid and to direct patients in achieving the desired goal or goals. In other words, the hypnotic technique serves only to induce a favorable setting in which to instruct patients in a more advantageous use of their own potentials of behavior.

Since the hypnotic technique is primarily a means to an end, while therapy derives from the guidance of the patient's behavioral capacities, it follows that, within limits, the same hypnotic technique can be utilized for patients with widely diverse problems. To illustrate, two instances will be cited in which the same technique was employed, once for a patient with a distressing neurotic problem and once for a patient suffering from intolerable pain from terminal malignant disease. The technique is one that the author has employed on the illiterate subject and upon the college graduate, in experimental situations and for clinical purposes. Often it has been used to secure, to fixate, and to hold the attention of difficult patients and to distract them from creating difficulties that would impede therapy. It is a technique employing ideas that are clear and comprehensible, but which by their patent irrelevance to the patient-physician relationship and situation distract the patient. Thereby the patients are prevented from intruding unhelpfully into a situation which they cannot understand and for which they are seeking help. At the same time a readiness to understand and to respond is created within the patient.

Reprinted with permission from *The American Journal of Clinical Hypnosis*, January, 1966, *8*, 198-209.

Thus, a favorable setting is evolved for the elicitation of needful and helpful behavioral potentialities not previously used, not fully used, or perhaps misused by the patient.

The first instance to be cited will be given without any account of the hypnotic technique employed. Instead, there will be given the helpful instructions, suggestions, and guiding ideas which enabled the patient to achieve his therapeutic goal and which were interspersed among the ideas constituting the hypnotic technique. These therapeutic ideas will not be cited as repetitiously as they were verbalized to the patient for the reason that they are more easily comprehended in cold print than when uttered as a part of a stream of utterances. Yet, these few repeated suggestions in the hypnotic situation served to meet the patient's needs adequately.

The patient was a 62-year-old retired farmer with only an eighth-grade education, but decidedly intelligent and well read. He actually possessed a delightful, charming, outgoing personality, but he was most unhappy, filled with resentment, bitterness, hostility, suspicion, and despair. Approximately two years previously, for some unknown or forgotten reason (regarded by the author as unimportant and as having no bearing upon the problem of therapy), he had developed a urinary frequency that was most distressing to him. Approximately every half-hour he felt a compelling urge to urinate, an urge that was painful, that he could not control, and that would result in a wetting of his trousers if he did not yield to it. This urge was constantly present day and night. It interfered with his sleep, his eating, and his social adjustments, and compelled him to keep within close reach of a lavatory and to carry a briefcase containing several pairs of trousers for use when he was "caught short." He explained that he had brought into the office a briefcase containing three pairs of trousers, and he stated that he had visited a lavatory before leaving for the author's office, another on the way, and that he had visited the office lavatory before entering the office, and that he expected to interrupt the interview with the author by at least one other such visit.

He related that he had consulted more than 100 physicians and well-known clinics. He had been cystoscoped more than 40 times, had had innumerable X-ray pictures taken and countless tests, some of which were electroencephalograms and electrocardiograms. Always he was assured that his bladder was normal; many times he was offered the suggestion to return after a month or two for further study; and "too many times" he was told that "it's all in your head," that he had no problem at all, that he "should get busy doing something instead of being retired, and to stop pestering doctors and being an old crock." All of this had made him feel like committing suicide.

He had described his problem to a number of writers of syndicated medical columns in newspapers, several of whom offered him in his stamped self-addressed envelope a pontifical platitudinous dissertation upon his problem, stressing it as one of obscure organic origin. In all of his searching not once had it been suggested that he seek psychiatric aid.

On his own initiative, after reading two of the misleading, misinforming, and essentially fraudulent books on "do-it-yourself hypnosis," he did seek the aid of stage hypnotists—in all, three in number. Each offered him the usual blandishments, reassurances, and promises common to that type of shady medical practice, and each failed completely in repeated attempts at inducing a hypnotic trance. Each charged an exhorbitant fee (as judged by a standard medical fee, and especially in relation to the lack of benefit received).

As a result of all this mistreatment, the medical no better than that of the charlatans and actually less forgivable, he had become bitter, disillusioned, resentful, and openly hostile, and he was seriously considering suicide. A gas station attendant suggested that he see a psychiatrist and recommended the author on the basis of a Sunday newspaper article. This accounted for his visit to the author.

Having completed his narrative, he leaned back in his chair, folded his arms, and challengingly said, "Now psychiatrize and hypnotize me and cure this —— bladder of mine."

During the narration of the patient's story the author had listened with every appearance of rapt attention except for a minor idling with his hands, thereby shifting the position of objects on his desk. This idling included a turning of the face of the desk clock away from the patient. As he listened to the patient's bitter account of his experiences, the author was busy speculating upon possible therapeutic approaches to a patient so obviously unhappy, so resentful toward medical care and physicians, and so challenging in attitude. He certainly did not appear to be likely to be receptive and responsive to anything the author might do or say. As the author puzzled over this problem, there came to mind the problem of pain control for a patient suffering greatly in a terminal state of malignant disease. That patient had constituted a comparable instance where a hypnotherapeutic approach had been most difficult, yet success had been achieved. Both patients had in common the experience of growing plants for a livelihood, both were hostile and resentful, and both were contemptous of hypnosis. Hence, when the patient issued his challenge of "psychiatrize and hypnotize me," the author, with no further ado, launched into the same technique employed with that other patient to achieve a hypnotherapeutic state in which helpful suggestions, instructions, and directions could be offered with reasonable expectation that they would be accepted and acted upon responsively in accord with the patient's actual needs and behavioral potentials.

The only difference for the two patients was that the interwoven therapeutic material for the one patient pertained to bladder function and duration of time. For the other patient the interwoven therapeutic instructions pertained to body comfort, to sleep, to appetite, to the enjoyment of the family, to an absence of any need for medication, and to the continued enjoyment of time without concern about the morrow.

The actual verbal therapy offered, interspersed as it was in the ideation of the technique itself, was as follows, with the interspersing denoted by dots.

You know, we could think of your bladder needing emptying every 15 minutes instead of every half-hour . . . . Not difficult to think that. . . . A watch can run slow . . . . or fast . . . . be wrong even a minute . . . . even two, five minutes . . . . or think of bladder every half hour . . . . like you've been doing . . . . maybe it was 35, 40 minutes sometimes . . . . like to make it an hour . . . . what's the difference . . . . 35, 36 minutes, 41, 42, 45 minutes . . . . not much difference . . . . not important difference . . . . 45, 46, 47 minutes . . . . all the same . . . . lots of times you maybe had to wait a second or two . . . . felt like an hour or two . . . . you made it . . . . you can again . . . . 47 minutes, 50 minutes, what's the difference . . . . stop to think, no great difference, nothing important . . . . just like 50 minutes, 60 minutes, just minutes . . . . anybody that can wait half an hour can wait an hour . . . . I know it . . . . you are learning . . . . not bad to learn . . . . in fact, good . . . . come to think of it, you have had to wait when somebody got there ahead of you . . . . you made it too . . . . can again . . . . and again . . . . all you want to . . . . hour and 5 minutes . . . . hour and 5½ minutes . . . . what's the difference . . . . or even 6½ minutes . . . . make it 10½, hour and 10½ minutes . . . . one minute, 2 minutes, one hour, 2 hours, what's the difference . . . . you got half a century or better of practice in waiting behind you . . . . you can use all that . . . . why not use it . . . . you can do it . . . . probably surprise you a lot . . . . won't even think of it . . . . why not surprise yourself at home . . . . good idea . . . . nothing better than a surprise . . . . an unexpected surprise . . . . how long can you hold out . . . . that's the surprise . . . . longer than you even thought . . . . lots longer . . . . might as well begin . . . . nice feeling to begin . . . . to keep on . . . . Say, why don't you just forget what I've been talking about and just keep it in the back of your mind. Good place for it—can't lose it. Never mind the tomato plant—just what was important about your bladder— pretty good, feel fine, nice surprise—say, why don't you start feeling rested, refreshed right now, wider awake than you were earlier this morning [this last statement is, to the patient, an indirect, emphatic, definitive instruction to arouse from his trance]. Then [as a dismissal but not consciously recognizable as such by the patient], why don't you take a nice leisurely walk home, thinking about nothing? [an amnesia instruction for both the trance and his problem, and also a confusion measure to obscure the fact that he had already spent 1½ hours in the office]. I'll be able to see you at ten A.M. a week from today [furthering his conscious illusion, resulting from his amnesia, that nothing yet had been done except to give him an appointment].

A week later he appeared and launched into an excited account of arriving home and turning on the television with an immediate firm intention of delaying urination as long as possible. He watched a two-hour movie and drank two glasses of water during the commercials. He decided to extend the time another hour and suddenly discovered that he had so much bladder distension that he had to visit the lavatory. He looked at his watch and discovered that he had waited four hours. The patient leaned back in his chair and beamed happily at the author, obviously expecting praise. Almost immediately he leaned forward with a startled look and declared in amazement, "It all comes back to me now. I never give it a thought till just now. I plumb forgot the whole thing. Say, you must have hypnotized me. You were doing a lot of talking about growing a tomato plant and I was trying to get the point of it and the next thing I knew I was walking home. Come to think of it I must of been in your office over an hour and it took an hour to walk home. It wasn't no four hours I held back, it was over six hours at least. Come to think of it, that ain't all. That was a week ago that happened. Now I recollect I ain't had a bit of trouble all week—slept fine—no getting up. Funny how a man can get up in the morning, his mind all set on keeping an appointment to tell something, and forget a whole week has went by. Say, when I told you to psychiatrize and hypnotize me, you sure took it serious. I'm right grateful to you. How much do I owe you?"

Essentially, the case was completed, and the remainder of the hour was spent in social small talk with a view of detecting any possible doubts or uncertainties in the patient. There were none, nor, in the months that have passed, have there occurred any.

The above case report allows the reader to understand in part how, during a technique of suggestions for trance induction and trance maintenance, hypnotherapeutic suggestions can be interspersed for a specific goal. In the author's experience such an interspersing of therapeutic suggestions among the suggestions for trance maintenance may often render the therapeutic suggestions much more effective. The patients hear them and understand them, but before they can take issue with them or question them in any way, their attention is captured by the trance-maintenance suggestions. And these in turn are but a continuance of the trance-induction suggestions. Thus, there is given to the therapeutic suggestion an aura of significance and effectiveness deriving from the already effective induction and maintenance suggestions. Then again the same therapeutic suggestions can be repeated in this interspersed fashion, perhaps repeated many times, until the therapist feels confident that the patient has absorbed the therapeutic suggestions adequately. Then the therapist can progress to another aspect of therapy using the same interspersal technique.

The above report does not indicate the number of repetitions for each of the therapeutic suggestions for the reason that the number must vary with each set of ideas and understandings conveyed and with each patient and each therapeutic problem. Additionally, such interspersal of suggestions for amnesia and posthypnotic suggestions among the suggestions for trance maintenance can be done most effectively. To illustrate from everyday life: A double task assignment is usually more effective than the separate assignment of the same two tasks. For example, a mother may say, "Johnny, as you put away your bicycle, just step over and close the garage door." This has the sound of a single task, one aspect of which favors the execution of another aspect, and thus there is the effect of making the task seem easier. To ask that the bicycle be put away and then to ask that the garage door be closed has every sound of being two separate, not to be combined, tasks. To the separate tasks a refusal can be given easily to one or the other task or to both. But a refusal when the tasks are combined into a single task means what? That he will not put away the bicycle? That he will not step over to the garage? That he will not close the garage door?

The very extent of the effort needed to identify what one is refusing in itself is a deterrent to refusal. Nor can a refusal of the "whole thing" be offered comfortably. Hence Johnny may perform the combined task unwillingly but may prefer to do so rather than to analyze the situation. To the single tasks he can easily say "later" to each. But to the combined task he cannot say "Later" since, if he puts away the bicycle "later," he must "immediately" step over to the garage and "immediately" close the door. This is specious reasoning, but it is the "emotional reasoning" that is common in daily life, and daily living is not an exercise in logic. As a common practice the author says to a patient, "As you sit down in the chair, just go into a trance." The patient is surely going to sit down in the chair. But going into a trance is made contingent upon sitting down, hence a trance state develops from what the patient was most certainly going to do. By combining psychotherapeutic, amnestic, and posthypnotic suggestions with those suggestions used first to induce a trance, and then to maintain that trance, constitutes an effective measure in securing desired results. Contingency values are decidedly effective. As a further illustration, more than once a patient who has developed a trance upon simply sitting down has said to the author, "I didn't intend to go into a trance today." In reply the author has stated, "Then perhaps you would like to awaken from the trance and hence, *as you understand that* you can go back into a trance when you need to, *you will awaken.*" Thus the "awakening" is made contingent upon "understanding," thereby ensuring further trances through association by contingency.

With this explanation of rationale the problem of the second patient will be presented after a few preliminary statements. These are that the author was reared on a farm, enjoyed and still enjoys growing plants, and has read with interest about the processes of seed germination and plant growth. The first patient was a retired farmer. The second, who will be called "Joe" for convenience, was a florist. He began his career as a boy by peddling flowers, saving his pennies, buying more flowers to peddle, etc. Soon he was able to buy a small parcel of land on which to grow more flowers with loving care while he enjoyed their beauty which he wanted to share with others, and in turn, to get more land and to grow more flowers, etc. Eventually he became the leading florist in a large city. Joe literally loved every aspect of his business and was intensely devoted to it but he was also a good husband, a good father, a good friend, and a highly respected and valued member of the community.

Then one fateful September a surgeon removed a growth from the side of Joe's face, being careful not to disfigure Joe's face too much. The pathologist reported the growth to be a malignancy. Radical therapy was then instituted, but it was promptly recognized as "too late."

Joe was informed that he had about a month left to live. Joe's reaction was, to say the least, unhappy and distressed. In addition he was experiencing much pain—in fact, extremely severe pain.

At the end of the second week in October a relative of Joe's urgently requested the author to employ hypnosis on Joe for pain relief since narcotics were proving of little value. In view of the prognosis that had been given for Joe the author agreed reluctantly to see him, stipulating that all medication be discontinued at 4:00 A.M. of the day of the author's arrival. To this the physicians in charge of Joe at the hospital courteously agreed.

Shortly before the author was introduced to Joe, he was informed that Joe disliked even the mention of the word *hypnosis.* Also, one of Joe's children, a resident in psychiatry at a well-known clinic, did not believe in hypnosis and had apparently been confirmed in this disbelief by the psychiatric staff of the clinic, none of whom is known to have had any firsthand knowledge of hypnosis. This resident would be present, and the inference was that Joe knew of that disbelief.

The author was introduced to Joe, who acknowledged the introduction in a most courteous and friendly fashion. It is doubtful if Joe really knew why the author was there. Upon inspecting Joe, it was noted that much of the side of his face and neck was missing because of surgery, ulceration, maceration, and necrosis. A tracheotomy had been performed on Joe, and he could not talk. He communicated by pencil and paper, many pads of which were ready at hand. The information was given that every four hours Joe had been receiving narcotics (¼ grain of morphine or 100 milligrams of Demerol) and heavy sedation with barbiturates. He slept little. Special nurses were constantly at hand. Yet Joe was constantly hopping out of bed, writing innumerable notes, some pertaining to his business, some to his family, but many of them were expressive of complaints and demands for additional help. Severe pain distressed him continuously, and he could not understand why the doctors could not handle their business as efficiently and as competently as he did his floral business. His situation enraged him because it constituted failure in his eyes. Success worked for and fully merited had always been a governing principle in his life. When things went wrong with his business, he made certain to correct them. Why did not the doctors do the same? The doctors had medicine for pain, so why was he allowed to suffer such intolerable pain?

After the introduction Joe wrote, "What you want?" This constituted an excellent opening, and the author began his technique of trance induction and pain relief. This will not be given in its entirety since a large percentage of the statements made were repeated, not necessarily in succession but frequently by referring back to a previous remark and then repeating a paragraph or two. Another preliminary statement needed is that the author was most dubious about achieving any kind of success with Joe since, in addition to his physical condition, there were definite evidences of toxic reactions to excessive medication. Despite the author's unfavorable view of possibilities there was one thing of which he could be confident. He could keep his doubts to himself and he could let Joe know by manner, tone of voice, by everything said that the author was genuinely interested in him, was genuinely desirous of helping him. If even that little could be communicated to Joe, it should be of some comfort, however small, to Joe and to the family members and to the nurses within listening distance in the side room.

The author began:

> Joe, I would like to talk to you. I know you are a florist, that you grow flowers, and I grew up on a farm in Wisconsin and I liked growing flowers. I still do. So I would like to have you take a seat in that easy chair as I talk to you. I'm going to say a lot of things to you, but it won't be about flowers because you know more than I do about flowers. *That isn't what you want.* [The reader will note that italics will be used to denote interspersed hypnotic suggestions which may be syllables, words, phrases, or sentences uttered

with a slightly different intonation.] Now as I talk, and I can do so *comfortably,* I wish that you will *listen to me comfortably* as I talk about a tomato plant. That is an odd thing to talk about. It makes one *curious. Why talk about a tomato plant?* One puts a tomato seed in the ground. One can *feel hope* that it will grow into a tomato plant that *will bring satisfaction* by the fruit it has. The seed soaks up water, *not very much difficulty* in doing that because of the rains that *bring peace and comfort* and the joy of growing to flowers and tomatoes. That little seed, Joe, slowly swells, sends out a little rootlet with cilia on it. Now you may not know what cilia are, but cilia are *things that work* to help the tomato seed grow, to push up above the ground as a sprouting plant, and *you can listen to me, Joe,* so I will keep on talking and *you can keep on listening, wondering, just wondering what you can really learn,* and here is your pencil and your pad, but speaking of the tomato plant, it grows so slowly. *You cannot see* it grow, *you cannot hear* it grow, but grow it does—the first little leaflike things on the stalk, the fine little hairs on the stem, those hairs are on the leaves, too, like the cilia on the roots, they must make the tomato plant *feel very good, very comfortable* if you can think of a plant as feeling, and then *you can't see* it growing, *you can't feel* it growing, but another leaf appears on that little tomato stalk and then another. Maybe, and this is talking like a child, maybe the tomato plant does *feel comfortable and peaceful* as it grows. Each day it grows and grows and grows, *it's so comfortable, Joe,* to watch a plant grow and *not see* its growth, *not feel* it, but just know that *all is getting better* for that little tomato plant that is adding yet another leaf and still another and a branch, and it is *growing comfortably* in all directions. [Much of the above by this time had been repeated many times, sometimes just phrases, sometimes sentences. Care was taken to vary the wording and also to repeat the hypnotic suggestions. Quite some time after the author had begun, Joe's wife came tiptoeing into the room carrying a sheet of paper on which was written the question, "When are you going to start the hypnosis?" The author failed to cooperate with her by looking at the paper and it was necessary for her to thrust the sheet of paper in front of the author and therefore in front of Joe. The author was continuing his description of the tomato plant uninterruptedly, and Joe's wife, as she looked at Joe, saw that he was not seeing her, did not know that she was there, that he was in a somnambulistic trance. She withdrew at once.] And soon the tomato plant will have a bud form somewhere, on one branch or another, but it makes no difference because all the branches, the whole tomato plant will soon have those nice little buds—I wonder if the tomato plant can, *Joe, feel really feel a kind of comfort.* You know, Joe, a plant is a wonderful thing, and *it is so nice, so pleasing* just to be able to think about a plant as if it were a man. Would such a plant *have nice feelings, a sense of comfort* as the tiny little tomatoes begin to form, so tiny, yet so *full of promise to give you the desire to eat* a luscious tomato, sun-ripened, it's so *nice to have food in one's stomach,* that wonderful feeling a child, a thirsty child, has and can *want a drink, Joe,* is that the way the tomato plant feels when the rain falls and washes everything so that *all feels well.* [Pause.] *You know, Joe,* a tomato plant just flourishes each day *just a day at a time.* I like to think the tomato plant can *know the fullness of comfort each day. You know, Joe, just one day at a time* for the tomato plant. That's the way for all tomato plants. [Joe suddenly came out of the trance, appeared disoriented, hopped upon the bed, and waved his arms; his behavior was highly suggestive of the sudden surges of toxicity one sees in patients who have reacted unfavorably to barbiturates. Joe did not seem to hear or see the author until he hopped off the bed and walked toward the author. A firm grip was taken on Joe's arm and then immediately loosened. The nurse was summoned. She mopped perspiration from his forehead, changed his surgical dressings, and gave him, by tube, some ice water. Joe then let the author lead him back to his chair. After a pretense by the author of being curious about Joe's forearm, Joe seized his pencil and paper and wrote, "Talk, talk."] "Oh yes, Joe, I grew up on a farm, I think a tomato seed is a wonderful thing; *think, Joe, think* in that little seed there does *sleep so restfully, so comfortably* a beautiful plant yet to be grown that will bear such interesting leaves and branches. The leaves, the branches look so beautiful, that beautiful rich color, *you can really feel happy* looking at a tomato seed, thinking about the wonderful plant it contains *asleep, resting, comfortable, Joe.* I'm soon going to leave for lunch and I'll be back and I will talk some more."

The above is a summary to indicate the ease with which hypnotherapeutic suggestions can be included in the trance induction along with trance-maintenance suggestions, which are important additionally as a vehicle for the transmission of therapy. Of particular significance is Joe's own request that the author "talk." Despite his toxic state, spasmodically evident, Joe was definitely accessible. Moreover, he learned rapidly despite the absurdly amateurish rhapsody the author offered about a tomato seed and plant. Joe had no real interest in pointless, endless remarks about a tomato plant. Joe wanted freedom from pain, he wanted comfort, rest, sleep. This was what was uppermost in Joe's mind, foremost in his emotional desires, and he would have a compelling need to try to find something of value to him in the author's babbling. That desired value was there, so spoken that Joe could literally receive it without realizing it. Joe's arousal from the trance was only some minutes after the author had said so seemingly innocuously, "want a drink, Joe." Nor was the reinduction of the trance difficult, achieved by two brief phrases, "think, Joe, think" and "sleep so restfully, so comfortably" imbedded in a rather meaningless sequence of ideas. But what Joe wanted and needed was in that otherwise meaningless narration, and he promptly accepted it.

During lunchtime Joe was first restful and then slowly became restless; another toxic episode occurred, as reported by the nurse. By the time the author returned Joe was waiting impatiently for him. Joe wanted to communicate by writing notes. Some were illegible because of his extreme impatience in writing. He would irritatedly rewrite them. A relative helped the author to read these notes. They concerned things about Joe, his past history, his business, his family, and "last week terrible," "yesterday was terrible." There were no complaints, no demands, but there were some requests for information about the author. After a fashion a satisfying conversation was had with him as was judged by an increasing loss of his restlessness. When it was suggested that he cease walking around and sit in the chair used earlier, he did so readily and looked expectantly at the author.

"You know, Joe, I could talk to you some more about the tomato plant and if I did you would probably go to sleep, in fact, *a good sound sleep.* [This opening statement has every earmark of being no more than a casual commonplace utterance. If the patient responds hypnotically, as Joe promptly did, all is well. If the patient does not respond, all you have said was just a commonplace remark, not at all noteworthy. Had Joe not gone into a trance immediately, there could have been a variation such as: "But instead, let's talk about the tomato flower. You have seen movies of flowers *slowly, slowly* opening, giving one *a sense of peace, a sense of comfort* as you watch the unfolding. So beautiful, *so restful* to watch. One can *feel such infinite comfort* watching such a movie."]

It does not seem to the author that more needs to be said about the technique of trance induction and maintenance and the interspersal of therapeutic suggestions. Another illustration will be given later in this paper.

Joe's response that afternoon was excellent despite several intervening episodes of toxic behavior and several periods where the author deliberately interrupted his work to judge more adequately the degree and amount of Joe's learning.

Upon departure that evening, the author was cordially shaken by hand by Joe, whose toxic state was much lessened. Joe had no complaints, he did not seem to have distressing pain, and he seemed to be pleased and happy.

Relatives were concerned about posthypnotic suggestions, but they were reassured that such had been given. This had been done most gently in describing so much in detail and repetition the growth of the tomato plant and then, with careful emphasis, *"You know Joe," "Know the fullness of comfort each day,"* and *"You know, Joe, just one day at a time."*

About a month later, around the middle of November, the author was requested to see Joe again. Upon arriving at Joe's home, he was told a rather regrettable but not actually unhappy story. Joe had continued his excellent response after the author's departure on that first occasion, but hospital gossip had spread the story of Joe's hypnosis, and interns, residents, and staff men came in to take advantage of Joe's capacity to be a good subject. They made all the errors possible for uninformed amateurs with superstitious misconceptions of hypnosis. Their behavior infuriated Joe, who knew that the author had done none of the offensive things they were doing. This was a fortunate realization since it permitted Joe to keep all the benefits acquired from the author without letting his hostilities toward hypnosis interfere. After several days of annoyance Joe left the hospital and went home, keeping one nurse in constant attendance, but her duties were relatively few.

During that month at home he had actually gained weight and strength. Rarely did a surge of pain occur, and when it did it could be controlled either with aspirin or with 25 milligrams of Demerol. Joe was very happy to be with his family, and there was considerable fruitful activity about which the author is not fully informed.

Joe's greeting to the author on the second visit was one of obvious pleasure. However, the author noted that Joe was keeping a wary eye on him, hence great care was taken to be completely casual and to avoid any hand movement that could be remotely misconstrued as a "hypnotic pass" such as the hospital staff had employed.

Framed pictures painted by a highly talented member of his family were proudly displayed. There was much casual conversation about Joe's improvement and his weight gain, and the author was repeatedly hard pushed to find simple replies to conceal pertinent suggestions. Joe did volunteer to sit down and let the author talk to him. Although the author was wholly casual in manner, the situation was thought to be most difficult to handle without arousing Joe's suspicions. Perhaps this was an unfounded concern, but the author wished to be most careful. Finally the measure was employed of reminiscing about "our visit last October." Joe did not realize how easily this visit could be pleasantly vivified for him by such a simple statement as, "I talked about a tomato plant then, and it almost seems as if I could be *talking about a tomato plant right now. It is so enjoyable to talk about a seed, a plant.''* Thus there was, clinically speaking, a re-creation of all of the favorable aspects of that original interview.

Joe was most insistent on supervising the author's luncheon that day, which was a steak barbecued under Joe's watchful eye in the backyard beside the swimming pool. It was a happy gathering of four people thoroughly enjoying being together, Joe being obviously most happy.

After luncheon Joe proudly displayed the innumerable plants, many of them rare, that he had personally planted in the large backyard. Joe's wife furnished the Latin and common names for the plants, and Joe was particularly pleased when the author recognized and commented on some rare plant. Nor was this a pretense of interest, since the author is still interested in growing plants. Joe regarded this interest in common to be a bond of friendship.

During the afternoon Joe sat down voluntarily, his very manner making evident that the author was free to do whatever he wished. A long monologue by the author ensued in which were included psychotherapeutic suggestions of continued ease, comfort, freedom from pain, enjoyment of family, good appetite, and a continuing pleased interest in all surroundings. All of these and other similar suggestions were interspersed unnoticeably among the author's many remarks. These covered a multitude of topics to preclude Joe from analyzing or recognizing the interspersing of suggestions. Also, for adequate disguise, the author needed a variety of topics. Whether or not such care was needed in view of the good rapport is a debatable question, but the author preferred to take no risks.

Medically, the malignancy was continuing to progress, but despite this fact Joe was in much better physical condition than he had been a month previously. When the author took his departure, Joe invited him to return again.

Joe knew that the author was going on a lecture trip in late November and early December. Quite unexpected by the author, a long distance telephone call was received just before the author's departure on this trip. The call was from Joe's wife, who stated, "Joe is on the extension line and wants to say 'hello' to you, so listen." Two brief puffs of air were heard. Joe had held the telephone mouthpiece over his tracheotomy tube and had exhaled forcibly twice to simulate "hello." His wife stated that both she and Joe extended their best wishes for the trip, and a casual conversation among friends ensued with Joe's wife reading Joe's written notes.

A Christmas greeting card was received from Joe and his family. In a separate letter Joe's wife said that "the hypnosis is doing well, but Joe's condition is failing." Early in January Joe was weak but comfortable. Finally, in his wife's words, "Joe died quietly January 21."

The author is well aware that the prediction of the duration of life for any patient suffering from a fatal illness is most questionable. Joe's physical condition in October did not promise very much. The symptom amelioration, abatement, and actual abolishment effected by hypnosis, and the freedom of Joe's body from potent medications, conducive only of unawareness, unquestionably increased his span of life while at the same time permitting an actual brief physical betterment in general. This was attested clearly by his improved condition at home and his gain in weight. That Joe lived until the latter part of January despite the extensiveness of his malignant disease undoubtedly attests to the vigor with which Joe undertook to live the remainder of his life as enjoyably as possible, a vigor expressive of the manner in which he had lived his life and built his business.

To clarify still further this matter of the technique of the interspersal of therapeutic suggestions among trance induction and trance maintenance suggestions, it might be well to report the author's original experimental work done while he was on the Research Service of the Worcester State Hospital in Worcester, Massachusetts in the early 1930s.

The Research Service was concerned with the study of the numerous problems of schizophrenia and the possibilities of solving some of them. To the author the psychological manifestations were of paramount interest. For example, just what did a stream of disconnected, rapidly uttered incoherencies mean? Certainly, such a stream of utterances must be most meaningful to the patient in some way. Competent secretaries from time to time had recorded verbatim various examples of such disturbed utterances for the author's perusal and study. The author himself managed to record adequately similar such productions by patients who spoke slowly. Careful study of these verbal productions, it was thought, might lead to various speculative ideas that in turn might prove of value in understanding something about schizophrenia.

The question arose of whether or not much of the verbigeration might be a disguise for concealed meanings, fragmented and dispersed among the total utterances. This led to the question of how the author could himself produce a series of incoherencies in which he could conceal in a fragmented form a meaningful message. Or could he use the incoherencies of a patient and intersperse among them in a somewhat orderly fashion a fragmented, meaningful communication that would be difficult to recognize? This speculation gave rise to many hours of intense labor spent fitting into a patient's verbatim, apparently meaningless utterances a meaningful message that could not be detected by the author's colleagues when no clue of any sort was given to them. Previous efforts at producing original incoherencies by the author disclosed a definite and recognizable personal pattern indicating that the author was not sufficiently disturbed mentally to produce a bonafide stream of incoherent verbigerations.

When a meaning was interspersed in a patient's productions successfully, the author discovered that his past hypnotic experimentation with hypnotic techniques greatly influenced the kind of a message he was likely to intersperse in a patient's verbigerations. Out of this labor came the following experimental and therapeutic work.

One of the more recently hired secretaries objected strongly to being hypnotized. She suffered regularly upon the onset of menstruation from severe migrainous headaches lasting three to four or even more hours. She had been examined repeatedly by the medical service with no helpful findings. She usually retired to the lounge and "slept off the headache," a process usually taking three or more hours. On one such occasion she had been purposely and rather insistently forced to take dictation by the author instead of being allowed to retire to the lounge. Rather resentfully she began her task, but within 15 minutes she interrupted the author to explain that her headache was gone. She attributed this to her anger at being forced to take dictation. Later, on another such occasion, she volunteered to take certain dictation which all of the secretaries tried to avoid because of the difficulties it presented. Her headache grew worse, and she decided that the happy instance with the author was merely a fortuitous happenstance. Subsequently she had another severe headache. She was again insistently requested by the author to take some dictation. The previous happy result occurred within 10 minutes. Upon the occurrence of another headache she volunteered to take dictation from the author. Again it served to relieve her headache. She then experimentally tested the benefits of dictation from other physicians. For some unknown reason her headaches only worsened. She returned from one of these useless attempts to the author and asked him to dictate. She was told he had nothing on hand to dictate but that he could redictate previously dictated material. Her headache was relieved within eight minutes. Later her request for dictation for headache relief was met by some routine dictation. It failed to have any effect.

She came again, not too hopefully, since she thought she had "worn out the dictation remedy." Again she was given dictation with a relief of her distress in about nine minutes. She was so elated that she kept a copy of the transcript so that she could ask others to dictate "that successful dictation" to relieve her headaches. Unfortunately, nobody seemed to have the "right voice," as did the author. Always, a posthypnotic suggestion was casually given that there would be no falling asleep while transcribing.

She did not suspect, nor did anybody else, what had really been done. The author had made comprehensive notes of the incoherent verbigeration of a psychotic patient. He had also had various secretaries make verbatim records of patients' incoherent utterances. He had then systematically interspersed therapeutic suggestions among the incoherencies with that secretary in mind. When this was found to be successful, the incoherent utterances of another patient were utilized in a similar fashion. This was also a successful effort. As a control measure, routine dictation and the dictation of "undoctored incoherencies" were tried. These had no effect upon her headaches. Nor did the use by others of "doctored" material have an effect, since it had to be read aloud with some degree of expressive awareness to be effective.

The question now arises, why did these two patients and those patients used experimentally respond therapeutically? This answer can be given simply as follows: They knew very well why they were seeking therapy; they were desirous of benefitting; they came in a receptive state, ready to respond at the first opportunity, except for the first experimental patient. But she was eager to be freed from her headache and wished the time being spent taking dictation could be time spent getting over her headache. Essentially, then, all of the patients were in a frame of mind to receive therapy. How many times does a patient need to state his complaint? Only that number of times requisite for the therapist to understand. For all of these patients only one statement of the complaint was necessary, and they then knew that the therapist understood. Their intense desire for therapy was not only a conscious but an unconscious desire also, as judged clinically, but more importantly, as evidenced by the results obtained.

One should also give recognition to the readiness with which one's unconscious mind picks up clues and information. For example, one may dislike someone at first sight and not become consciously aware of the obvious and apparent reasons for such dislike for weeks, months, even a year or more. Yet finally the reasons for the dislike become apparent to the conscious mind. A common example is the ready hostility frequently shown by a normal heterosexual person toward a homosexual person without any conscious realization of why.

Respectful awareness of the capacity of the patient's unconscious mind to perceive meaningfulness of the therapist's own unconscious behavior is a governing principle in psychotherapy. There should also be a ready and full respect for the patient's unconscious mind to perceive fully the intentionally obscured, meaningful therapeutic instructions offered them. The clinical and experimental material cited above is based upon the author's awareness that the patient's unconscious mind is listening and understanding much better than is possible for his conscious mind.

It was intended to publish this experimental work, of which only the author was aware. But sober thought and awareness of the insecure status of hypnosis in general, coupled with that secretary's strong objection to being hypnotized—she did not mind losing her headaches by "taking dictation" from the author—all suggested the inadvisability of publication.

A second secretary, employed by the hospital when this experimental work was nearing completion, always suffered from disabling dysmenorrhea. The "headache secretary" suggested to this girl that she take dictation from the author as a possible relief measure. Most willingly the author obliged, using "doctored" patient verbigeration. It was effective.

Concerned about what might happen to hypnotic research if his superiors were to learn of what was taking place, the author carefully failed with this second secretary and then again succeeded. She volunteered to be a hypnotic subject, and hypnosis, not "dictation," was then used to meet her personal needs. She also served repeatedly as a subject for various frankly acknowledged and "approved" hypnotic experiments, and the author kept his counsel in certain other experimental studies.

Now that hypnosis has come to be an acceptable scientific modality of investigative and therapeutic endeavor and there has developed a much greater awareness of semantics, this material, so long relegated to the shelf of unpublished work, can safely be published.

SUMMARY

Two case histories and a brief account of experimental work are presented in detail to demonstrate the effective procedure of interspersing psychotherapeutic suggestions among those employed to induce and to maintain a hypnotic trance. The patients treated suffered respectively from neurotic manifestations and the pain of terminal malignant disease.

29. Hypnotic Training for Transforming the Experience of Chronic Pain

Milton H. Erickson and Ernst L. Rossi

E: You have a patient that comes to you for chronic pain. He has been in the waiting room and then comes into your office. You put him in a trance, tell him to walk back into the waiting room, leave his pain there, and come back into the office. Tell it to him as if you were telling him to take his jacket into the other room and leave it there.

R: You tell it to him that casually?

E: Yes. When he comes back you tell him, "Now I want to awaken you while your pain is still in the waiting room." You talk casually about various things, and when the hour is over you have him leave by the other door out of the office because he says he doesn't want to go back through the waiting room where the pain is. He doesn't know why he says that because he doesn't know he left his pain there.

R: I wonder if this is a form of literalness where the patient follows your casual suggestion and treats the pain as a reified or concrete thing that can be left behind like a jacket?

E: It is. But bear in mind that the patient's pain will seep back.

R: How do we prevent the pain from seeping back? You will recall the patient of mine who has the back pain. Her X-rays showed an organic source of the pain, and the medical recommendation was an operation to fuse her vertebrae. She comes into my office and goes into trance beautifully and becomes completely free of pain while with me. For a brief period of time, after awakening from the trance and while still in my office, she remains free of pain. Then it begins to seep back when she leaves the office. Now I would like to prevent that pain from seeping back so quickly. I've trained her in self-hypnosis so she can be free of pain by herself when in trance at home. It works for her while she's in trance. As soon as she comes out of the trance, however, her pain is there again. How can we extend the relief for her?

E: One of the best measures for teaching extended pain relief is to teach the patient to let catalepsy persist.

R: In the painful part of the body?

E: No!

Unpublished dialogue between Erickson and the editor, 1973.

R: In any body part.

E: You saw the demonstration I did with the visiting psychiatrists who did not believe they could experience catalepsy.

R: Yet they did experience it bit by bit and even discussed all their sensations in detail as they learned the cataleptic experience of an arm becoming rigid and immobile.

E: You establish a belief in catalepsy that can persist and *resist* the person's efforts to remove it.

R: You mean to actually let the patient leave the office and go about daily life with, say, a little finger cataleptic?

E: No, you let the catalepsy persist for some time in the office.

R: You have the patient test it to see how it lasts and to see that it can be a real and persisting experience even when he comes out of trance?

E: Yes, and then later you bring in an analogy with pain. You extend time by saying your catalepsy can extend 10 seconds just as it can last 11. If 11, then 12. If 12, then 14 seconds is possible. If 14, then 17 is possible. If 17, then *certainly* 27 seconds! You then extend that to a few minutes and eventually hours.

R: While the patient's hand is cataleptic?

E: Yes, you let him discover he can extend the catalepsy—but he can also lose his catalepsy. He can lose his pain, but he can also get it back. He can lose his catalepsy, but he can get it back. People can learn so simply to turn pain, catalepsy, or any other subjective experience on and off.

R: You give patients hypnotic training to extend in time just about any hypnotic phenomena they are skillful in experiencing. You then establish a new learning set (*dentero*—learning) for turning that subjective experience on and off. In dealing with the problem of chronic pain it would be especially useful to train the patient in whatever subjective phenomena would interfere with or transform the pain. Since most people are highly idiosyncratic in their personal psychosomatic interactions (see the section on Psychophysiological Processes in Volume Two of this series), this kind of hypnotic training for pain relief would always proceed on an exploratory basis. For some patients a hypnotic experience of warmth or coldness, numbness, pressure or itch, hallucinatory taste, smell, or whatever might be found useful in learning to displace or relieve in some way their pain. Pain relief by hypnosis is not some sort of vague magic; it is based on essentially irrational associative patterns, but it is very definitely a valid empirical process. With careful training it becomes a reliable way of cultivating and transforming all sorts of subjective experiences—including that of pain.

V. Hypnotherapeutic Approaches in Rehabilitation

The papers in this section illustrate the manner in which Erickson utilizes a patient's emotions, interests, and personality to provoke rehabilitative efforts to cope with organic problems. The papers are all particularly poignant because the reader can be certain that Erickson was utilizing a personal perspective in these cases, since he himself was twice faced with such extensive rehabilitative efforts: He was stricken with polio at the age of 17 and again at the age of 52. His self-rehabilitative efforts on both occasions (see "Autohypnotic experiences of Milton H. Erickson," Volume One of this series) led him to an understanding of the use of sense and kinesthetic memories for the recovery of lost muscular functions.

The cases reported in this section are illustrative of numerous such cases treated by Erickson in his many years of therapeutic work. One case in particular, previously published with this editor's commentary (Case 13: "Hypnotherapy in organic spinal cord damage: New identity resolving suicidal depression," in Erickson & Rossi, 1979), belongs with the spirit of this section. When faced with the massively catastrophic consequences of sudden brain or spinal cord damage, the patient is confronted by an overwhelming threat to his integrity as a total personality. Along with physical rehabilitation, therefore, Erickson takes great care to help patients create new mental frameworks and identities that can support their new status. These new frameworks always utilize values and motivations intrinsic to each patient's personality. The organic accident that led to physical impairment is thus integrated into the patient's life in a manner that facilitates the evolution of new and broader patterns of awareness and self-understanding. The rehabilitative effort provokes a greater maturation of the total personality than may have been possible without the organic impairment. There is a deep religious and philosophical tradition that views suffering as a major provocation for the development of consciousness ("On the discourses of the Buddha" in Jung, 1976). While this editor has never heard Erickson speculate about these issues, it is evident that his personal life and his rehabilitative work with others lends some credence to this deep view.

30. Hypnotically Oriented Psychotherapy in Organic Brain Damage

Milton H. Erickson

Ordinarily brain damage with continued evidence of organic changes and destruction presents a seriously difficult problem for psychotherapy. In the following case history a rather detailed report is given of the use of a multitude of psychological measures, forms of instruction, direct and indirect hypnosis, and the manipulation of patterns of responsive behavior and reactions, all to effect therapeutic gains after a failure of conventional medical and surgical procedures. Considerable detail is given in presenting this case history instead of summarizing it by a simple statement of pertinent medical facts. An effort is made in this more detailed account to give the reader the "feel" of the psychological as well as the organic picture that confronted the author, both of which had a determining role in the therapy he devised.

On July 20, 1955, this 38-year-old college-bred woman who had been a brilliant student and who had a master's degree was returning with her husband and three children from a happy vacation trip. On the way she complained of a developing headache which rapidly grew worse and led to a state of coma.

She was hospitalized, and examination disclosed fresh blood in her spinal fluid, a right hemiparesis, a severe aphasia, and an aneurysm at the division of the left internal carotid artery just before its division into the middle and anterior cerebral arteries.

Treatment was conservative until August 2, when her symptoms became much worse and she developed sever hyperalgesia over her entire right side, which was diagnosed as a "thalamic syndrome." She was given numerous medications to control her pain, but since she appeared to receive no benefit, surgery was employed August 8th to clamp off the common carotid artery slowly and completely. This relieved her headache and some general symptoms but left some of her right-sided hemiparesis and hyperesthesia. A month later she developed extreme pain over her right side, which was diagnosed as "central in origin—the thalamic syndrome."

Reprinted with permission from *The American Journal of Clinical Hypnosis*, October, 1963, *6*, 92-112. This article was published simultaneously in translation in *Ceskoslovenská Psychologie*, Prague, Czechoslovakia.

She had regained her ability to walk fairly well although unsteadily, but her increased thalamic symdrome pain and the failure of analgesic medication and sedatives led in a few months to hospitalization in a well-known clinic in January, 1956.

General examination there confirmed the previous diagnosis of thalamic syndrome, disclosed numerous additional neurological findings concerning right-sided muscular and sensory dysfunction as well as the aphasia. The recommendation was offered that no further laboratory studies or general examinations were needed for diagnostic or other purposes. The previous failure of medications was noted, and the final recommendation was made that various untried experimental drugs *might* be considered. The prognosis offered was most unfavorable. This was rejected by the family, and in March, 1956, at her husband's insistence and because of his wife's completely vegetative course during her illness, she was admitted to another well-known neurological institute. The findings there confirmed the persistence of considerable hemiparesis, severe aphasia, and a continuance of the right-sided hyperalgesia. As in the previous neurological studies, she was found to have normal sensations and normal muscular functioning on the left side of her body. Her thalamic syndrome of generalized right-sided continuous pain and hypersensitivity was considered to have continued as possibly unchanged. No specific recommendations were made, and her prognosis was again stated as most unfavorable.

She entered a third neurological institute in June, 1956, and underwent neurosurgery for her thalamic syndrome. Report was made to her family physician that "we interrupted the spino-thalamic and quinto-thalamic tracts on the left side and succeeded in producing a definite hemi-hypalgesia without side effects. This diminished the dysesthesia that she experienced on stroking the skin, while the deep diffuse spontaneous pain is still preserved." In further discussion of the patient mention was made of the frequent association of a vegetative state associated with thalamic pain, and the increase of the potentials for sensory disturbances following thalamic injury. Her prognosis was given as most unfavorable, and mention was made of a possible continued vegetative state.

Therefore, recommendation was made that the patient be discharged and subsequent treatment be instituted by X-ray irradiation of the hypothalamus in an area posterior and dorsal to the sella turcica as a possible means of decreasing her hyperalgesia and perhaps a lessening of the vegetative state.

Upon the patient's return home, it was found that she had not retained the benefit noted immediately after the operation, and the neurological institute was again queried. Explanation was given further that such an operation as had been done was often unsuccessful; they again advised X-ray treatment, and in case of failure of that, they stated that they would consider re-operation. On July 3rd the institute, in response to further inquiries about increasing symptomatology in the patient, suggested the possibility of further attempts by new trial medications. They obviously were not interested in another operation and considered the situation as hopeless.

Her family physician then sent her to a general practitioner, who noted upon physical examination a remarkable anomaly not mentioned in all previous examinations—namely, an exact anatomical midline distribution from the scalp to the perineum of the hyperalgesia of the right side of her body and of the normal sensation on the left side, in addition to her vegetative state and the obvious numerous neurological evidences of brain damage. This peculiar anatomical midline demarcation of normal and abnormal sensations he regarded as a hysterical overlay, especially when the patient nodded her head affirmatively to the effect that the right side of her vagina and rectum were also both continuously painful.

As an outcome of his examination and recommendations the family and the family physician decided to refer the patient to the author for hypnotherapy since, in the 11 months that had already elapsed, there had occurred only a diminution of her hemiparesis and the development of a profoundly vegetative state from which the patient could be aroused only by unusual stimuli, and then only briefly, despite months of continued effort by her family and numerous friends.

The husband hopefully accepted the suggested referral, and the patient was brought to the author on July 14, 1956.

Her husband gave her history; communications sent by the family physician served to give summaries of the patient's four separate hospitalizations—the findings made, the services rendered, and the various respective recommendations suggested. He then proceeded to describe her progressive vegetative decline.

The patient entered the office somewhat unsteadily and haltingly, slumped into the chair, but now and then nodded her head vigorously when her husband stated that she really wished to get well. She presented a most discouraging appearance. Her hair was just beginning to grow out after neurosurgery, the right side of her face drooped, all right-sided movements were awkward, and she gave good evidence by her behavior and manner that she seemed to be suffering severe pain throughout the entire right side of her body. Examination disclosed that gentle touches were less well tolerated than hard slaps or deep pressure on the right side. It was also noted that she showed marked pain reactions to any stimulus of the right side of her body from the midline of her scalp, down the face and upper chest. Her entire right leg was painful, and she nodded her head toward the right when asked if her vagina and rectum were painful. When asked if she meant only the right side of those parts, she nodded affirmatively. Closing of her eyes during tests or testing the sensation of her back and scalp did not alter the rather remarkable exact anatomical midline division of left-sided normal sensations and the hyperalgesia of the right side. A brief test also disclosed a severe alexia which had not been noted in any of the previous examinations. The history, the appearance, and the obvious physical handicaps, including her aphasia and alexia, left no doubt as to the organic nature of her illness and of actual brain damage, despite the seeming "hysterical" character of her sensory disturbances, which did not allow for the normal interdigitation of sensory nerves from one side of the body to the other.

Inquiry about her clinical course was described by the husband as characterized by brief definite interest on the part of his wife whenever discussion of the possibility of further medical study was mentioned and a hopeful attitude at each clinic, only to be followed by tears, despondency, and apparently profound disappointment each time she returned home unimproved. For several months she had endeavored laboriously to talk to her husband and children and to participate somewhat in the home life. Sometimes it would take her 15 minutes to say haltingly "I can't talk" or "it hurts," referring to the right side of her body. Repeatedly she tried to take an interest in the visits of numerous friends, especially those of her family physician who was also a close family friend, but she seemed to find this impossbile. While her paralysis had lessened greatly, she experienced much difficulty ascending or descending stairs or in stepping backward. The patient indicated that in using stairways she had to use the banister because her eyes did not seem to measure the steps correctly, and that stepping backward was a slow, laborious "thinking" process since her feet would lag behind the backward movement of her body, with a fall resulting.

Coldness and increased humidity also increased her physical distress, and her right-sided hyperalgesia as well as increasing the right-sided muscular dysfunction, sometimes severely, depending upon the degrees of cold and the humidity.

The patient's reaction to her condition at first was one of severe fright and concern. Her first hospitalization was marked by cooperation and an attitude of full confidence in her physicians and the future. The exacerbation of her symptoms that led to her second hospitalization at a nationally famous clinic was accompanied by a reaction of complete hopefulness and certainty. The recommendation there of trial medications and new drugs and the implied hopelessness of her condition resulted in a feeling of despair and, at the same time, a desperate determination to do everything possible to help herself. She did succeed in improving so far as her hemiparesis was concerned, but ascending and descending stairways, her difficulty in stepping backward, the cold winter weather in her home state, and her aphasia and alexia constituted serious obstacles. Codeine and empirin and barbiturates were progressively less effective.

She would struggle vainly and laboriously to talk to her children and husband, but her aphasia gave her so helpless a feeling that she despaired each time. Also, she did not recognize what her alexia really was. She merely felt it to be a peculiar visual impairment of blurring, although objects in general seemed to be clearly outlined.

She made numerous but futile efforts to respond to the almost daily visits of friends, but often found her attention severely distracted from them by surges of pain. There resulted a progressive withdrawal from everything. She would sleep until 10:30 A.M., then arise and take a shower despite the severe pain it caused her. (Her explanation later was that, aside from personal cleanliness, she hoped such a procedure might help her to get accustomed to her constant right-sided hyperesthesia and hyperalgesia.)

She would then eat a combination breakfast and lunch, lie down on the couch, stare at the ceiling, and smoke. At 6:00 P.M. she would arise, eat dinner, return to the couch, stare at the ceiling, smoke and now and then, but with decreasing frequency, try to talk to her husband or to listen to her children, but with less and less success.

Her third hospitalization and the possibility that neurosurgery might be done aroused her intense interest and hope, which turned rapidly into despair. At the fourth hospitalization she had cooperated with new confidence and enthusiasm but was severely disappointed that only hemihypalgesia was secured. She looked forward to a return to the hospital for a second neurosugical operation and further benefits, but with not too hopeful an attitude. The transiency of the improvement resulted in black despair and a feeling of hopeless frustration, a feeling that had been present for many months but now seemed to dominate her completely. She passively agreed to see the general practitioner recommended by her family physician, but even his discussion of the anatomical midline division of normal and painful sensations as a hopeful evidence of benefit from hypnotherapy did not arouse much active interest. She passively accepted the referral to the author and, upon meeting him, handed him a slip of paper reading, "Help me," very poorly, almost illegibly written.

This special, personally made plea despite the fact that her husband was with her, and the peculiar, seemingly hysterical character of her anatomical midline demarcation of her body sensations, impressed the author most favorably as hopeful indications that the patient would be cooperative in every effort at therapy, and they seemed to represent not hysterical reactions but an extensive somatic overcompensation. Such an explanation was made to her, to her husband, and written in a letter to her family physician. To give her some feeling of faith she was carefully told, with intense emphasis and much elaboration, that such a midline distribution of sensations could very well be interpreted not as hysterical but as an utterly intense compensatory effort by her body to improve and by itself to effect "normal" sensations. This rather specious explanation appeared to give her some faith and hope.

Nevertheless, the problem presented appeared far from hopeful to the author. The first hour's interview exhausted her, and she seemed to have lost interest within 15 minutes, even though her husband did the talking. There was not question of the husband's interest and intense desire to see his wife benefitted, but all general understandings indicated that the question of any improvement, if at all possible, would be dependent upon the intensity and persistence of her efforts. Hence, before they left the office, a solemn vow was extracted from the patient to the effect that she would cooperate in every detail with the therapist, and she was warned that "good medicine often tastes bad" and that she would not always enjoy executing therapeutic instructions. She shrugged her shoulders and, after many futile halting attempts, finally managed to say, "I——I—— do——what——" and when finally asked if she meant that she would do what was asked of her, she nodded her head vigorously.

She was dismissed from the room, which she left rather unsteadily to the alarm of her husband, and certain arrangements were made with him since his business required prolonged frequent absences. These arrangements included the patient's staying with a companion who would serve as an assistant in any way the author demanded. A relative who had accompanied the patient volunteered, and the interview with her led to the conclusion that she would be an ideal person for any therapeutic plan developed.

Three days of intensive thinking of what to do with an obviously brain-damaged patient with definite residuals of a hemiparesis from a hemorrhage within the skull, a severe aphasia, an alexia, a thalamic syndrome for which the patient had undergone thalamic surgery without recognizable benefit, a history of nearly 11 months' vegetative living in a state of frustration and despair, and an agreed-upon poor prognosis by outstanding neurological clinics led to a decision to investigate experimentally the possibilities of helping the patient by combining hypnosis, hypnotic techniques, the patient's own well-developed pattern of frustration, and the implications of Lashley's work, which, within certain wide limits, demonstrated through experiments of cortical destruction upon rats and monkeys that the loss of learning was largely dependent upon the amount of cortical destruction, rather than the location, and that the learning is carried in the form of neural patterns that in some way preserve their identity in spite of variations in sensory, motor, and cortical elements.

The results the author began achieving led later to a modified adaptation of similar but much less complicated techniques for behavioral retraining under hypnotherapy of a 70-year-old woman previously diagnosed as suffering from a circumscribed irregular arteriosclerotic condition of the brain (Erickson, 1963). In the case now being reported the rationale of the author's decision was that the patient had a well-developed pattern of frustration and despair which, properly employed, could be used constructively as a motivational force in eliciting responses with a strong and probably compelling emotional force and tone leading to actual new learnings of self-expression or possibly to a restoration of some learnings.

The plan devised was complex and involved; sometimes it varied not only from day to day but within the day itself, so that, outside of certain items, the patient never knew what to expect, and even what was done often did not seem to make much sense to her. As a result, the patient was kept in a striving, seeking, frustrated, struggling, and emotional state in which anger, bewilderment, disgust, impatience, and an intense, almost burning desire to take charge and do things in an orderly and sensible manner became overwhelming. (During the writing of this paper the patient was interested in what was being included and pointed out that many times, "I hated you horribly, you made me so furious, and the madder I got, the more I tried.")

Since the problem was clinical in nature and no conventional therapy was known, therapy had to be experimental, but since it was the patient's welfare at stake, there was no way nor attempt at evaluation of the actual usefulness and validity of any single one of the procedures employed. Recognition can only be given to the agreement of competent outstanding clinics in their evaluation of the patient's prognosis as decidedly poor—in fact, hopeless—and the actual eventual outcome of the therapy devised.

Fortunately, the patient's first companion was a highly intelligent, deeply interested, wholly cooperative person with an amazing flow of language and fluency of speech. This was seized upon as the first therapeutic approach, but without acquainting the patient with essential details or purposes.

At the first session the patient was told by the author with painful exactitude and emphasis that she was to extend herself to the very fullest extent of her physical and mental ability to listen carefully to each question the author asked her and to make every effort to reply, however arduous she found the task to be. She nodded her head vigorously, and she was asked her husband's full name. Before she could complete the first partial efforts to frame his name with her lips, the companion, as previously instructed, replied with great rapidity with his name, age, and birthplace, all of which was gravely recorded by the author as if furnished by the patient.

Equally carefully and slowly, the patient was asked her full name, including her maiden name. Again the companion, while the patient was struggling with her mouth, gave the name, age, street address, etc. On and on this went, the author gravely and earnestly asking the patient questions, recording as if they were the patient's replies each of the companion's answers, some of which were purposely approximations or even wrong. Slowly the patient's early wonderment turned to obvious anger and infuriation, especially at the erroneous answers and misinformation.

At the end of the hour the author remarked casually to the patient, "You're as mad as a wet hen, aren't you?" in response to which the companion verbosely reassured the author that the patient was not in the least angry. The author continued, "And you really don't want to come back either, do you?" Again the companion solicitously reassured the author, while the patient, apparently in an utter fury, with trembling lips, stammered, "I prom——prom——prom——[ised]" and stalked out of the room much more steadily and easily than she had entered.

The next day, as soon as the patient, Anne, was seated, she was asked for her entire history. Immediately, the companion Jane, began a rapid-fire summary of Anne's purported personal history such as date and place of birth, schooling, teachers' names, years of attendance at college, and much family data, many of which were merely approximations or often in actual error. Anne glared at Jane in increasing anger and also at the author, who was hastily making notes and behaving as if it were Anne who was speaking. All of the time Anne's lips and mouth were struggling to reply, to make corrections, and when the hour was concluded by the author's announcement of the hour for the next appointment, Anne stalked out of the office even more steadily than she had before, only to be called back and told gravely that a daily schedule of activities had been arranged for her and that the companion's responsibility was to keep a chart on Anne's cooperativeness. Anne nodded her head vigorously and angrily, turned quickly with a single backward step, and left, still angry. She was called back, and with great intensity, after fixating her gaze rigidly upon the author's face, she was told slowly, repetitiously, that she was to be fully and completely obedient in relation to the schedule. She was then allowed to leave the office, departing at first slowly as if in a trance state and then gradually more briskly. As she turned to leave the office her appearance and manner indicated that she was in a trance. No effort was made to test her for hypnosis. The reasons for this are no more than the author's clinical experience in securing hypnotic responses from subjects without letting them know at first, lest the conscious awareness lead a patient to try to be overhelpful in the therapeutic procedures.

Much later Anne remarked to the author, "I was sent to you for hypnosis, but you never even seemed to try to use hypnosis. When I look back, though, I'm sure you must have had me in a trance many times when I didn't know it. When I get mad at people, I stay mad—maybe for years. But it was different with you. I'd get mad, really mad, but the next day when I was still mad, something in me made me want to come back.

Maybe that just means you were getting through to my subconscious mind, and that was why. Did you have me in a trance a lot of times?" To this question, since she had not made all the progress the author felt to be possible, his standard evasive reply was given: "I like to help patients, but I often don't try to explain what I'm doing. The answer to your question is, you can guess any way you want to, and either way is all right with me." Such a reply closes the question without answering it, yet leaves the author free to elicit trance states or selected or isolated hypnotic phenomena without the patient's awareness of what is really occurring. Much more readily do patients look upon them as their own conscious intentional effort rather than a passive responsive act elicited by the operator. Leading the patient to "See what I [the patient] can do," is much more effective than letting the patient see what things the therapist can do with or to the patient.

Jane showed Anne a typewritten schedule, but Anne actually could not read it because of her alexia. After many vain struggles by Anne to read it, Jane read it to her several times, but with specified and different errors. Anne listened intently, and her facial expressions indicated that she recognized some of the variously read items and was annoyed. It included bedtime, shower time, meal times, swimming hours, medical appointments, etc., and, most emphatically, the declaration that whatever Jane said or did was to be obeyed scrupulously regardless of what Anne thought, understood, knew, or wanted. There were to be no exceptions of any sort.

This schedule was intended only as another means of stimulating the patient without letting her realize what was happening. Thus, in spite of the clock in full sight and the radio announcing the time as 9:00 o'clock, Jane declared it to be 10:00 P.M. and "bedtime." Anne sputtered inarticulately, and Jane read from the schedule the author's emphatic declaration that Anne was not to dispute or disobey Jane's instructions, all of which were listed on the schedule furnished Jane by the author.

At breakfast time Anne was awakened early and asked if she wanted scrambled eggs, toast, and coffee. Anne nodded her head affirmatively, then noticed that the clock indicated she was being awakened 1½ hours too soon, and pointed at the clock. It was later learned that she recognized the time of day by the position of the hands, not the clock face numerals. Jane cheerfully remarked that it was a lovely morning, and Anne furiously dressed, came angrily into the breakfast room, and was dumbfounded to find oatmeal and a lettuce salad for her, while Jane had fruit, dry cereal and coffee. Immediately after the breakfast, which Anne ate with resentment while Jane cheerfully commented on every topic that came to mind—including the author's absolute order that Anne should always clean up her plate—Jane abjectly apologized for not having told Anne to take her shower before breakfast. Cheerfully and with much light chatter she took Anne back to the bedroom and saw to it that Anne took a shower, completely ignoring all of Anne's efforts to tell Jane by sign language that she had showered, that the shower floor was wet, that the towels proved that she had showered, etc. Jane merely chatted fluently on a wealth of topics. Jane's sense of humor and zest in following this type of instruction was extremely helpful, and she easily used her own ready ingenuity to execute the author's wishes.

At a later session Anne attempted to communicate effectively by writing a note with her left hand, which she did poorly, and handed it to the author who vainly attempted to read it upside-down and gravely handed it to Jane, who followed suit. Shrugging of shoulders and helpless looks led Anne to say "turn, turn, turn." Obediently the author and Jane turned back toward Anne with further shoulder shrugging. Anne burst into tears and said, "Turn paper round."

This was done, and the request was read "Can she take me diner out?" It was obviously slowly, painfully, and laboriously written.

Immediately consent was given, and Anne unhesitatingly but stumblingly asked, "Breakbreakfast lunchtoo." Ready consent was given, and Anne looked happy and triumphant. Jane had really enjoyed frustrating Anne at every meal by such measures as presenting her with a carrot instead of a banana while Jane cheerfully ate a banana herself. More and more at meals now and then Anne would explosively utter some article of food she wanted, and she was always properly rewarded in an entirely casual matter while Jane chattered endlessly on minor casual topics, always interspersing unimportant minor errors, to Anne's obvious annoyance. Thus a birthday present would be suggested for Anne's oldest child when it was the youngest child's birthday. (Incidentally, Anne was greatly underweight, but she rapidly gained weight in being obedient about cleaning up her plate.)

The request to go out for meals gave new opportunities for Anne's frustration since Jane drove the automobile. It did not take Anne long to discover the need to start to say "Right," meaning "Turn right" a block or so in advance, and shortly to say "Right" at the intersection, since Jane invariably turned the wrong direction or continued straight ahead if not instructed at the proper time.

The menus at the restaurant were another source of instruction and frustration. Since Anne could not read, Jane would order foods that she knew Anne did not like, and always the author inquired if she cleaned up her plate regularly.

Anne attempted to point out to the waitress the items she wished, but Jane stopped that by telling the waitress "Doctor's orders" and reaching for the menu. Shortly Anne began pointing out specific times on the menus, but unless she named it, Jane ordered wrongly. This led shortly to pointing and naming and the getting of some of the foods she wished. Her reading ability soon reached the point where she could read but not always name the item completely. This Jane handled by such a measure as ordering "potato salad" when Anne had pointed to "baked potato" but said only "potato." It was not long before Anne could say "steak me medium" or otherwise make her wishes clear.

Almost from the beginning the author had taught Anne and Jane the rhyme of "Pease porridge hot, pease porridge cold" and the accompanying hand and arm movements. This game was played regularly with the patient a dozen or two times a day, with Jane reciting the rhyme at first slowly, then with increasing speed. This was done at varying times during the day, sometimes in the middle of a meal or even during a shower bath. Gradually Jane began to make the wrong movements, eliciting corrections from Anne who would spontaneously correct her by saying irritatedly "no, no," "this this" or "no, this way." Without comment Jane would make the correction, only to make other errors later. Also Jane began reciting the rhyme with variations in tempo. This occasioned considerable annoyance to Anne, who soon began to mouth partially the various words of the rhyme. As Jane noted this, she would make deliberate errors in the words, and frequently Anne would explosively utter the correct words. Often this game was made a part of the therapeutic session with the author so that her progress could be noted and further instructions could be given to Jane about errors to be made.

Direct hypnosis seemed to the author to be impossible; therefore Anne was told impressively within the first two sessions that it would not be employed. (Many months later Anne explained, "You really fooled me when you said 'no hypnosis,' that I couldn't be hypnotized. Remember, I asked you before and you just talked and didn't really answer").

Instead, Anne was told in a most painstaking, laborious way, holding her attention in a most rigid, fixed fashion, "As Jane says that rhyme ["Pease Porridge Hot" was not the only one employed; there were many others], listen carefully, hear every syllable. Give it your full attention, notice each sound, all vowels and consonants. Remember each word. Think each word. Remember each word. Think each word. Remember carefully when you were a little girl, when you first learned those rhymes. Where were you sitting or standing? Who taught you? Remember how hard, when you were a little girl, it was to get the words just right. Remember who taught you, where you stood or sat and how, when you learned the onesies and twosies, how happy you were."

The preceding is a brief but representative example of the indirect method of fixating the patient's attention, regressing her in her thinking and remembering to earlier times and situations, and literally inducing through attention-fixation a trance state and possibly some hypnotic age regression through careful use of her actual past history obtained through extensive inquiries of the husband or Jane.

Also, very early in therapy an attempt had been made to capitalize upon infantile utterances such as "goo," "da," "ma" as a measure of teaching the patient to talk. This, however, hurt her feelings and served only to emphasize her infantile helplessness in speaking. This was apparently too threatening a measure, though Anne later told of doing it when alone because she had "promised" to do as told. Also, the author was the only person who seemed to have a genuine hope for her, and she wished not only to please but also to get "even with him for his silly tricks." Thus, a peculiar state of ambivalence, of mixed dislike and liking, existed in the patient, along with a compelling, highly emotional motivation to learn.

Each such session appeared to be followed by improved performance, and Jane's enthusiasm waxed anew each time she made her report preceding each session with Anne.

Rhymes were paraphrased and were fitted into the situation to personalize them to fit Anne's past experience. Thus, mention was made in a session of a certain street address, and at a signal from the author Jane obligingly in a singsong fashion recited "Annie and Willy sitting in a tree, k-i-s-s-i-n-g." The flush on Anne's face disclosed Anne's full remembrance of that specific childhood experience, and the situation was immediately seized upon again to fixate Anne's attention, to emphasize the time, the place, the difficulties in learning childhood rhymes, and the need always to listen to every word and sound. Numerous other little, more-or-less embarrassing experiences of Anne's past were used similarly.

One morning, when Jane had prepared an atrocious breakfast for Anne, Anne pushed Jane aside and, as she walked into the office first, said, "I'm mad——at you——at her too——she helping——can't help get mad—sorry—much sorry."

Anne's facial expression indicated that she was angry, that she regretted it, that she sensed some legitimate purpose on the part of the author and wished for some kind of reassurance.

In reply, with Jane joining in at once, the following rhyme was chanted to her: "Anne is mad and we are glad and we know how to please her; A bottle of wine to make her shine and (husband's name) to squeeze her."

Anne's reaction was a joyous response "He's coming, he's coming." By coincidence, her husband was coming into town that weekend, a fact known to the author, and the session was spent planning a pleasant weekend for Anne and her husband with an occasional spontaneous word or phrase from Anne suggesting other possibilities.

She was also complimented on the adequacy of her remarks and speech and told amusedly that however angry or mad she got, the worst was yet to come. Her surprising answer came unhesitatingly, "I'm game." She was beginning to realize her improvement.

Jane was then thoroughly drilled in saying the "Pease Porridge" rhyme in a halting, hesitant, and stuttering fashion.

She learned this in a phenomenally fast manner, and then Anne, who knew nothing of this special measure, was asked to recite with Jane the Pease Porridge rhyme, however hesitantly she had to do it.

Slowly the two began, Anne slowly, while Jane began to increase the tempo and then to stutter the words in a painfully annoying fashion. Anne glanced at the author, was sternly instructed to listen to Jane and to continue the joint recitation. Anne turned to Jane and her lips and face showed the ideomotor, therefore involuntary and uncontrollable, efforts on Anne's part to correct Jane's stutter. On and on, over and over, Jane continued, with Anne's lips twitching, and finally Anne was haltingly prompting Jane throughout the whole rhyme. This particular session lasted about two hours, and Anne's speech became increasingly better. The same measure was employed with other rhymes, and Anne was obviously pleased and confident though often immensely annoyed.

At the next session Anne made the pitiful plea, "Now Jane is my——best——friend——I——like her——much, very much. She—she——she does everything—you tell her. I don't want to hate her. Do—do——do—do—something else."

The author told her sternly, after fixating her attention rigidly by his manner, that he was conducting the therapy, that he would please or displease her as he felt best, but that her obvious improvement warranted a change. She was thereupon instructed to take Jane out to dinner and to put in the order for both of them, asking Jane each item she wished, and doing the ordering and she was assured that Jane would eat it, but she was warned to speak slowly, carefully, or that the situation would be reversed. Several evenings later Jane ate a dinner that was a mess, to Anne's intense merriment and the waitress's bewilderment, since both women were obviously amused and sober (e.g., mustard on lemon meringue pie!).

Interspersed with all of the above therapy was another variety of therapeutic endeavor. This was the beating of time to music, at first to slow music and then to rapid, lilting melodies, although Anne preferred either classical or dance music such as "The Blue Danube." This beating of time followed various patterns: right hand and left hand separately at intervals, then together, then alternately at every other beat; right and left hand separately at intervals, then together, then alternately at every other beat; right and left feet separately at intervals, then together, then left and right feet at alternate beats; left hand and left foot together, then alternate beats for the hand and foot similarly; then left hand and right foot jointly, then separately at alternate beats, then both hands and feet together, separately and alternately and then alternation of left hand, right foot, with right hand, left foot.

Jane was an excellent taskmaster and arbitrarily interrupted meals, showers, television and radio programs at will to ensure "enough practice to satisfy the doctor."

The final step of this measure was to have Anne beat time with the right hand on the left knee, the left hand on the right knee, each time alternating the position of the arms so that first the right arm would be in front of the left, and then vice versa.

As Anne progressed in variously beating time to music, she was instructed to hum. Jane would join in, softly singing out-of-time and off-key, to Anne's annoyance, and then, as Anne began singing the tune, Jane dropped out. In fact, Anne's only protection from Jane being out-of-time or off-key was to hum or sing the tune herself.

Family duties took Jane away, and in her place was put a shy, young, timid girl, extremely sweet and lovable, unwilling to offend and yet obviously afraid not to do exactly as instructed, and easily flustered by sharp criticism.

Anne's reaction was excellent. She liked the girl immediately, adopted at once a protective maternal role, and was constantly springing verbally to the girl's defense at the slightest threat of the author's displeasure directed to the girl.

The excellent progress Anne had made under Jane's care was not only maintained but enhanced by Anne's protective attitude toward the young girl, who was exceedingly conscientious despite her timidity and gentleness, and actually just as competent a taskmaster as was Jane.

More and more improvement occurred; Anne was taught to "relax" as a means of resting from the summer heat of Phoenix, and the girl, an excellent hypnotic subject, would posthypnotically relax with her and in rapport with Anne. Thus, Anne was exposed over and over to the hypnotic situation without ever needing to know she had been hypnotized. She was left no opportunity to wonder and to question and perhaps to doubt her own capacity to improve. Instead she had to attribute her responses and changes not to passive responses to the author and the task he assigned, but to her own efforts explained in part above.

Remembering Jane's conduct at the table, Anne was most careful to spare the young girl the distress Anne felt certain that the girl would experience in obeying the author's instructions if she patted her slice of bread to indicate she wanted the butter and being handed a stalk of celery. Also Anne soon learned that the girl, with obvious distress would reply to a patting of a slice of bread and say haltingly, "But—but—but——" would elicit the verbal response of, "Ask me not but's and I will tell you no lies," or when Anne asked for water by saying "wat—wat—wat" as she lifted her water glass would elicit from the girl a flush of embarrassment and the simple utterance, "What, when, where, and why are parts of speech." Thereby Anne readily realized the competence of Jane's reports, the author's own careful observations during therapeutic sessions, and the thoroughness of the instructions to this girl who aroused so strongly her protective maternal urges. (Incidentally, the young girl, now a mother of several children, and Anne are still the warmest of friends.)

When the author felt that Anne had gained as much as was possible from this protective maternal situation with the girl, a third companion was then secured, after a careful survey of possibilities with Anne's husband concerning friends and relatives who might be willing to serve. The woman selected by the author was oversolicitous, worried, mistrustful, very eager, in fact too earnestly eager to execute whatever instructions she had been given about Anne's daily program, though she did not like them or even understand them. These instructions were carefully limited to what Anne could do either easily or with some little effort. For example, the woman was instructed, "When Anne starts to butter a slice of bread, watch carefully, and when it is half buttered, you butter the other half, or if you see Anne reaching for her glass of water (or coffee cup or glass of iced tea) nearly empty, you are to jump up and tell Anne, 'You don't need to say a thing, I'll fill it,' or tell Anne to cut her meat or to put lemon in her iced tea, etc." The husband had most emphatically told this companion to obey the author's instructions, however nonsensical they might seem, such as making Anne take a dozen shower baths in a single day or at 2 A.M. or to put the right shoe on the left foot. (This had been done repeatedly by Jane more than once just before bringing Anne to the office.) The first time this happened, Anne angrily extended her feet and pointed at her shoes. The author complimented the appearance of the style of the shoes and the low heels. She shook her head angrily, and the author very rapidly recited the well-known jingle of "goats eat oats, mares eat oats, does eat oats, and little lambs eat ivy."

After a few moments of confusion both women recognized the jingle, but Anne unwittingly went through a mental process of sorting out words and identifying them and differentiating them from the auditory impression given by the rapid utterance.

Later, when Anne was beginning to correct somewhat her alexia, the same measure was employed somewhat differently. Slowly she was taught to recognize the words of similar jingles such as "Nation mice lender ver says knot" (Nay, shun my slender verses not) and then later to be told or to discover the words. This served not only to interest and amuse both women but to effect for Anne possibly a new ordering of her attitude toward words both written and spoken.

This companion's oversolicitude, overeagerness, and overhelpfulness aggravated Anne intensely, and she did every possible thing to prevent being helped. Also, Anne learned to retaliate. Anne herself sought from the author a number of such jingles written out with which to annoy this companion, who seemed to lack much of a sense of humor. Yet, Anne was a sweet personality, and the general relationship between the two women was good. The companion did recognize that in some inexplicable way the author was accomplishing therapy. This companion thus aided greatly in literally compelling more effort on Anne's part in order to escape the oversolicitious aid that served to motivate her to still greater effort. Also this companion could not comprehend what the author was attempting, and was worried and mistrustful of the author. Anne's favorable rapport with the author literally compelled her to demonstrate to this companion that the author's methods, however incomprehensible, were good and most helpful.

However, Anne tired of this companion, and earnestly told the author one day. "She good—do right [obeys author's orders]—not happy job— she have go." This was an exhausting effort at communication because it distressed Anne for two reasons: the discharge of the companion and distress at seeming to oppose the author. Her request was acceded to only after an extensive review over several hours of all the learning she had which had been frustrated by this woman, and then the author made clear to Anne some of his reasons for considering that frustration as desirable, and also why it was not previously explained to her. Additionally, many amused comments were made by the author over the woman's lack of a sense of humor, of Anne's half-resentful, half-amused plaguing of the woman with jingles and in other ways, and he pointed out that the woman always evened the score in some way. Anne did not realize how closely the author checked the daily course of events with that woman and gave instructions to her to help keep the score even and not to disturb the ties of a distant relationship that existed.

Accordingly, both women were much pleased by the author's termination of her employment, since a new venture in motivating and learning processes seemed in order.

A fourth companion was then secured after intensive questioning of the husband. She was a young girl, obedient but on the whole not too interested or impressed by the various procedures and the monotonous reports and activities at the office. Anne was frequently displeased and disgruntled with her, could find no direct fault with her except her lack of enthusiastic, intelligent interest. She did repeatedly tell the author that she would be glad when she was sufficiently improved to get rid of "that girl with her mind elsewhere." There was no question of where Anne's "mind was." Anne's interest was in her improvement, and she did not like to have anybody, however conscientiously obedient, disinterested. Thus Anne was forced into a position of validating her improvement by being irked, even angered, by her companion's lack of interest and meaningless (to the companion) obedience.

A fifth companion was then secured. This was an older woman, rather absorbed in her own interests, rather "slack about doing things" as Anne complained, and who obviously regarded the author's whole procedure as bizarre, purposeless, and without meaning—even silly and ridiculous. However, care was taken to make sure that she executed her duties, and Anne particularly enjoyed the author's assignment of special bizarre tasks. She also enjoyed the older woman's general dislike of the situation and duties and took particular pride in improving even more extensively just to demonstrate to that woman that the author, whom Anne had now come to like greatly, was correct in his methods and that the companion was wrong (Anne's opinion and emotional reaction to this companion were probably more vital than the author's procedures, which were to intensify Anne's own motivation).

One particular item thought of by Anne at this time was that when she could not say a word, she would "walk around it." The author agreed and pointed out that she could count and stop at the right number when she could not give her son's age. But Anne herself devised the method, when blocked on a word—for example, *butter*—of getting up from the table and elaborately walking around in a tortuous path about the furniture in the room, sitting down and saying, "Pass the yellow stuff there," pointing to it. What Anne did not realize was that, when blocked in saying a word and then walking a tortuous path in and out and around the furniture, she was indirectly and unwittingly adding to her vocabulary and lengthening her sentences. Thus, blocked on saying *butter,* she had, in the procedure she devised, to say to herself mentally, without realizing it, "I must get up and first walk around that chair and then over the end table and past the davenport and open and close the refrigerator door and then go back to the table and say, Please pass that yellow stuff." That this is what actually did occur is not known, nor was any inquiry made. She had suffered brain damage and she was improving by nonconventional methods. Experimentally, it would have been scientific to have inquired of her, but the goal was one of therapy, not of controlled scientific experimentation. However, a number of normal subjects were deliberately asked to do as Anne and her companion had described as the walking about the room in a random, tortuous path. This done, they were asked to relate the thinking they had done as they did so. Naturally they prefaced their explanation with, "I couldn't help wondering what your purpose was, but I decided to walk around the coffee table, and then over to the book case, and then around the throw rug and then past the radio." Anne's aphasia was a motor asphasia. Presumably her thinking processes were like those of the normal subjects. At all events, she would return to the table with some remark such as, "Pass that yellow stuff there," instead of limiting her utterances to "Butter, pass," or "yellow stuff, pass."

This particular companion was always bored by the sessions in the office, did not try to conceal the fact, and the author took advantage with

Anne's half-resentful half-amused attitude toward the companion, to delight in having them go through the various "exercises" that had been assigned. Particularly did Anne enjoy the author's discounting of her inability to talk originally by the bald assertion, which the companion resented, that any little baby could say "goo" and "ga" and "da," and so could Anne. These particular exercises Anne had resented at first. They had been used sparingly in the office, though it was later learned that they had been done secretly by Anne in her apartment. But Anne enjoyed going through them with this companion, even enlarging them from meaningless syllables to baby talk, a measure Anne did deliberately and without prompting to irritate the companion for her criticisms of the author. An excellent, constructive example is, "en—ee—bah—dee," and this intentionally transformed into "anybody."

One other step that seemed to the author of importance was the institution of a measure to correct, if possible, the alexia. This the patient was almost irrationally certain could not be corrected despite the considerable progress with menus and jingles, and hence a completely indirect measure was taken. She was furnished pencils and paper and told to sign her name. It was reasoned that, since aphasia involved motor elements and visual word memory and that the alexia was a matter of visual perception, a motor skill might be employed, one that was not related as such to ability to read which is naturally followed or accompanied by reading.

She signed her name in an almost illegible fashion. She could spell her name verbally but could not identify the letters when only one letter at a time was exposed to her. She could recognize her name and her husband's nickname. She could not recognize her last name or even such a simple word as *cat*.

She was instructed to take a pencil in each hand and, holding the pencils in the correct writing fashion, simultaneously to write with both hands her own name. She spontaneously noted that her left hand wrote backward and was spontaneously interested in figuring out the probable individual letters in both writings, since the right and left hand writings compared fairly well because of the poor writing caused by the residuals of the hemiparesis of the right arm.

This was one special exercise the author devised which the patient delightedly modified to confound the author while still abiding by instructions. The assignments were her name, those of her family, her birthplace, and then, knowing that she was an ardent baseball fan, she was instructed to write simultaneously with both hands numerous pages filled with the statement that she hoped her favorite team would lose each game. This she did reluctantly—in fact, resentfully. Then one day she entered the office with a broad, triumphant smile with a whole handful of sheets of paper covered with remarkedly improved script. Apprised by

Anne's facial expression, the author accepted the sheets most carefully, with only a casual careless look. At first then disappointment, then fury showed in Anne's face, whereupon she demanded imperiously of the author, "You read them." The reply was given that the author had trouble enough reading his own script without attempting someone else's. Since her secret plan was so easily defeated, Anne furiously snatched the papers back and read freely, "I hope the X team wins. I hope other teams lose." in all, she had written and read aloud easily a dozen different statements negating the author's original demand that her team lose, etc.

She was most elated over this, and the author promptly expressed his demand that she write various uncomplimentary things in relation to persons or objects she liked. She took much pleasure in defiance of this by simultaneously writing right- and left-handedly complimentary remarks, and, with less and less halting speech, reading them. She enjoyed this defiance greatly as well as taking much pride in her improved handwriting and ability to identify individual letters and words.

A newspaper was shown her, and she was asked to read an account of her favorite baseball team. She futilely attempted to do so, whereupon the author read it aloud to her, actually paraphrasing it into a most derogatory account. She snatched the paper from the author and haltingly and imperfectly reread the article aloud correctly, half amused, half angry at the author. This measure served to convince her that she could read "if you make me real mad."

There were, of course, numerous other measures essentially variations of those already described, that were employed to prevent boredom or slackness and to keep the patient continuously alert and yet annoyed, frustrated, and at the same time hopeful and pleased by recognizable yet often not immediately realized progress.

By November 1956 she was sent home for two months, returning for further therapy in January and February. She had lost considerable ground, which she attributed to the coldness of her home state. Improvement was rapid and quickly surpassed the previous gains.

She returned home again, and her friends noted no aphasia, although the family physician noted occasional evidences. The alexia persisted, although considerably decreased. Weekly letters from her were demanded, a laborious task often written with many errors. Some of these were arbitrarily sent back with peremptory demands for corrections without the errors being marked. She resented this disdainful handling of her correspondence but invariably found the errors, corrected them, and would append the statement, "This makes this week's letter." (One manupmanship is a potent therapeutic force.)

Very slowly she began to read short stories to her youngest child. Currently her alexia is far from being corrected, but she can and does read some of the newspaper.

She has been exhibited to a considerable number of physicians as a former patient and has joined the author in challenging them to guess her original diagnosis. Almost all have noted that her right leg is slightly edematous and have offered a diagnosis of thrombophlebitis. On one such occasion she laughingly replied, "You're right, only you are wrong. Just listen to me try to say that word and you will know." She then attempted to say "thrombophlebitis" and laughed at the guess of "speech defect," saying, "No, aphasia," even adding "from a hemorrhage."

She still is very slightly awkward from hemiparesis residuals, experiences considerable hypersensitivity and some deep pain of the right side; and cold weather and high humidity greatly increase the deep spontaneous pain and her hemiparesis residuals. She is still taking a minimum dosage of codeine and empirin and an occasional sedative. It was she who persuaded her husband to move to Arizona, but to Tucson, not Phoenix, where the author lives. Thus she is too far away for an emergency call, but she does see the author for occasional visits at irregular intervals of one to four months. For a family physician she was referred to an internist in Tucson, for whom she developed an immediate respect and liking.

She follows a good general daily program except on unusually chilly winter days. That period of the year she is most likely to want to see the author once a month, as "insurance that I am staying all right and it is just the cold that makes things more difficult." She entertains freely, drives the family car, picnics in the mountains with her family, does the family shopping, but has a housekeeper do routine household tasks.

The specific difficulty in stepping backward had been corrected by having her learn to dance, something she had always enjoyed, and which the first two companions had enjoyed doing with her, the first companion with considerable difficulty, the second with ease, while no trouble was later experienced by the patient in dancing with her husband. Posthypnotic suggestions to the second companion ensured certain awkwardness that Anne helpfully corrected.

Her stair climbing and descending difficulty persists, but the move away from her home state permitted living in a one-level house. However, a climb of two, three, and even four or five steps is easily managed by the measure of carefully noting the number and height of the steps. A larger number necessitates actual assistance.

Cold, if intense, and high humidity, besides increasing the symptoms of her thalamic syndrome and the paralytic residuals, have the peculiar effect of decreasing her sense of taste. This was confirmed by her over- and underseasoning of foods, an item of fact discovered by her family, since she is an excellent cook. At such times she carefully loads her plate and "cleans it up" so that she will not lose weight because of definite lack of appetite.

DISCUSSION

To discuss the therapy employed and its rationale is difficult. The patient had been rendered suddenly and distressingly helpless at a most happy period of her life but without any loss of her intellectual capacities. The helplessness of her situation, the frequent surges of hope occasioned by trips to nationally famous clinics, the black and hopeless despair that followed, the meaningless, well-intentioned, obviously false and uninformed assurances by all of her friends, associates, and her relatives that "everything is coming along fine," left her more hopeless and despairing than ever, to say nothing of her actual pain and physical difficulties. She recognized her vegetative state, felt helpless to do anything about it, and found herself facing a completely wretched future for which she could see no remedy nor any way to hope for one.

She knew that the diagnosis of "hysterical reaction of her partial hemiparesis" was wrong because she knew she did have pain explained to her as "thalamic syndrome," but she did recognize that the general practitioner actually had made a finding he could recognize as new and different from any made by all the other physicians and that he was obviously positive that it signified hope. This had encouraged her briefly, but then all of her hopes had been dashed on previous occasions of optimism.

She had consented to see the author, was again encouraged by his interest in the peculiar midline sensory demarcation and his prompt discovery of her alexia, which he seemed to recognize understandingly, although none of the famous clinics had seemed to pay any attention to it (nor do their reports make any mention of it). Next she was, as she later explained, "fearfully and powerfully" affected by the author's frank and open statement in her presence that she was a totally hopeless case unless she wanted, *really wanted,* to get well, that every possible opportunity would be given to her, that no effort would be made to spare her feelings at the sacrifice of her welfare, and that the case would be accepted only under an absolute promise of full cooperation despite the fact that therapy would not seem reasonable, nor even sensible nor considerate; that all reasonable, conventional things had been done to no avail for an intelligent adult now reduced to a state bordering on infantile incapacity. Therefore, she would be handled and treated accordingly without regard for her intelligence, her master's degree, or her social background.

Therapy would be oriented about her helpless condition, and use would be made of every possible pattern of reaction and response that she had retained without regard for banal social conventions, and a demand was made that she give her solemn promise to abide by whatever therapeutic measures the author might propose. It was pointed out simply and emphatically that to date all conventional therapies had failed, that there would be no loss entailed by new measures, and that a therapy devised to meet the actual reality she represented instead of the *lost realities of the past* might conceivably serve a useful purpose. (Later the patient stated that this frank, nonreassuring offer to give help, but a refusal to promise it, influenced her to take hope and to give and to keep her promise of cooperation despite the anger, frustration, and displeasure the author's methods occasioned. As she explained later, "It didn't make sense most of the time, but I couldn't help noticing that I was doing better. But you did make me just awful mad, and after awhile I discovered it [being angry] helped. Then I didn't mind how mad you got me. But it was awful at first."

Although it cannot be positively stated as factual, one may speculate that the treatment accomplished gains for the patient according to the following utilization of procedures:

1. Her vegetative state was corrected not by sympathetic care and attention nor by patient instruction, but was rendered intolerable by cheerful and obvious stupidity intentionally executed that refuted every intellectual understanding she possessed, and stimulated an actual desire to understand and to learn—but what to learn she did not know. Only a strong and compelling motivation was there, compelling her to seize upon anything offered. It intensified her need to avoid such unmistakably given misunderstandings of her needs, which then led to a frustration state quite different in character from the frustration of incapacity to which she had become so well accustomed. Instead, it was a frustration that compelled her to take action to avoid it by one means or another, and there was no fixed, set, or rigid pathway, nor any opportunity for passive withdrawal, by which she could escape. Each new measure employed by the author placed slightly new and different demands upon her, most of which frustrated her in some new and different way and in a fashion which was intended to lead to effort rather than to a vegetative state. In fact, "cleaning up her plate" when served weird combinations of good, nutritious foods often served to give expression to her innermost emotions of resentment, "which somehow made me feel better."

The emotions accompanying each new demand upon her were something more meaningful than useless despondency and the desperation of the past. There was a desire to retaliate, to do something, to change things, and for varied reasons—anger, amusement, bewilderment, confusion, disgust, etc. There was no one dominant emotional state causing a generalized rejection of things or a withdrawal as had derived from her despair and despondency and depression over her incapacities.

2. General knowledge indicates that verbal learning is based upon a

variety of experiential processes. Consider children learning to count. They can learn by rote repetition to count to 10 accurately. Given a good sample of children and various methods employed to teach them to count by verbal instruction and, at the same time, having them touch the instructor's fingers on the nails one by one in proper sequence from one little finger to the next makes the task easier. Hearing, seeing, tactile experience and verbalization combine to facilitate the process of verbal learning. Transfer to a task of counting the fingers without touching them is then easily accomplished. Then the child can be given the task of counting the fingers with the hands turned palms up and counting in sequence from one thumb to the next but without touching the fingers. The task suddenly is more difficult for the child unless he is allowed to touch the fingers. Then the hands can be held up, the palm of one, the back of the other, facing the child, and he counts readily without touching the fingers.

Transfer of this learning to the counting of 10 marbles in sequence is then easy. Then place one large marble anywhere, but usually best at the end of a row of marbles, and ask the child to count them visually. The answer too frequently is "nine little marbles and a big one," not the simple reply of 10. Then have that child count the marbles by touching each as he looks at them and counts; the answer is "10, but one is big."

Also, how does one learn to read without moving the lips? And the rhythmic person (as the author knows by personal experience and inquiries of similar persons) has intense difficulty in counting the rapid, rhythmical drumming on a table but can count more rapidly and more accurately when a few marbles are dropped from the hand to a tabletop in as rapid but nonrhythmic fashion.

Throughout therapy innumerable items and speculative ideas were kept in mind and revised at each session to fit any immediate changes in the patient's situation and to add new or to arouse old associations to all relearnings and any new learnings.

The Pease Porridge rhyme was ideal for this: it demanded attentiveness, an anticipatory span of attention, coordination of hand, arm, and eye movements, auditory attention, an active motor set and participation; too, presumably, it would arouse some ideomotor and ideosensory and hence involuntary speech movements, possibly, perhaps undoubtedly, including subliminal speech.

Certainly the painful stuttering so deliberately and well—though laboriously—done by her companion would serve to, and almost be sure to, elicit ideomotor and ideosensory speech experiences. (Consider the overwhelming natural tendency to say words for a stutterer). These would include quite possibly, even probably, subliminal speech and affectively reinforced speech memories, particularly associated motor memories. Also, it would serve to elicit strong self-protection tendencies, a desire to get away from something unpleasing to the self—even as her speech problem was unpleasing to her and it demonstrated that there is an escape from a speech problem—an item of vital general significance.

3. The rhythmic beating of time to music and listening while beating time to lilting songs would lead to ideomotor and ideosensory speech experience, and the peculiar and complex combinations of right and left-sided beating of time and the constant shifting of the beating pattern from left to right and vice versa were deemed to aid in the development of new alternative neurological pathways of response to auditory stimuli. Additionally, the tendency to hum, to anticipate the next words of the song already heard many times, the tendency to join in the singing, and the frustration by the companion's out-of-time humming and off-key singing appeared to offer a most compelling eagerness and motivation to use her vocal cords out of sheer self-protection, since she did have an excellent ear for music.

4. The patient's markedly underweight state and the authoritative demand that "she clean up her plate" served not only to correct her weight, an item she could sense and appreciate as a visible proof of her improvement, but put her into an eager state of mind of wanting to have her choice of food instead of the nutritious but unwanted selections by her companion. Her appetite, her long-established tastes in food, and her need to protect them served to motivate her desire to speak and also to read the menu so that she could be certain of having her wishes met.

5. The alexia, a distinct problem in itself, is nevertheless related closely to speech. (Watch little children's lips, even those of some adults, as they try to read silently.) Thus, the restaurant menu served the dual purpose of compelling not only speech but reading also. (As reported by Anne later, the first restaurant meal ordered for her, taking advantage of her hopeless speech condition and alexia, aroused not only her anger, but a tremendous desire for doing a turnabout on Jane, something she planned for weeks before the opportunity arose. And such a plan had to be based on actual and inclusive expectations).

Thus the diet frustration, despite her gain in weight, filled her not only with a wealth of mixed emotions but literally forced her into a position anticipative of the correction, but not so recognized, of both the alexia and the aphasia as a means to an end rather than an end in itself.

6. The selection of the first companion was a fortunate act of fate, but it suggested the use of different companions, each to call forth progressively and more assertively the various natural patterns of response that characterized Anne. The first companion by her quickness in seizing upon situations and taking advantage of them while obeying orders forced Anne from a state of frustration and black despair into a state of intense desire to frustrate the companion—hence to do and not to yield hopelessly.

The second companion was picked as a measure of evoking Anne's own deep maternal urges. She missed her family greatly, seized upon the second companion as a substitute, and to the very extent of her ability attempted to do things to prevent the author from rebuking this girl. Also, the girl was a good hypnotic subject and could be given posthypnotic suggestions creative of special situations such as the radiating joy at every success of Anne's and her eyes brimming with tears whenever she mistook Anne's helpless pointing at something instead of naming it and therefore proffering something wrong, which Anne's vigorous negative shake of her head disclosed it not to be wanted. Thus, by virtue of the girl's excellent posthypnotic amnesias, she and Anne would attribute events to situational developments which could not appear in any way to have stemmed from the author's instructions. Also Anne, in her maternalism, would have another type of aversion toward her difficulty, an aversion having its origin in its distress not to her but to someone else. Thus, a set of circumstances could be created in which Anne could take charge spontaneously and not feel that it had been arranged by the author. Anne knew full well that Jane and the author worked hand in hand, but with this girl Anne was inspired to take charge herself. Additionally, the afternoon siesta which posthypnotic suggestion made so easy for the girl served to set an almost irresistible example leading to "joint relaxation," and Anne delighted in following the example set with the development of an intensely warm interpersonal situation in which Anne was the dominant personality, which was not hitherto the case with Anne's friends during her illness at home nor with Jane. And she is definitely a strong character.

7. The third companion served the significant purpose of compelling Anne to reject emphatically any effort at oversolicitude and to compel a determination to be as self-reliant as possible. This continued unrecognizedly the work initiated by the previous girl and compelled Anne to strengthen it.

8. The fourth girl, by virtue of her feeling of boredom and disinterest, served a most important role of compelling Anne to recognize that much was yet to be done, that much had already been accomplished, and that she herself would have to undertake the responsibility to do all that was requested and even more.

9. The fifth and last companion, absorbed in her own thoughts and troubles, with her tendency to scorn and belittle the author, was actually exceedingly helpful. She powerfully reinforced Anne's assumption of self-responsibility, placed Anne in the position of appraising and recognizing the extent of her improvement, and aroused intense emotional desires to protect the author from criticism of his methods. Thereby Anne unwittingly placed herself in the position of not only justifying and validating the methods, but the forcing of recognition by this companion that the methods were right and that she was continuing to improve.

10. The handwriting exercise in itself was an added special measure of

peculiar complexity. Anne knew that she could write only illegibly, and the simultaneous right- and left-handed writing intrigued her curiosity and interest.

At first her left hand wrote more legibly than her right. This pleased her, but although she did not realize it, it also forced her unwittingly into taking *a reading attitude* toward her handwriting. Then having her write derogatory things about her baseball team gave her the golden opportunity to retaliate with much amusement against the author for all the things he had done directly or indirectly against her. By such amused execution of an assigned task, abiding by the essence of the task and yet seemingly defying the author, there was established an easy, comfortable, interpersonal give-and-take relationship between two adults rather than an impersonal physician-invalid relationship. Thus there could be a sense by the patient of sharing significantly and pleasurably in both a joint and a separate accomplishment conducive to her welfare.

As she continued the writing, she realized progressively her capacity to read more and more, and this was assumed by her to be her own spontaneous development. Thus, her faith in herself was greatly strengthened. The impersonally critical treatment of her weekly letters compelled her not only to read while writing them but to read them with searching care *to correct errors.* She enjoyed receiving letters, but cold impersonal criticism of errors noted but not marked in an otherwise friendly newsy letter, coupled with a peremptory demand reminiscent of her original promise to the author, compelled her not only to read while writing them but to read with seaching care to prevent errors. Thus, the return of her letter with a peremptory demand for corrections not indicated for her gave her a golden opportunity to retaliate by searching out the errors and then returning the corrected letter with the triumphant statement that it was the letter for the current week. And one or two occasions in which she missed errors she had made taught her to ensure her triumphant escape from a letter every week because a letter twice returned for correction was accorded no value. Moreover, Anne was strongly competitive, and her need to win was of utmost value in this manner of dealing with her letters. (She now dictates letters by tape recorder—it is more convenient since there are residuals of hemiparesis in her right arm and her alexia is far from corrected so far as writing is concerned.)

11. The recitation of childhood rhymes, little experiences from her childhood, embarrassing or semi-embarrassing incidents, served not only to awaken past memories but to reinforce all associated mechanisms of behavior and learning responses.

12. It is true that the patient's progress might be attributed simply to the increased individual attention she received. However, it is also true that she had received an immense amount of individual attention from numerous relatives, friends, and her family, all of which did not prevent

the development of a vegetative state. Also, she received extensive and highly skilled nursing and medical care and attention, all to no avail. But all such care and attention had been based upon concern, sympathy, fear, worry, helpful protective attitudes and a despairing concept of her as helplessly and hopelessly invalided, despite the diminution of her hemiparesis. Such attention was always accompanied by sympathetic and encouraging assurances in the face of obvious and unmistakable disability and therefore was patently false and expressive only of the wishes of others and an unintentional emphasis upon her invalidism. The patient's *own retained intellectual capacities* permitted her recognition of the falsity of the assurances and the significance of the sympathetic concern as actual expectation of a continuance of her invalidism. As was mentioned early in her medical history, she had a master's degree and possessed excellent intelligence.

The therapeutic attention devised for her and described in this report was of another character entirely. There was no fear, concern, anxiety, or sympathy offered. Instead, there was literally a peremptory demand for cooperation and the exacting of such a promise. Instead of gentleness and sympathetic consideration, there was the annoying assignment of seemingly meaningless tasks and the deliberate devising of situations which would lead to feelings of frustration accompanied by intense emotions of a motivating character rather than of hopeless despair. She was not encouraged to talk, but a situation was created that could lead to involuntary ideomotor efforts of speech and quite possibly to subliminal speech. Frustration was used deliberately to prevent despair by compelling the patient, in self-protection, to strive to secure some satisfaction of ordinary, reasonable, and legitimate desires. For example, being handed a carrot instead of a banana not only infuriated her but tremendously intensified her desire to talk and a need to reject her helplessness so that she might retaliate in kind, as indeed she later did. Yet she had not been asked to talk, which she knew she could not do. Instead, a situation was created which, through the intensity and welter of her emotions, would impel her to seek some measure or means of meeting her wishes and needs. Neither was she asked to learn to step backward without falling. Instead, her maternal urge to protect the second companion from the author's seeming displeasure about the companion's inability to dance well was used. (A posthypnotic suggestion to the companion ensured a certain awkwardness.) Hence, stepping backward easily and readily was only an incidental and unrecognized part of her emotional relationship to that young girl.

Likewise, the simultaneous writing with her right and left hands, especially of statements offensive to her personal loyalties, could not be recognized by the patient as a form of speech corrective of alexia. To her it was a motor task, repetitious and monotonous, that inspired her to confound and defy the author finally by angrily reading aloud the exact opposite of what he had deliberately misread.

So it was with all of the other individual attentions she received. They were all deliberately and intentionally controlled and directed *toward the evoking of whatever capacities for all kinds of responses which she might have or could develop,* without regard for courtesies or social niceties *but only for whatever responsive behavior might be conducive to restoration of previous patterns of normal behavior.* However, the nature of her specific reactions was not and could not always be anticipated. *Her welfare* was the governing purpose of the therapy devised—not sympathy, consideration, or even common courtesy. Perhaps the best example to illustrate this was the occasion on which Anne had laboriously, slowly and with apparent distress crossed her legs in an effort to relieve her deep spontaneous pain. When she had completed this difficult task, the author amusedly chanted the old childhood rhyme, "I see London, I see France, I see somebody's underpants." The celerity and ease with which Anne embarrassedly uncrossed her legs with no apparent recognition of painful feelings was a startling revelation both to herself and to her companion. Later Anne recalled this incident by saying haltingly, "member——underpants—move——move leg fast——no hurt."

Numerous other little incidents like this, conducive to strong emotions and automatic responses, unquestionably served to restore and to reinforce normal responsive patterns of behavior and to compel a confident realization of her own recovery of latent capacities of response awaiting adequate stimulation.

13. Hypnosis and hypnotic techniques, usually indirectly and unexpectedly, were frequently employed to arrest and to fixate her attention rigidly upon therapeutic ideas and understandings. By so using hypnosis, her attention was directed and controlled and possible demands for conventionally "sensible" instructions were forestalled. The liking she had developed for the author, the slow but continuing progress which she could see and sense, served with the hypnosis to prevent an intermingling in her conscious daily thinking of conscious doubts, fears, anxieties, and uncertainties with the authors' carefully given helpful ideas. Instead, she became the author's ally, and any questioning doubts were left to the companions.

Even now, seven years later, she feels "different" in the office, and much of her behavior is highly suggestive of a hypnotic state. (For therapuetic reasons no effort is made to test her.) However, this seemingly hypnotic behavior is absent in the waiting room, and she socializes easily and well with the author and others. Another comment in this connection is warranted. About a year ago she met the author at the Tucson airport and took him to her home for some additional therapy. However, she first acted as a hostess, displaying her home and her garden and making inquiries of a purely social character for about an hour. Then when the author remarked, "I believe you have some questions to ask me," there developed a fixed, rigid attentiveness and a seemingly unwareness of her surroundings similar to that of her behavior in the office.

14. In brief, the therapy developed to meet Anne's manifold problems may be best summarized as: (a) The devising of measures to negate her passive withdrawal and her vegetative state dominated by a sense of hopeless, helpless frustration; (b) Employment of measures, sometimes directly, sometimes indirectly, capitalizing upon her frustration and despair by employing measures which might conceivably make use of resulting strong emotional drives as a basis of evoking a great variety of response patterns and of motivating learning; (c) Arousal of motivational forces and memories that had played a part in her development from infancy to normal adulthood; and (d) Inducing and compelling an open-mindedness or mental receptiveness to new, inexplicable, curiosity-evoking ideas in settings causing the patient to look forward with hopeful anticipation and not to expend her energies in despondent despair over the past. Always and ever-changing challenging activities of the present and the future occupied her mind, and thus there existed a mental frame of reference conducive to recovery of lost learnings and the development of new learnings, possibly by new and alternative associative neural pathways.

31. Hypnotically Oriented Psychotherapy in Organic Brain Disease: An Addendum

Milton H. Erickson

In the report presented in the October 1963 issue of this Journal, the fact was not specifically emphasized but is nevertheless obvious that underlying the entire procedure was the utilization of the patient's emotions. Each new measure in some manner elicited emotional reactions, attitudes, and states—sometimes pleasant, but more often of special personal displeasure—and these were employed to intensify and promote her learnings and to stimulate her to greater effort. In some degree, and progressively more and more so, she recognized this through the therapeutic course and endured it willingly, though with frequent reluctance.

At that time thought was given only to the possible effect upon the patient of any sudden catastrophic emotion in relation to family matters of illness and death, which were dealt with adequately as actual probabilities. The patient proved able to cope with this type of stress. However, there was no thought of provision for an overwhelming emotion at a catastrophe of national importance such as she experienced at the announcement of the assassination of President Kennedy. She was an ardent supporter and admirer of the late president, and the announcement of his death had a sudden and detrimental effect upon her. Within a few hours the pain of her thalamic syndrome had increased greatly; she experienced a marked sense of weakness and motor instability; within three days she lost 20 pounds and found the process of eating a laborious task, "I swallow a few bites, then something happens—my appetite—it's gone—I try to eat another bite—I get sick to stomach—try to eat another bite—lose everything. I just eat a bite or two—wait a while—try to eat another—eat all time little bit—mustn't lose weight—but lose fast—awful fast—I'm so weak—so tired—so much pain—no sleep—almost like when I came to you—I'm scared, but still I just want to lie down and give up."

She was brought to see the author after the passage of one week of progressive deterioration. After securing the history, a rapid testing for speech and reading ability was made, which showed no appreciable losses.

Reprinted with permission from *The American Journal of Clinical Hypnosis,* April 1964, *6*, 361-362.

Her motor ability and ease of walking were definitely impaired. Her right-sided hyperalgesia was severely increased.

Her interest in food, once an item of intense desire and frustration, was gone. Even slight discussion of her previously favorite foods elicited reactions of nausea.

Her previous companions during therapy were indirectly mentioned in a seemingly casual conversation without arousing interest in her, except for the mention of the second companion, the shy timid girl who had stirred her protective maternal emotions. She otherwise showed marked indifference or an astonishing dislike, but this dislike was found to be related to the course of events in their later lives since the time that they had been her companions. (She and her husband had maintained casual contact with them). More astonishing was the change in her emotional attitude toward her husband and children. Contrary to her usual maternal concern, she showed disinterest in all except her youngest child, but even this was barely more than mild interest. Her attitude toward her husband was cold, unsympathetic, and indifferent, seriously in contrast to the vividly warm affection in which she had held him.

Her husband's spontaneous statement was most informative. It was, "You have just got to do something. I went through this once before, losing hope and faith, just watching her go downhill for almost a year. Except for being able to talk, she's just about where she was when we first brought her to you (1956). I can't go through that again, and she can't either. Now do something and do it fast. Make her eat. She tries, but she can't. Maybe you can teach her some way, but do it fast. Make her feel alive and real."

In lieu of any well-formulated or even carefully considered plans, and because the patient was rapidly becoming listless and apathetic, the husband was dismissed, and the author began an exhaustive but vivid discussion of the assassination and its possible immediate meanings and those of historical perspective. The patient's interest was slowly but effectively aroused, at first by a deliberate use of morbidness in the discussion, and then was maintained by as thoughtful and meaningful a discussion as could be offered.

Gradually a shift was made to the youngest child's interest in the same topic, and then to the question of that child's tendency toward overweight and faulty and demanding eating habits, particularly of foods with high carbohydrate content. Then, by extremely cautious indirection, the patient was slowly but intensely inspired (but this was seemingly not noticed by her) to set that child a pattern of table behavioral conduct of such tact and good example as to lead him effectively away from previous indulgence in a large portion of dessert before meat and vegetables and toward a proper approach to kinds and qualities of food. All this was done in a guarded, prolonged, and indirect fashion, and the patient finally left the office more stable physically than she had entered it. Her purposeful attitude and almost peremptory demand that her husband hurry up and get home so that she could prepare dinner for the youngest child was in marked contrast to her behavior upon arrival.

Her husband was promptly and secretly told to be matter-of-fact and noncommittal, to make neither inquiries nor suggestions.

Subsequent information disclosed that the patient had made excellent progress, her thalamic pain had again decreased to its previous low level, and there was little evidence of untoward reaction to the national tragedy. Apparently the appeal to her maternal instinct, so effective in relation to her second companion, again proved a remarkable effective measure of reviving her previous learnings and attitudes.

A month later the patient was again in good condition, although she had not yet gained back all of her weight loss. Her appetite was excellent, but it was noted by her husband that now and then she would seem to have momentary difficulty in swallowing. At such times her husband reported, "Her face gets blank, she seems to forget where she is, doesn't even seem to see us; then she seems to wake up and she doesn't know what just happened to her and keeps on eating. I suppose she just goes into a momentary trance, so none of us say a thing. But she is really doing something about the boy's eating.

"She is not upset anymore, and her pain is greatly reduced. I'd say she's back to where she was except she still lacks 10 pounds, maybe more. She is O.K."

In all, less than four continuous therapeutic hours had been spent with her.

DISCUSSION

The significance of emotional trauma to individual adjustment is universally recognized. But it is noteworthy that in this particular case of the effects of organic brain damage, corrected in large part by new learnings having marked personal emotional components, the adjustment was seriously threatened by a national tragedy with strong personal emotional overtones, even though a death in her immediate family and two other serious family disasters had not caused more than normal grief.

32. An Application of Implications of Lashley's Researches in a Circumscribed Arteriosclerotic Brain Condition

Milton H. Erickson

A 70-year-old woman had been repeatedly and separately diagnosed by several different groups of competent neurologists. The findings of each examination were essentially the same. In essence, these were to the effect that the patient was suffering from what appeared to be a peculiar circumscribed irregular arteriosclerotic condition of the brain, resulting in manifestations suggestive of Parkinson's disease which were limited to her face and which affected her speech. Her mental functioning otherwise appeared in no way to be affected. All agreed that no effective medication was known and that the condition was untreatable.

The patient reacted by becoming a dependent, inactive, rather despondent recluse, but after several years of urging by her family, she and her husband consented to attempt again to secure treatment, and she came to the author for hypnotherapy.

Examination of the patient's face disclosed: (a) tremors of the lips; (b) spasmodic, erratic movements of the entire facial musculature; (c) faulty, interrupted verbalizations; (d) athetoidlike movements of her lips and jaw.

Both the husband and his wife were assured of the organic character of her difficulty and of the dubiousness of the effectiveness of therapy except for a possible amelioration of her emotional withdrawal and despondency. They were asked to consider seriously the organic nature of her condition, her age, and the duration of her problem before requesting hypnotherapy. No promise of therapeutic benefits was given and doubt was expressed even concerning emotional benefits, but it was agreed to make an attempt.

Seeking a possible basis and rationale for treatment, the writer called to mind Lashley's research on maze learning in rats, with subsequent relearning after surgical destruction of various areas of the brain, as well as the implications of his research for the utilization of alternate neurological pathways after brain damage. The possible applications of this type of relearning led to the formulation of the following experimen-

Reprinted with permission from *Perceptual and Motor Skills*, 1963, *16*, 779-780.

tal proposal to which they agreed when they returned for a therapeutic session.

The proposal made was that she undergo hypnosis (a) to learn relaxation and (b) to develop motivation to ensure long-continued posthypnotic adherence to all the instructions given her. These were that three times daily, a half-hour each time, she would study her facial image in the mirror and carefully, concentratedly, and repetitiously move her chin up and down and from left to right and back to the midline. Also three times a day, midtime between her jaw exercises, she was to make deliberately the one syllable sounds of infantile articulations such as goo, da, etc., also for half-hour periods.

As she progressed in this task, she was to begin talking slowly to her mirror image, carefully observing and endeavoring to make correct facial movements, giving her mirror image such simple instructions as, "Now open [close] your mouth. Now move your chin to the right [left, midline]. Now smile." As soon as she learned this to her satisfaction, she was to explain to her mirror image carefully and systematically the numerous, often complicated, recipes for food which she once had greatly enjoyed preparing.

The patient was most conscientious for some months, during which she developed normal facial movements and speech and returned to her normal home and social activities. This led gradually to a progressive neglect of her daily "exercises," which had been reduced to once a day because of her complete self-confidence. Shortly she experienced a progressive and rather rapid return of her symptomatology, and she was dismayed to learn that she had forgotten her instructions.

She returned for further therapy, was given the same instructions again, and within a month regained her normal facial behavior and speech.

Since then she has been given "permission to skip exercises" two or three times a week. She now lives and has lived for more than a year a full normal home and social life, much more like that of an energetic 40-year-old woman than one nearly 80. Her recovery has withstood several family tragedies and a progressive slow hearing loss.

Previous to this study a similar experimental reeducative procedure was employed successfully with another patient with brain damage which is yet to be reported. Since then, there has been reported by Slater and Flores in *The American Journal of Clinical Hypnosis* (1963, *5*, 248-255) a study of "Hypnosis in organic symptom removal: A temporary removal of an organic paralysis by hypnosis."

The important question raised by these reports concerns the value of hypnosis in organic disease, the need to recognize the possible potentiating of natural corrective body processes by hypnosis, and the possibility of the establishment of new learning pathways in cases of organic brain disease.

33. Experimental Hypnotherapy in a Speech Problem: A Case Report

Milton H. Erickson

Eight years previously a woman in her mid-sixties had been diagnosed as suffering from "Parkinsonism." She had been dissatisfied with the diagnosis and had sought the opinion of a second and a third neurological clinic. She resigned herself then to the fact that all three clinics independently gave the same diagnosis and offered the same unhappy prognosis. She visited a medical library and read extensively concerning her affliction. This led to a decision to resign herself to her affliction except for one symptom, which she had been told at all three neurological clinics was "atypical" and for which there was no accounting. This symptom was a peculiar harsh, deep-tone, grating, rasping speech, which the author learned to imitate by tensing his neck and thoracic muscles and then tensing his entire abdomen as if he were trying to force air out of his lungs under great pressure while speaking. The patient was noted to behave somewhat similarly but not to the extreme degree to which the author had to resort to match the patient's speech.

She resented her speech difficulty. It was difficult; it tired her; it was unpleasant even to her ear; and she felt that such an atypical symptom could be treated. For the past eight years she had sought all manner of speech therapy to no avail. She finally read about hypnosis and sought therapy from the author.

After securing her history, noting the character of her speech and observing her intensely vigilant attitude and suspicious manner, she was informed that hypnosis was not applicable and that she was not hypnotizable. (This was correct at the time.) Verbally she expressed great regret, but her manner indicated a sense of profound relief, and her entire behavior became much more friendly and cooperative.

She was given a second appointment and a promise that consideration would be given to possible therapeutic measures.

At the next session she was told with impressive emphasis that she might be able to correct her speech if she "concentrated absolutely

Reprinted with permission from *The American Journal of Clinical Hypnosis*, 1965, 7, 358-360.

completely upon a course of relearning" that the author had devised. This was involved and difficult and would require the utmost of mental effort on her part. (The utter confidence and simplicity with which she was so instructed gained her full attention.)

To lay the groundwork for an experimental approach to her problem, all effort at scientific accuracy of problem description or explanation was discarded in favor of securing the patient's full cooperation. Also the author kept in mind his previous experimental speech therapy with a woman with a localized arteriosclerotic condition of the brain (preceding article in this section). Hence, it was explained that her voice was too deep; that is, her affliction had resulted in the use of muscles deep within her body to give rise to speech. Therefore, it was proposed to create a form of speech that could be located completely above her shoulders. Over and over this explanation was repeated, in varying words and phrases, until her attention was so fixated that she developed a hypnotic trance. (New hope had made her accessible to indirect hypnosis. That such an indirect induction was employed, after her previous relief upon being told that she was not hypnotizable, was entirely legitimate. Her reason for coming to the author was for hypnotherapy despite whatever unfavorable reactions she had toward hypnosis.) Slowly the author went on to explain that this change of speech could be accomplished if she would paste on her bureau, dressing table, and full-length mirrors, typed in large letters, all the nursery rhymes she could discover that she possibly might or could have known in her childhood. Additionally she was told to paste up the alphabet as well. Then she was instructed that she was to listen intently to special explanations and instructions that the author would give her concerning how she was to perform a certain important task. This task was the assignment as a duty for her to *think and read visually* the alphabet forward letter by letter while *saying it backward* letter by letter. Thus she would be in a state of great mental strain. This mental strain would all be above her shoulders, hence her voice would be above her shoulders because all strain and effort would be primarily in her head. Similarly she was to think and read visually the rhyme of "Mary had a little lamb . . ." forward while repeating it all word by word backward.

She was told to sit or stand in front of her various mirrors from 20 to 30 minutes three times a day, concentrating laboriously on reading visually all the various typed material forward while she laboriously matched each visually read word or letter by softly pronouncing its corresponding place-mate in the end-to-beginning progression of her verbalizations. The reading and the verbalization were to be simultaneous. Thus, as she read the letter A she would pronounce the letter Z, and this she was to practice with such utter intensity that she would hear or see nothing else, unless absolutely important, during each practice session until she developed fluency. In order to avoid the limitations deriving from the trance state that she had unwittingly developed in the office while being given instructions, she was told that she would execute her task with conscious learning as well as with unconscious learning, every day, whether awake, dozing, sleeping, dreaming, hungering, or thirsting. In fact, she would perform her task regularly and happily in whatever mental state would serve to allow her to learn to talk normally in the ordinary course of the day's events and in all personal situations, and that she would do so even if she never in her life—past, present, or future—developed a trance and that under all circumstances whatsoever she would have a full, effective conscious and unconscious awareness of her task. (This all-comprehensive statement, despite the inclusion of the absurd reference to the past, was both reassuring to her and a posthypnotic suggestion reinforced by the emotional comfort suggested.)

She was seen for eight additional one-hour appointments to reinforce her understandings and to give her an opportunity "to practice" in the author's presence to permit further guidance if necessary, but very little was needed. There was no question about the good quality of her trance states, though no formal induction was employed. Also, she never recognized the fact that she developed a trance each visit. These appointments were spread over a period of two months.

At the end of two months only one or two words out of ten were spoken in the former faulty fashion. The patient was highly elated, and though she moved out of the state, she kept in correspondence with the author to assure him that her problem had diminished to an almost vanishing point, although her other symptoms persisted.

CONCLUDING REMARKS

The therapy devised was patterned with the experimental speech therapy study cited above in mind. It was based in part on the assumption that there could easily be large psychogenic elements in her speech problem. Even if it were completely organic in origin, over the years there had been added a strong emotional reaction to it. Therefore it was reasoned that it would be well to create a learning situation that would bypass the possible psychogenic elements. This could be done with a newly created learning situation which could then be associated with childhood learning situations involving vocalization. By an enforced alteration of a simple visual-vocal reading task, there could be effected a strong divergence of her attention from her speech problem and the learning of vocal reading associated with visual reading as difficult as that combined task had been in her early childhood.

Perhaps this is the explanation of the patient's eventual recovery of better than 90 percent of her disability. This was far beyond all original hopes. However, one experimental instance such as this constitutes proof of nothing more than that many more experimental ventures are warranted in seemingly hopeless problems which are encountered so often in medical practice.

34. Provocation as a Means of Motivating Recovery from a Cerebrovascular Accident

Milton H. Erickson

Karl was in his fifties, an energetic, hard-working man incapable of working for others because of his "German stubbornness," but fully competent to develop and successfully conduct his own business. Karl seldom wasted a moment; he engaged in numerous incidental projects that developed profitably, or else he spent his spare time in extensive reading of a definitely educational character, most of it at a postgraduate level. His personality was that of a "hard-headed stubborn, bullheaded German who insists on having his own way and always works hard enough so that he proves that he's right, even if he has to do things the hardest way first." He was sharp-tempered but essentially kind and most enthusiastically approving of the endeavors of others to work hard, to better themselves, and to achieve. He always had a helping hand to lend any hard-working person who wished to accomplish something, but he would never give more help than was actually needed. Self-reliance, as much as possible, was his guiding personal principle.

Then unexpectedly an unbearable calamity struck Karl, a cerebrovascular accident that paralyzed him and rendered him physically a completely helpless bed patient, capable of understanding but unable even to read or to talk. His communications were limited to head movements, most of them nothing more than an enraged shaking of his head when spoken to or questioned about his needs. As his wife explained, "Karl has always been so capable. He could do just anything, and if he couldn't, he would read up on it and then do it. He just never let himself fail in anything. He is a proud, determined man, and now he is so pitifully helpless. He feels so ashamed because we lost our savings in medical bills and our shop because he couldn't run it and I couldn't. It kills him to have me work. And he is a stubborn, impatient man. He always wants to do things right now and make them perfect. They kept him a whole year at the University on the neurological ward, trying to help him, doing a lot of things. But he was a 'teaching case,' and Karl would go half out of his mind when the medical students would come in and one after another examine him. Then they would hold clinics on him and talk about 'irreparable damage,'

Unpublished manuscript, circa 1965.

'hopeless prognosis,' and talk about the parts of his brain he had lost because he can't talk and can't read, and Karl would get madder and madder and shake his head so furiously and sweat so they told me they might have to put him on the psychiatric ward. So I took him home, but I can't do much for him except massage and feed and bathe him. He has learned a little use of his one leg and arm, and he can use a cane a little, and if I practically carry him, we can get from one room to another. You saw how he got out of the car and how we came into the office. That's the best he can do." (Watching this activity had been most painful, but it did present good clear evidence of extreme physical disability somewhat lessened by laborious, awkward, frequently useless efforts at self-help.)

All of this history and further elaborations of the above were taken in the patient's presence. As parts of the history were given, he would nod or shake his head in agreement, or shake his head in anger, perspiring freely as he did so, and he would make grunting and snorting noises expressive of bitter anger and rage when mention was made of the year's thoughtless treatment as a "hopeless teaching case" on the neurological ward (confirmed by the author's personal inquiry while lecturing there).

The purpose in seeing the author, his wife explained, was to have hypnosis employed to reeducate new neural pathways so that he could learn new ways of functioning, new ways of using his arms and legs by employing newly developed neural pathways. A family friend, a physician, had studied an article by the author on the reeducation of a patient with brain damage (Erickson, 1963) and had urged them to consult the author and have the possibilities of reeducation under hypnosis explored for Karl.

A prolonged history was taken from his wife in the patient's presence. The same questions were asked repeatedly in slightly different form. Unnecessary and pointless questions were asked. Throughout this time-consuming procedure the patient was carefully watched, chiefly by peripheral vision so that he would not realize how extensively he was being scrutinized.

Finally the author began asking repeated questions about the patient's willingness to accept help. His wife replied that there would be one serious handicap—namely, however much Karl wanted help, he would insist that it be done his way, "that man can't help bossing everything." She was asked what would happen if "a bigger boss than your husband takes over, then what will he do?" She replied that on a few occasions her husband had had to bow to greater forces than he could muster, that he did so ungraciously and resentfully, but "no matter how mad he gets when he is forced to bend under, he always sees to it that he benefits or profits in some way, and he never holds a grudge very long. He is really too sensible-minded."

The patient listened to all of this, manifesting variously agreement, impatience, resentment, even anger, and boredom. More than once his wife commented, "Look at him now. He is disgusted with all this talk. He wants to get started right now," to which remark Karl vigorously nodded his head in assent.

When the author finally concluded that he had observed the patient long enough and had evoked enough emotional responses and a sufficient number of erratic physical movements expressive of disgust, impatience, and eagerness to permit a somewhat favorable assessment of the therapeutic possibilities, the situation was cautiously outlined to her. Karl listened with mounting impatience, breathing heavily, snorting, grunting, perspiring, and making many minor spasmodic movements with the one leg and arm over which he had gained some slight control. His wife stated in explanation, "Karl wants to start right now. He can't tolerate waiting until tomorrow for another appointment." Karl nodded a most emphatic assent. His wife added apologetically, "I know Karl, he wants things always his own way, and he wants to start now, so I suppose you will have to cancel the rest of your patients today and work with him." To this Karl nodded an emphatic affirmation.

The author's reply was simply that, as a physician, he was in charge of the patient, and any further work would be started the next day. Karl leaned his head back and stiffened his neck and back, whereupon his wife explained, "Karl means he won't leave your office."

In reply she was told to bring Karl back at 11:00 A.M. the next morning, and then the author summoned two grown sons and instructed them to pick up Karl, to carry him outside, and to load him into the car gently but most firmly. This they did while his wife wrung her hands, sobbed, and fearfully declared that Karl would never come back. She was reassured, "Not so; that man wants absolute proof that he can be handled, and he will probably make one more test. You say nothing. Disregard everything that Karl tries to communicate to you. Do not be disturbed by anything that occurs. Let Karl seethe in his anger all he wants to. And tomorrow morning at the right time get the car and pull it up to the door on the simple assumption that Karl is going to keep his appointment. Now, dry your tears, straighten your face, talk and act cheerfully."

Karl refused to eat that evening, refused to be undressed, refused breakfast, snorted, and seemed to be in a continuous rage from the time he left the office. His wife managed to play her part until 10:00 A.M. the next morning, when she asked him if he would keep his 11:00 A.M. appointment. Karl grunted, snorted, and managed to throw his cane on the floor. Then he began perspiring, and he shook his head negatively in a furious fashion. She burst into tears and retreated into the next room. However, at 10:30, when she drove the car up to the front door, she was astounded to see Karl opening the door. In some way he had managed by the use of his cane, chairs, and furniture to work his way from the bedroom to the front door; getting him into the car as well as out of it and into the office had proved easier than she had believed to be possible.

This information was secured while Karl sat alone in the office, apparently raging because the author had left him alone in order to question his wife about the above account of his behavior.

"Well, Karl, I see that you are still mad, but the important thing is that you are here. The rest of the session I will spend merely explaining various things to you, not doing anything, just making clear to you what kind of a job we have to do, how we will have to start at it, and how you are going to take orders and obey them without question whether you like them or not."

At this point he grunted loudly and shook his head negatively in a violent fashion. "You mean, Karl, that you want to start today?"

Most vigorously he nodded his head affirmatively.

"Well, unless you change your mind rapidly, very rapidly, and decide to let me state how things are to be done, today's interview will be concluded and you can return tomorrow for the explanation I intended to give you today."

For a moment he glared angrily at the author, then resignedly and slowly he nodded assent.

An explanation was then offered that:

1. Hypnosis would be utilized only to the extent considered useful for the varied therapeutic purposes in the author's mind.
2. Hypnosis would definitely be excluded in certain relationships to be determined solely by the author.
3. Prompt and complete obedience would be imperative.
4. All judgmental assessments would be made by the author, and Karl's opinions would be disregarded completely.
5. The author's medical knowledge would govern all matters and Karl's wishes and desires would not be considered.
6. The first evidence of disobedience or hesitation in regard to the author's orders would terminate that particular session.
7. The only information desired from the patient would be the author's own observations and whatever information was requested of his wife.
8. Additional instructions would be formulated as progress was made.

The interview was then terminated by the peremptory measure of stating in a most dictatorial fashion, "Now, get up out of that chair. Stagger your way to the office door and get out of here and get to your car and give your wife's tired arms and back a little rest on the way. Get going!"

Karl's startled look was replaced by a flash of anger, followed by an expression of utterly intense effort as he proceeded, grabbing a chair, then a bookcase to haul himself to the door already opened by the author. Karl's wife came rushing to Karl's assistance but was firmly cautioned to give him only enough help to keep him from falling. Clumsily jerking, twisting, using his wife only to balance himself, Karl made his way to the outside steps, where the author's sons wordlessly picked him up and set him at the bottom of the stairs to make his own way to the car. This he did with increasing clumsiness, and by the time he reached the car he was obviously fatigued. Without a word the author's sons picked him up and placed him in the car, while the author advised his wife to go for a scenic drive so that Karl could rest enough to help her get him out of the car. She was also told that if he grunted to get her attention, she was to tell him, "The doctor says I am to tell you to shut up, so shut up."

TRANCE INDUCTION BY AN AUTHORITARIAN APPROACH

The next day she related that she had to tell him to "shut up only twice" in the 24 hours that had elapsed. She also reported, "He's improving. He let me read the newspaper. He got to the breakfast table alone. He got to the front door alone. I think he wants to tell you about it by having you ask questions so he can nod his head."

Instead, as Karl dragged, jerked, and stumbled with a minimum of help to his seat in the office, he was told peremptorily, "Close your eyes. Lower your head toward your chest. Relax as much as you can. Listen to the clock on my desk ticking. Spend the next 15, 20, 30, 40, 50, or 60 minutes going asleep in a hypnotic sleep. Take the whole hour if you want to. I know you can do it in 15 minutes, but you can take the whole hour and the next hour tomorrow we can spend time doing what could have been done in the 45 minutes left. I'll know when you are in a trance. All you have to do is just go to sleep listening to the clock and waiting for me to talk to you and remaining asleep while I talk to you. Get going!"

Within 15 minutes the tension of his facial muscles had altered in the characteristic hypnotic fashion, his swallowing reflex had disappeared, his respiratory rhythm had greatly changed, and he presented an acceptable appearance of a deep trance. He was told, "Now listen to me. If you are deep asleep, just nod your head gently up and down." Five minutes later he was still perseveratively nodding his head gently in affirmation. This was taken to signify a deep trance, and the noisy dropping of a heavy paperweight on the floor did not elicit a startle reflex or any alteration in his respiratory rhythm.

From here on in the trance state I told him that I reserved the privilege of using invective whenever I pleased, but *that his cure was in his hands.* He was to walk more and more each day. Within three months he was walking well. On the day he walked 15 miles in the desert areas around the city, he visited me and told me about it in speech that was very clear. He reversed the anger he had had, and used it up in directing his energy into walking and all the other aspects of his rehabilitation. His wife was astonished when she heard him tell me, "I love you as a brother."

R: How often did you see him in that three-month period?

E: Usually when he came to see me he would try to proudly tell me of his progress, but I would make disparaging remarks and accuse him of laziness and giving up too soon. He'd come back a week later and tell me how many more blocks he had walked, but I continued to be unkind in all my remarks, goading him into further effort. When he was in trance, I was very gentle and would only tell him how I was going to act when he was conscious.

R: So when he was in trance, you prepared him for your goading behavior when he was conscious. You were working on his unconscious at one level, preparing him for the motivating provocations you would later hurl at him on the conscious level. How do you explain that?

E: The man really wanted to do things. I carefully told his unconscious that his conscious mind did not yet have the new brain patterns that he needed. So I'm going to keep his conscious mind angry and resentful so he will work while you (his unconscious) help him build up more and more brain patterns. Karl was a tool-and-die maker who had his own factory. He was inventive.

R: So you utilized this inventiveness and the metaphor of making "more brain patterns" because that was particularly apt for a tool-and-die maker who was used to carefully making new "patterns."

E: Yes. Karl did well returning to his factory and supporting his family until he had a much more massive stroke 10 years later. When his wife brought him to me then, she said the stroke was so bad he could not even get mad anymore.

R: He no longer had the motivation to fuel the rehabilitation process?

E: It was unfortunate that when he went back to his factory after his initial recovery, he was even more angry and impatient. He took out some of my assumed anger and impatience and tried to drive his employees too hard. I did not know that at the time.

R: That was an unfortunate side-effect you had not counted on. You helped him live 10 more years of useful life, but his unresolved anger could have been instrumental in that final massive stroke. But we cannot know for sure; in practical clinical work we are usually handicapped by insufficient knowledge.

Do you believe the explanation you gave Karl's unconscious during the trance state was a pseudo-argument, or do you really believe his unconscious was manufacturing new brain patterns? Are new brain patterns being constructed during such rehabilitative efforts?

E: Yes. In my own experience with myself it seems to be a matter of learning to use muscles in a different way. When I was 60, I went for a physical, and the examining neurologist found that I had divided some muscles into halves, some into thirds. One-third of a muscle was realigned to pull against the outer two-thirds of itself. One-half of a muscle was pulled against the other half.

R: You believe that new brain patterns do develop in physical rehabilitation and that these can be manifested by all sorts of readaptations in muscles to recover lost functions. There is greater plasticity in both the central nervous system and our actual musculature than most of us have dared believe. You would definitely encourage more strenuous rehabilitative efforts and greater expectations for recovery?

E: Yes, Karl was told he was a hopeless case, and so was I when I had polio the first time at the age of 17.

VI. Hypnotherapy with Psychotics

One of the enduring misconceptions about hypnotherapy is that it is either dangerous or ineffective with patients experiencing a psychotic episode. Certainly there are special dangers and difficulties in applying any therapeutic approach with psychosis because we still know so little about it. Hypnotherapeutic principles are particularly useful with psychotics, however, when they are applied with sense and sensibility.

The cases in this section come from an early period of Erickson's career. Like much of his later work, they involve exploratory-clinical approaches. The major problem, as in all therapeutic approaches with psychotics, was in securing attention and rapport with the patient. This is particularly evident and is described in detail in the first case of Laskarri, where Erickson uses some traditional approaches in an innovative manner. There are some interesting similarities between this early case and the later case of Edward (see "Hypnosis: Its renascence as a treatment modality" in Section 1 of this volume). Both men were catatonics, and both manifested superficially similar ward behavior. But their educational levels and family structures were different. Both were able to work out their essential inner life problem by dreaming it over and over again under hypnosis with a different set of characters and situations that gradually provided growing insight that led to an eventual resolution of their psychotic process.

A particularly interesting theoretical analysis of Erickson's work is provided by Zeig in his presentation of the second case in this section. This analysis in terms of "symptom prescription" is another way of understanding Erickson's utilization approach, which is found to be as useful with psychotics as it is with any other diagnostic category of patients.

35. Hypnotherapy with a Psychotic

Milton H. Erickson and Ernest L. Rossi

Laskarri had been diagnosed on the psychiatric ward as suffering from schizophrenia of the mixed catatonic-hebephrenic type. He was moderately disturbed in his behavior; several times a day he would shout gibberish apparently at hallucinatory figures and race back and forth and around and about the dormitory beds or scramble frantically under and over them. Or in the dayroom comparable behavior might be manifested in relation to the chairs and tables. Otherwise, he merely mumbled and muttered when questioned, despite the fact that he had a college education. Another item of great interest was his alert, intelligent gaze when not disturbed emotionally. He seemed to be intently studying his fellow patients and the interpersonal relationships between patients and the nursing and medical personnel. Yet when approached directly, his interest seemed to vanish and his gaze became veiled.

INDIRECT TRANCE INDUCTION

Made curious by "this" Laskarri's behavior, the writer approached a passively obedient, rather stuporous patient and maneuvered him into a chair nearby so that Laskarri would have a full view of him. The writer then took a chair slightly to one side so that his primary view was of the stuporous patient but his secondary, somewhat sidelong glance permitted an adequate view of Laskarri. In effecting this seating arrangement the writer spoke earnestly and intensely to the unresponsive stuporous patient, but was well aware of Laskarri's intent observations. The writer then gave the stuporous patient a series of suggestions to induce attentiveness, relaxation, a state of restfulness, a state of attentive sleep, restful sleep during which one might hear, understand, wish to respond, to communicate, to tell things of interest, to need to tell one's thoughts and feelings, to express one's need to ask for help, to do so comfortably even while asleep and without fear.

Previous experimentation with the mildly stuporous patient, who

---

Unpublished manuscript, circa 1940s, edited by E. L. Rossi.

tended to stand about immobile with a vacuous expression in his eyes, had disclosed that he would, if seated in a chair, loll comfortably and seemingly go to sleep. No interpersonal contact had yet been made with him, but he could be used as a suggestive example for Laskarri.

Peripheral vision and sidelong glances soon disclosed that Laskarri, as is common among normal people, was responding to the suggestions he apparently thought were addressed to the subject. Shortly Laskarri gave every appearance of being in a trance, and he manifested catalepsy upon being tested. Slowly the tempo of the hypnotic "sleep" suggestions was decreased, and there was a gradual replacement of them by increasingly urgent suggestions that sometime, somewhere, somehow, courage be found to tell a little, just a little about what happens when you run, you twist, you turn, you crawl over, crawl under, run, twist, shout, sometime soon, somehow, must some way . . . will . . . must . . . can . . . must . . . tell what happens when crawl, run, rush, shout, go over, go under.

These suggestions were repeated many times—softly, gently, insistently, urgently—and they were followed with cautious slowness, ". . . and head will nod, nod, nod, yes . . . yes . . . yes . . . yes . . . slowly nod yes . . . slowly . . . will do . . . will do soon."

Shortly Laskarri's head nodded "yes" gently, perseveratively, and further suggestion was offered that he sleep restfully for a while, since he might want to say something that afternoon. The afternoon of that same day the writer slowly made ward rounds, finally seating himself in a chair beside Laskarri and waited patiently. Within 20 minutes Laskarri leaned over slightly and murmured, "Big Joe—you—put Joe asleep—put him asleep—different way."

What Laskarri meant was readily recognized. Some 10 days previously Big Joe, six feet five inches tall and 275 pounds, had become increasingly restless and had announced finally, in the writer's presence, his intention of "singing and yelling for about an hour" and then "smashing the ward and everybody in it." There had been previous such experience with him. Immediately the writer secured a syringe with 15 grains of sterile intravenous solution of sodium amytal and took a seat in front of Big Joe's chair. Suspiciously Big Joe inquired if an intravenous injection was planned. He was told that none was planned, but that if he were to sing and yell for about an hour, his mouth would get dry, but the writer could squeeze a small stream into his mouth without interrupting his singing and yelling and his mouth would not get dry and sore. Big Joe nodded his head agreeably, tipped his head back, and began his bellowing. Little by little the sodium amytal was squirted into Joe's mouth. He swallowed it as he sang and soon lapsed into sleep.

Having thus oriented the writer to his needs, Laskarri's requests now became more personally meaningful. The writer moved his chair closer and Laskarri said, "Sleep—I dream awful dreams—you help." Suggestions of hypnotic sleep were offered, and soon Laskarri was in a trance. He replied to questions of what he should do by answering, "Just let me sleep here in chair—awful dream—hurt—hurt." Taking a chance, I told him, "Sit here in chair, don't move, don't wake up, just don't hurt—just dream awful dream and then tell me."

He seized my wrist, shuddered, perspired, and kept on shuddering and moaning. After some 15 minutes he aroused, stating, "My dream—I had it—I got to keep dreaming until I find out." What it was he had to find out he could not tell. But the next day he could tell the content of the dream, and he begged for further help because he must dream until he found an answer. The content of the dream was that he was being forced, shoved, pulled, yanked, twisted, and thrown through an endless, lightless corridor crowded and filled with bramble bushes, thorny bushes, crucifixion thorns, barbed wire, jagged spikes, long, penetrating slivers of glass, swords, daggers, all manner of painful lacerating, cutting things—a journey that would come to a sudden end with the knowledge that again he would have to traverse that painful way until he "found it." Though approached many times, Laskarri never had revealed anything verbally to any of the hospital personnel.*

R: What was the next step of your therapy with Laskarri?

E: The next dream was of a similar character. I then told him to dream the same dream again with a different set of characters. In his next dream, instead of bramble bushes, he found himself dealing with a net full of fishhooks.

R: This variation of the dream indicated that his unconscious was receiving your suggestions and that he had enough control within his inner processes to actually modify them in accordance with your suggestions.

E: He repeated that dream with a number of people in it. He did not know who they were or even their sex, but they were fishing. Somehow or other they would snag him in that net full of fishhooks. In the next dream it was the same situation with another cast of characters on a grassy bank of a river with four people there all fishing. Three of them (two women and a man) kept catching him with their fishhooks. The fourth person, a man, caught a fish. He then fried this fish, and it smelled good.

The final dream was of an older brother of his who protected him; he was the one who caught and fried the fish that smelled so good in the previous dream. The other three people who caught Lascarri were his mother, father, and sister. These three were the hurtful people in his earlier life.

*MHE's original manuscript was left in an incomplete form at this point. Questioning by the editor completed the case history in 1978.

R: Did you interpret that dream to him?

E: No, he interpreted it to me! He said he could never get along with his father, mother, or sister, but he could get along with his brother, who always did good things for him. Then we discussed what he ought to do when he left the hospital.

R: Most of his personality was intact; he just needed this insight. The bad dreams of the dark corridor with sharp cutting things were symbolic of the hurt arising from his early family situation. Do you agree that insight was the curative factor in this case? This was a case where the unconscious did have to be made conscious, as Freud believed.

E: Yes. Familiarity breeds contempt. When you go through a painful situation again and again in a dream, changing it a bit each time, it becomes less painful.

R: Yes, that is the desensitization technique of behavior therapy.

E: I got into a lot of trouble over that case. The staff said I had no right to engage in the "unethical and unprofessional act" of sedating Big Joe that way while he was singing.

R: But that act not only protected the ward, it also helped Laskarri gain a positive transference to you as that protective older brother.

E: When he saw the difficulty I got into with the nurses and doctors over my undignified way of sedating Big Joe, that also helped him sympathize and establish rapport with me. The hospital staff did not realize I was actually carrying out Laskarri's first request to put Big Joe asleep in a "different way."

36. Symptom Prescription for Expanding the Psychotic's World View

Milton H. Erickson and Jeffrey Zeig

This example is from my initial meeting with Milton Erickson in 1973. It is the first case that Erickson discussed with me in explaining his therapeutic approach. The case description contains some of Erickson's own rationale for his technique, and is quoted directly:

E: Concerning psychotherapy, most therapists overlook a basic consideration. Man is characterized not only by mobility but by cognition and by emotion, and man defends his intellect emotionally. No two people necessarily have the same ideas, but all people will defend their ideas whether they are psychotically based or culturally based, or nationally based or personally based. When you understand how man really defends his intellectual ideas and how emotional he gets about it, you should realize that the first thing in psychotherapy is not to try to compel him to change his ideation; rather, you go along with it and change it in a gradual fashion and create situations wherein he himself willingly changes his thinking. I think my first real experiment in psychotherapy occurred in 1930. A patient in Worcester State Hospital, in Massachusetts, demanded he be locked in his room, and he spent his time anxiously and fearfully winding string around the bars of the window of the room. He knew his enemies were going to come in and kill him, and the window was the only opening. The thick iron bars seemed to him to be too weak, so he reinforced them with string. I went into the room and helped him reinforce the iron bars with string. In doing so, I discovered that there were cracks in the floor and suggested that those cracks ought to be stuffed with newspaper so that there was no possibility (of his enemies getting him), and then I discovered cracks around the door that should be stuffed with newspaper, and gradually I got him to realize that the room was only one of a number of rooms on the ward, and to accept the attendants as a part of his defense against his enemies; and then the hospital itself as a part of his defense against

This paper is a portion of "Symptom Prescription and Ericksonian Principles of Hypnosis and Psychotherapy" presented by Jeffrey Zeig, Ph.D., to the 20th Annual Scientific Meeting of the American Society of Clinical Hypnosis, October 20, 1977, Atlanta, Georgia.

his enemies; and then the Board of Mental Health of Massachusetts as part, and then the police system—the governor. And then I spread it to adjoining states and finally I made the United States a part of his defense system; this enabled him to dispense with the locked door because he had so many other lines of defense. I didn't try to correct his psychotic idea that his enemies would kill him. I merely pointed out that he had an endless number of defenders. The result was: the patient was able to accept ground privileges and wander around the grounds safely. He ceased his frantic endeavors. He worked in the hospital shops and was much less of a problem.

There is a discernible pattern to Erickson's series of interventions. A comparable pattern can be seen in many of Erickson's cases (cf. Haley, 1973). This pattern can be divided into three major elements, which occur in the following sequence: (1) meeting the patient where the patient is; (2) establishing small modifications that are consistent with, and follow from, the patient's behavior and understandings; and (3) eliciting behaviors and understandings from the patient in a manner that allows the patient to initiate change. These elements are discussed below in relation to the case that Erickson describes.

Initially, Erickson meets the patient where the patient is. In an "anxious and fearful" manner the patient has demanded protection. By assisting the patient in the process of reinforcing the iron bars with string, Erickson provides protection in a manner that is consistent with the patient's frame of reference and indirectly communicates a number of powerful messages. For example, he implicitly establishes a high degree of empathic rapport. The patient is given the opportunity to experimentally understand that Erickson really realizes his dilemma. (The importance of empathy in the psychotherapeutic process has been addressed by researchers [e.g., Carkhuff & Berenson, 1967]. Such researchers have traditionally emphasized the importance of overt and verbal empathic responses on the part of the therapist.) Erickson incorporates a style of using indirection to demonstrate empathic rapport to the patient.

In assisting the patient in reinforcing the bars with string, Erickson enters the metaphor that the patient is living, thereby showing the patient that he respects the patient's integrity and behavior. There is no attempt to interpret the patient's delusion or force him to change his behavior immediately. Rather, Erickson goes along with the patient and thereby begins the therapy on the patient's level of behavior and understanding. If such an initial intervention were made in a sarcastic manner, or from a frame of reference of trying to trick the patient out of his symptom, the positive outcome would be limited. An attitude of empathy and respect on the part of the therapist is crucial to ensure successful change.

After meeting the patient at his level, Erickson makes use of the patient's psychotically based behavior to increase rapport and establish a base for future change. Erickson begins a process of making modifications (finding the cracks in the floor and door) that are in accord with the patient's view of the situation (i.e., the need to protect himself from his enemies). Erickson even seems to immerse the patient more deeply in his psychotic understandings by pointing out the other possible weaknesses in his defense (e.g., the cracks in the floor). However, this maneuver has a paradoxical effect, because by pointing out weaknesses in the patient's attempts to defend himself, Erickson becomes an undeniable defender. He then builds on this small change and subtly aids in the transfer of the protector role to other persons and institutions, until the patient himself can come to the conclusion that he is safe. Moreover, the modifications that Erickson makes seem to have the effect of reframing institutions that the patient may once have feared by emphasizing their protective nature in a manner the patient can account and realize.

The establishment of small modifications by the therapist paves the way for future understandings on the part of the patient that can be oriented in a more positive direction. It can be assumed that most patients have some desire to function in a more effective and enjoyable manner. Through the use of the small modification technique, the patient can avail himself of his desire to function more effectively.

It can further be assumed that the patient has resources in his personal history that can be used to effect change. These resources (past learnings) can be elicited by the therapist in such a way that the patient can avail himself of them. Erickson does not have to teach this patient overtly how to behave in a nonparanoid manner. Rather, he can trust that the patient has years of experience with nonparanoid behavior, and that given the right circumstances, the patient can discover that he can again behave in a nonparanoid manner. In this way the cure is elicited from within the patient.

The initial process of psychotherapy with this patient was based on meeting the patient within his frame of reference and then establishing modifications that the patient could use to establish a new level of functioning. This process is akin to a dance in which one partner begins by synchronizing his steps to the steps of his partner and then (and only then) by beginning to take the initiative and lead.

Overall, the cornerstone of the therapeutic process with this patient is built around the symptom prescriptive approach. In a manner that is basically implicit the patient is encouraged to continue symptomatic behavior until, on the basis of new understandings promoted in part by the modification provided by the therapist, the patient changes his own behavior. While some therapists might engage in such therapeutic practices in a way that is based on trickery or coercion, that is not the case here. Rather, the patient is given the opportunity to recognize and change his behavior to a more constructive and less self-defeating pattern.

VII. Sexual Problems: Hypnotherapeutic Reorientations to Emotional Satisfaction

The papers of this section on sexually related problems are illustrative of the extremely wide range of approaches the hypnotherapist has available to him. The roots of many of these papers are to be found in the experimental work on psychodynamics presented in Volume Three of this series, particularly that on experimental neuroses. Many of the previously unpublished sexual cases in this section were actually written up during that earlier period of experimental work. Because of this the editor has endeavored to formulate something about the psychodynamics of how experimental neuroses or "therapeutic implants" can facilitate the resolution of psychological problems. As with all hypnotherapeutic suggestion, we are navigating here precariously between the Charybdis of open-ended indirect suggestions that may be so tangential as to have no evocative power for a particular patient's unconscious processes, and the Scylla of hard-and-fast direct suggestions that cannot be accepted by the patient's individuality.

THE PSYCHODYNAMICS OF HYPNOTHERAPY WITH EXPERIMENTAL NEUROSES: HYPOTHESIS ABOUT "THERAPEUTIC IMPLANTS"*

What are the psychodynamic processes whereby the evocation of an experimental neurosis effects the resolution of a related and real neurosis or personality problem? We hypothesize that a four-stage process may be operative:

First Stage: The therapeutic implant, the "experimental neurosis," exists as a semiautonomous, temporary complex that is integrated within

*Formulated by the editor and received with interest by MHE.

the total personality but in a very tenuous manner. The experimental complex shares a few crucial associative connections or common contents with the patient's real neurosis. The experimental and real neuroses have just enough ties to allow a psychodynamic connection.

Second Stage: Because of these intimate psychodynamic connections, the central emotional content or charge (cathexis) that holds the real neurosis together as an isolated, self-perpetuating complex is able to spread itself over to the experimental neurosis. It is as if the chief conspirator of a robber band (the patient's real neurosis) has been fooled into visiting a new hamlet (the experimental neurosis) he thought was in complete sympathy with him.

Third Stage: Once integrated with the experimental neurosis, however, the real neurosis now finds other possible means of discharge that may bypass neurotic symptom formation. These healthier means of discharge were already built into the experimental neurosis when it was accepted by the patient's total personality. With these new channels of expression now available, the neurotic content (cathexis) can be discharged and the neurosis resolved. The inner psychodynamic supports for symptom formation are weakened, and the symptoms collapse.

Stage Four: The energy that was formerly bound up in the real neurosis is suddenly freed. The patient is relieved and excited. He experiences a heightened period of emotional reactivity and learns new ways of living life in a more meaningful way.

What are the means of creating therapeutic implants? They can be as elaborate and carefully constructed as the techniques illustrated in Erickson's papers on experimental neuroses in Volume Three of this series, or as casual as the period of hypnotic role-playing he evoked in the case of latent homosexuality in this section. Sometimes the therapeutic implant is a loose set of open-ended, posthypnotic suggestions, as in the first case of premature ejaculation in this section. Sometimes it is a jumble of pseudo-logic presented in impressive scientific jargon; or it may be a single idea that is intriguing to the patient. All these possibilities are illustrated in the cases that follow. Success is probably related to four major factors paralleling the four stages described above:

1. An important common content or common denominator between the real neurosis and the temporary therapeutic implant (the experimental neurosis, role-playing, etc.).

2. An acceptance of the temporary therapeutic implant by the total personality. The implant is acceptable as an interesting and worthwhile (though temporary) "play." *Its relation to the neurosis is not obvious.* The new therapeutic channels it opens to the personality are *certainly not obvious when it is first accepted.* The usefulness of the new channels becomes obvious only after the

patient has accepted them. These hidden or *unrecognized implications* of the therapeutic implant are the essence of Erickson's "indirect approach."
3. An incubation period during which significant internal psychodynamic processes integrate the real problem with the therapeutic implant. Of particular importance are the presence of available channels within the therapeutic implant that can permit the real problem to realign or discharge itself.
4. A supportive environment (therapy, a sympathetic mate or family, etc.) that allows the patient the needed freedom and acceptance to explore the new channels of self-expression.

Most of the papers of this section as well as the next two sections (Self-Exploration in the Hypnotic State, and Facilitating New Identity) illustrate varying aspects of the above hypothesized formulation.

37. Posthypnotic Suggestion for Ejaculatio Praecox

Milton H. Erickson

A 30-year-old unmarried man sought therapy because of premature ejaculation. It had first occurred at his initial sexual experience at the age of 20. His reaction had been most unhappy, and he had then felt that it was punishment for his immorality. He felt damaged and incompetent as a result and rationalized that he would have to correct the condition before he could ever undertake marriage. He became tremendously obsessional on the subject and read everything he could find on sex, searching for some explanation of his specific problem. Additionally, he constantly sought new and different women from every strata of society, age groups, racial groups, and physical types, all to no avail. All efforts had proved futile.

Aside from his obsessional-compulsive search for sexual achievement, he had adjusted satisfactorily. He graduated from college, secured a position as a certified public accountant, and was well regarded by his associates. When asked for a complete description of his behavior in the sexual act, he declared that it was invariably the same regardless of whether his partner were an aging, drunken prostitute or an attractive, charming, well-educated young girl. He never had difficulty in securing and maintaining an erection, even after ejaculation. However, upon an attempt at insertion, ejaculation occurred first. Many times he had disregarded the premature ejaculation and engaged in active coitus, but this gave him neither pleasure nor satisfaction. Rather, he regarded it as an unpleasant effort in a "desperate" desire to achieve sexual competence. Usually he would persist in the intravaginal masturbation until ready for a second ejaculation, whereupon he would invariably and unwillingly but compulsively withdraw. He would then be unable to gain insertion until he had completed the second ejaculation externally. This would always enrage him, and he disliked making the second attempt, but he often felt compelled to do so.

Some months previously he had read this writer's experimental study on *ejaculatio praecox** and had promptly attempted to apply it to himself,

---

Unpublished manuscript, circa 1930s.

*Editor's Note: See "A study of an experimental neurosis hypnotically induced in a case of ejaculatio praecox," in Volume Three of this series.

since he did not want anybody to know about his problem. He had spent much effort in an endeavor to fantasy himself in the experimental therapeutic situation described in that study, but failed completely.

Finally, as a last resort, he sought out the writer. He expressed his willingness for therapy but stipulated that the procedure reported upon in that publication not be used, since he had proved its inefficacy to himself. Nevertheless, he declared his full willingness to leave matters in the writer's hands completely if that method were not employed. Inquiry promptly disclosed that he regarded hypnosis as permissible; his objection concerned the implantation of an artificial neurosis.

A half-dozen sessions were spent letting him expatiate in endless detail upon his innumerable but futile attempts at intercourse. Throughout each session, in an indirect, unobtrusive, but repetitious fashion, he was induced to emphasize over and over the fact that he never had difficulty in securing and maintaining an erection, until he regarded any inquiry in that direction to be as stupid as repeated inquiries about the number of feet on a biped.

TRANCE INDUCTION WITH POSTHYPNOTIC AMNESIA

With this fact about his competence in relation to tumescence rigidly established in his thinking, he was hypnotized during the next two sessions. He developed a fair trance—not deep, but sufficient for therapeutic purposes in that he experienced considerable posthypnotic amnesia.

In the next therapeutic session, while in a trance state, he was questioned extensively about his current liaisons, which had not been interdicted. It was learned that he was assiduously courting a clandestine prostitute who lived on the second floor of an apartment court, in a suite above the entrance to the court. Access to her apartment was gained by walking the full length of the court, climbing a rear stairway, and then circling back on the balcony. Although the two of them had a full understanding of the intended nature of the relationship, the woman demanded a number of dinner and theater engagements before she fulfilled her "obligations," a not uncommon arrangement in his past experience and one that he liked. The suggestion was offered that, thenceforth, in visiting her, he would develop an erection immediately upon enternng the court and maintain it until he left the court, either alone or in her company. This suggestion he accepted readily.

AN ASSOCIATIVE NETWORK OF INTERSPERSED POSTHYPNOTIC SUGGESTIONS FOR NEUROTIC PROBLEMS

Then, for about two hours, a long rambling discussion was offered him. In it were numerous poorly organized comments about his past history, vague speculations about possible meanings and significances of various incidents, and various pleasing but essentially meaningless generalizations. However, systematically and unobtrusively interwoven into that monologue was a whole series of posthypnotic suggestions. These were given at first in random order, with confusing, vague elaborations, until the entire list had been presented. Then they were presented again, over and over, always with much interspersed, seemingly pertinent, but actually irrelevant discussion intended to distract and confuse any attempt at analysis of what was being said. Finally, these posthypnotic suggestions were presented in fairly close succession and in a progressive fashion to build up, without his awareness, certain significant ideas. The possible effectiveness of the suggestions was the primary consideration, not their actual or theoretical validity. These posthypnotic suggestions were as follows:

1. Neurotic ideas and symptoms serve a purpose for the personality.
2. Neurotic manifestations are often seemingly constant but are fundamentally inconstant, since the purposes they serve change as time passes. Circumstances change and personality needs alter.
3. Neurotic symptoms can actually reverse and resolve themselves when the need arises.
4. Correction of neurotic problems can occur as effectively by accidental and coincidental measures as by deliberate effort.
5. No neurotic can really know what will happen to his problem at a given time.
6. Replacement of a neurotic problem can occur by the development of another, and this in itself is beneficial.
7. A specific neurotic symptom such as a premature ejaculation could, without warning, be reversed into a frightening delay of ejaculation, a delay of half an hour to an hour.
8. He would really have something to worry about if that ever happened to him.

9. He really knew how to worry both consciously and *unconsciously*.
10. Such a development would undoubtedly result in a totally unexpected internal ejaculation.
11. Then he would be confronted with the *tremendous problem of accomplished sexuality, which would require constructive utilization*.
12. For the next few days or week or 10 days there would be a growing unrest in him, *presaging an impending change in him*.

The interview was closed with further vague discussion, and he was awakened with instructions to feel excessively tired and to want to go home and to sleep and to do nothing for a while—not even to think—but just to rest comfortably. He was given appointments for the next day, which was Tuesday, and for Wednesday, and Friday. On Tuesday he was seen briefly but not allowed to talk. He was told that he would be given, in return for the briefness of the interview, a very special appointment on Sunday. (The writer was well aware of his Saturday-night regularity.) The Wednesday appointment was similarly handled, with further and extensive emphasis on the Sunday appointment to the effect that he would really have to "give out" for that interview. Friday's interview was also brief, and again emphasis was placed upon the special character of what he would have to relate on Sunday.

All of this maneuvering appeared to bewilder and confuse him. However, on Sunday morning he explained immediately and urgently that, whatever the writer had in mind for the appointment, it would have to be postponed because of certain developments he had experienced. His story was that the three previous brief interviews, or "brush-offs" as he termed them, had made him restless, unhappy, and uncertain. He had been so ill-at-ease after the Friday interview that he sought out his female associate, whom he had been seeing frequently, but with whom he had not yet had sex relations, and suggested a date for dinner and the theater. However, during the evening he had been inattentive to his companion and preoccupied. Recurrently the question "popped into" his mind of whether or not he actually could ejaculate intravaginally. Almost at once the idea would elude his mind, and he would try to remember what he had been thinking. Shortly the idea would again "pop into" his mind, only to elude him once more. Over and over this occurred, with continued preoccupation on his part throughout the evening.

As he was returning with his companion to her apartment, he developed an erection upon entering the court. This persisted, although he was still so preoccupied with his thoughts, which he could not define to himself, that he did not contemplate sex relations. Nevertheless, upon entering the apartment, his companion manifested such aggressive, amorous behavior that he promptly went to bed with her. Because his preoccupation still persisted, he allowed her to take an aggressive role, and his reaction to insertion was one of sudden fear that he would not be able to have an ejaculation. So absorbing was this fear that "I forgot completely all my past popping off. All I could think of was that I wanted to pop into her, and I was afraid I couldn't."

He responded to his fear by active coitus, and "for some unknown reason watching the minute hand on my wristwatch, which I never wear to bed." As the end of a half-hour approached, he became increasingly excited and, at the same time, more anxious and fearful. Then suddenly, but without noting the time until some 20 minutes later, he experienced a satisfying intravaginal ejaculation. His erection continued, and after a short rest without withdrawal, he engaged in active coitus and had a second satisfying intravaginal ejaculation. Completely satisfied, he waited for detumescence before withdrawal. They slept comfortably and the next day went for an automobile trip. That night there occurred further normal sexual activity.

Upon completing this story, the patient asked if there were any explanation of why he had become normal. Reply was given that neither he nor the writer need explain the normal, that it was infinitely more pleasurable simply to accept the normal unquestioningly as something to which everybody is entitled. (There seemed to be no good reason to permit him to break down his posthypnotic amnesia and thus perhaps vitiate his therapeutic gains.)

His relationship with the woman continued for about three months before they drifted apart. Several other liaisons were formed before he became seriously interested in marriage. At this writing he is engaged to be married, and he and his fiancee are speculating upon building a home. Following his first successful sexual experiences, he was seen professionally a few times, but with no significant communications resulting except his continued adjustment. Thereafter he was seen occasionally on a casual social basis.

38. Psychotherapy Achieved by a Reversal of the Neurotic Processes in a Case of Ejaculatio Praecox

Milton H. Erickson

This author has repeatedly stressed the importance of utilizing patients' symptoms and general patterns of behavior in psychotherapy. Such utilization renders unnecessary any effort to alter or transform symptomatology as a preliminary measure to the reeducation of patients in relation to the crucial problems confronting them in their illness. Such problems cause a distortion of their thinking, feeling, and patterns of living, thereby causing them to seek therapy. By using the patients' own patterns of response and behavior, including those of their actual illness, one may effect therapy more promptly and satisfactorily, with resistance to therapy greatly obviated and acceptance of therapy facilitated. Indeed, it often seems absurd to attempt to reeducate patients when all that may be needed may be a redirection of their endeavors, rather than a change or a correction of their behavior. Particularly so is this true when a patient has a circumscribed type of neurosis.

The fact that a patient has symptoms signifies that some kind of an effort at some psychological or physiological level is being made to alter a troublesome state of being. That patients are disturbed in their behavior means that they are distressed and that they have a desire to put forth effort to alter the situation, but that they do not direct that effort correctly. Furthermore, therapy should be a cooperative venture, the therapist contributing his skills and understandings and the patients contributing their own kind of responsiveness and their own capacities to utilize what can be proffered to aid them. Therapy is never and can never be a simple matter of the patient reacting solely in accord with how the therapist, with his own understanding of what is right and good, might expect the patient to respond. Quite otherwise, the experienced therapist makes clear to patients that responses must be in accord with their own potentialities, even though those potentialities may as yet be unrealized, misused, or misunderstood. What the therapist knows, understands, or believes about a patient is frequently limited in character and often

Reprinted with permission from *The American Journal of Clinical Hypnosis,* April, 1973, *15*, 217-222.

mistaken. What he is willing to let patients discover about themselves and to use effectively is of exceedingly great therapeutic importance.

The following experimental hypnotherapeutic handling of a patient's problem of extensive duration will illustrate the above discussion.

THE PROBLEM

A single man, aged 38, had suffered from premature ejaculations since his first attempt at sex relations at the age of 20. This experience had frightened and humiliated him, and it had deterred him from another attempt for several years. He then sought to resolve his doubts by a visit to a brothel, reasoning that in this way he would experience less humiliation should he again fail. And, as might be expected, he did fail. After a brief period of days he revisited the brothel, this time selecting the least attractive inmate, thinking for some unclear reason that such a choice might be helpful. This endeavor failed also.

He then resorted to casual pick-ups, sometimes on the frank basis of an explanation of his difficulty and an agreement of "no success, no pay." This procedure netted only failure despite assorted varieties of stimulation, some of which led to unpleasant brawls. Liquor was resorted to as a "calming" measure. This too proved to be useless. He finally decided that his problem derived from an overactive conscience. He sought out an eligible, attractive young woman and began a most cautious, chaste courtship. After about six months he realized that he desired to marry the girl, and he asked her for a kiss. A premature ejaculation occurred as he kissed her. Even meeting the girl thereafter resulted in the same unfortunate contretemps.

He discontinued the relationship with that girl and sought out a woman definitely his inferior socially and educationally and "began a slow careful cultivation of her so I could have relations with her. I knew she was promiscuous and that she couldn't understand what I wanted since I only bought her dinners and went to the movies with her until finally I got so sick of her I couldn't stand her. Then I tried it [meaning sex relations]. Same thing! Same old thing."

All of this enraged him and at the same time made him feel so inferior that he sought out prostitutes with great frequency, but always he failed to achieve his goal. The years went by, and he became increasingly fixated upon correcting his problem, first by his own efforts, then by medical and pseudo-medical aids. He was cystoscoped, given prostatic massage and injections of testosterone; he was furnished with various prescriptions, and he purchased many kinds of patent medicines and mechanical aids advertised in magazines. He reacted unfavorably to two physicians who advised him to seek psychiatric aid, insisting that his trouble was organic, noticeably so, and that "it certainly is not in my head."

At long last he learned through the lay press about hypnosis and reached the conclusion that hypnosis was the destined means of putting to an end his obsessive-compulsive search for therapy. He resolved "not to fumble or bumble" in this regard. He rejected lay hypnotists as unquestionably untrained in medical problems and hence charlatans because of the unqualified promises of their advertisements. Physicians consulted too often admitted to ignorance of hypnosis or denounced it, often without actual knowledge, as he realized from his "reading about hypnosis in an encyclopedia and some recent books written by medically trained men."

Eventually he sought out the author, to whom he related his story in extensive, systematic detail. Efforts to get him to abbreviate or to summarize his story were futile. He insisted on doing things his own way. He was unconcerned about how many hours it required to give an exact, orderly history of his problem. He simply wanted "to be sure that everything is understood . . . so that there can't be any failure . . . so that I know you know everything."

This rigid, compulsive narration in minute detail of his many failures gave the author adequate time not only to appraise the patient's obsessional-compulsive personality and behavior, but also to speculate upon possible psychotherapeutic measures. The patient's rigidities, his compulsiveness, the fixity with which he had conducted his search for symptomatic relief, the comprehensiveness (according to his understandings) with which he pursued his goal, his perseverance in the face of all difficulties, and the absolute, fixed belief he manifested in the incurableness of his disability all seemed to offer little promise of therapeutic results. When the patient finally concluded the narration of his search for hypnotherapy and his investigation of hypnosis as a possible cure, it became appallingly apparent that the patient was convinced in his own mind that, while hypnosis might readily be an effective cure for others, it was not such for him. He was beyond the pale of hope, and he was merely determined to prove this fact beyond any shadow of doubt. Then he could resignedly abandon his quest for potency and be at peace with himself.

Such was his purpose in seeking out the author and requesting that hypnosis be employed therapeutically upon him. Hypnosis would constitute, so he explained, the utmost, the final superlative method of therapy. Nevertheless, it would fail, since he was at last fully aware of his complete incompetence, and he wished only to put an end to his endless compulsive search for therapy. He felt himself unable to control his obsessive-compulsive searching for an unreachable goal. Once he had tried the ultimate in therapeutic procedures and had encountered failure, then and only then could he resign himself to his fate. This purpose was explained as elaborately as he had given his history.

It was only at this time that the author became fully aware of the nature of the problem confronting him—namely, that the patient had involved himself in an ever-increasing maze of contradictions that was governing his entire personal life.

The realization of this psychological import of the patient's communications suggested an experimental therapeutic approach to the patient's problems that might conceivably be effective. Such an experimental therapeutic approach would of necessity include obsessive-compulsive behavior, actual uncertainty and fear, even a complete expectation of failure. Against this expectation he would be induced to strive desperately and, in so doing, would actually achieve the success so long believed to be impossible. But there would need to be a doubting of the success and many repetitions until he could accept success as a valid reality for him.

This actually simple but seemingly most involved plan of therapy had been roughly formulated by the author by the time the patient had completed his lengthy narrative and argument. During the course of these communications the patient had been induced to disclose a great wealth of details about his present living arrangements, particularly the apartment in which he lived and where he had "tried" with so many women. A useful fact was that it was reached by following a long outdoor board walkway, a stairway, and a long upstairs balcony walkway; there were other details, many of which were incorporated in the therapeutic plan. The author secretly paid a visit to that series of apartments to be certain of the terrain where the patient had battled so futilely.

THERAPEUTIC PROCEDURE

Therapy was begun by inducing a light trance in the patient and impressing upon him, most tediously, that the "light trance" was a most important measure. Its purpose, he was told repetitiously, was to ensure that he had both a conscious and an unconscious understanding of the fact that a deep hypnotic trance would settle once and for all time whether or not he could ever succeed in sex relations. Two hours of repetition of these general ideas resulted in a deep trance, but no effort was made to give him an awareness of this fact. An amnesia, spontaneous or one indirectly suggested, was desired for therapeutic purposes.

Then, as a posthypnotic suggestion, he was told that he must, absolutely must, get a wristwatch. If at all possible, this wristwatch should have an illuminated dial and illuminated hands. Absolutely imperative was the fact that the watch should have a second hand. The second hand, it was stressed over and over, would be absolutely necessary.

A second posthypnotic suggestion was given that he must, and could, and would thenceforth sleep with a night-light at his bedside so that he could tell time to the very second at any time during the night, since he must, absolutely must, and would wear his wristwatch whenever he should happen to be in bed.

Solemn promises in relation to these demands were secured from the patient with no effort on his part to question the author's reasons for his various insistences.

It was then explained to him that he would continue his "useless inviting of girls to spend the night" with him. To this he also agreed, whereupon it was emphasized that only in this way could he find out what he "really really really would want to learn."

The next posthypnotic suggestion was presented most carefully, in a gentle yet emphatic tone of voice, commanding, without seeming to command, the patient's full attention and his full willingness to be obedient to it. This suggestion was a purportedly soundly based medical explanation of the expectable development, on an organic physiological basis, of his "total problem." This was the fact that his premature ejaculation, by virtue of body changes from aging processes, would be diametrically changed. The explanation was the following posthypnotic suggestion:

> Do you know, can you possibly realize, can you genuinely understand, that medically all things, everything, even the worst of symptoms and conditions, must absolutely come to an end— *but not, but not, I must emphasize, not in the way a layman would understand?* Do you realize, do you understand, are you in any way aware, that your premature ejaculation *will end in a failure,* that no matter how long your erection lasts, no matter how long and actively you engage in coitus, you will fail to have an ejaculation for 10, for 10 long, for 15 long minutes, for 20, for 25 minutes? Even more? Do you realize how desperately you will strive and strive, how desperately you will watch the minute hand and the second hand of your wristwatch, wondering, just wondering if you will fail, fail, fail to have an ejaculation at 25 minutes, at 25½, at 26, at 26½ minutes? Or will it be at 27½, at 27½ minutes—at 27½, at 27½ minutes? (this last said in tones expressive of deep relief.)
>
> And the next morning you still will not believe, just can't believe, that you won't fail to have an ejaculation, and so you will have to discover again, to discover again, if you really really can have an ejaculation, but it won't be, it can't be, at 27½ minutes, nor even at 28, nor even at 29 minutes. Just the desperate hope will be in your mind that maybe, just maybe, maybe at 33 minutes, or 34, or 35 minutes the ejaculation will come. And at

the time, all the time, you will watch desperately the wristwatch and strive so hard lest you fail, fail again, to ejaculate at 27 minutes, and then 33, 34, 35 minutes will seem never, just never, to be coming with an ejaculation.

And now this is what I want you to do. Find one of the girls you are used to. Walk her to your apartment. When you come to the corner at 8th, even as you turn right (all of this was said with the utmost of intensity), try so very hard to keep your mind on the conversation, but notice that you can't help counting one by one the cracks in the sidewalk until you turn into the courtway and step upon the boardwalk. With complete intensity you are to try hard, very hard to keep your mind on the conversation, but keep desperately counting the cracks, the cracks between the boards, the cracks under you (to the unsophisticated, slang often gives opportunities for double meanings), all those cracks all along the way to your apartment until it seems that you will never never never get there, and what a profound relief it will be to enter, to feel comfortable, to be at ease, to give your attention to the girl, and then, and then, to bed, but not the usual—but the answer, the real real real answer, and from the moment you enter [pause] the apartment [pause], your mind will be on your wristwatch, the watch that, as time goes by, can, at long last, bring you the answer.

Quickly now, keep all that I have said in your unconscious mind—locked up, not a syllable, not a word, not a meaning forgotten—to be kept there, used, obeyed fully, completely. You can even forget me, all about me—just obey fully—then you can remember just me and come back and tell me that the wristwatch was right when it read 27½ minutes and when it read 33, 34, and 35.

Arouse now, completely rested and refreshed, understanding in your unconscious mind the completeness of the task to be done." The patient aroused, seemed puzzled, and departed hurriedly.

THE RESULTS

Three days later the patient telephoned to state, "I would like to see you, but I don't need an appointment. I just want to tell you that everything's all right and pay my bill."

He came at the suggested time, stated that the long, detailed account he had given the author of his problem had apparently served as some kind of mental catharsis, that he was fully competent sexually, and that he had proved it to himself repeatedly during the last three nights and mornings. Then, with considerable embarrassment he asked if it were "normal and proper" to prolong coitus "to, let us say, maybe as long as half an hour or more." He was reassured and dismissed, apparently with the hypnotic amnesia still present.

However, from time to time he arranged to meet the author "casually" to exchange a few remarks. About 18 months later he married a woman nine years younger than himself. He announced this to the author over the telephone, and then three months later he asked for an appointment. The reason was simply that he had recovered trance memories. He now had a "full understanding" of what had happened, and he stated his appreciation for the therapy. Actually he had only a general memory of the therapeutic procedure, but he was satisfied with it. He also reminisced about the number of times he "happened to be passing by" when the author came out of his home, and he speculated about the purpose of those meetings.

He explained further that he was certain he had obeyed instructions which had been given to him and that he had been profoundly elated by an ejaculation at 27½ minutes despite intense, despairing fears preceding it. The next morning he had again engaged in coitus with the same distressing fears of failing to ejaculate only to be relieved of those fears by an ejaculation at 33 minutes. He was then convinced that his problem "had reversed itself" and that it had been corrected on some organic basis. He felt a need to retest his "recovery" several times. This had finally given him full confidence in himself, and his self-confidence had never lessened.

He was asked what he thought the author's purpose had been in having him count the cracks in the sidewalk, the boardwalk, etc. His reply was, "I didn't know it then, and I didn't know until you asked me just now. You were having me look at all the useless 'cracks' under me before I entered where I succeeded." He flushed as he said this and added, "I think that answer came straight out of my subconscious mind."

Seven years have passed, and the marriage has continued successfully.

DISCUSSION

To analyze exactly what was done is rather simple. The patient had told his story, and note had been taken of the patterning of his behavior as was revealed by that story. Then came the problem of devising a therapeutic procedure employing symbolic language expressive of his story. It would need to encompass the same sort of labored, obsessive-compulsive, repetitious behavior, and be provocative of comparable emotions of desperation and defeat, but so organized that the culmination of his behavior would be a success each time. At no time was he assured of therapy. He was not told that he would have the "real" answer; instead, he was told that the "real real real" answer would become known, and "real real real" is different from "real," as any child knows.

The purpose of the wristwatch was to emphasize, as he had for years, the element of time but in an opposite way. To the wristwatch was attached the same despairing emotion pertaining to time as he had experienced in relation to his long history of failures. The author simply recognized that "failure equals failure," so time (a wristwatch) was equated with failure (failure to ejaculate). "But all things come to an end, even failure." Hence, at the rather peculiar time of 27½ minutes (the oddness of that specified period of time precluded any analysis and compelled rigid attention to the passage of time) the "failure" to ejaculate came to an end. This, of course, could not be a final answer, hence coitus occurred the next morning with the "end" of the "failure" to ejaculate occurring at 33, 34, or 35 minutes. Why such a time specification? Simply to lead him into a situation where he could choose his own time to ejaculate. Remember the patient's guarded inquiry about the duration of intercourse "to, let us say, maybe as long as half an hour or more."

What was the purpose of the hypnotic amnesia? The patient's memories could not be erased, but his immediate awarenesses pertaining to his problem needed redirection and reorganization. By "locking his memories" in his unconscious mind there resulted an amnesia of the therapeutic suggestions and a delayed "remembering" of the therapist but nothing more. Thus, he was given a burden of unconsciously remembered ideas which he was to execute in an obsessive-compulsive, desperate endeavor to prevent the failure of the very thing that had constituted the failures of his past. But in the new time setting the "failure" constituted a success that had to be doubted and repeatedly achieved until its successfulness could be accepted as such. This is the kind of thinking which many patients do and which often serves to present an opportunity to turn or to reverse the illogic of their conceptions of themselves into new and better understandings.

39. Modesty: An Authoritarian Approach Permitting Reconditioning Via Fantasy

Milton H. Erickson

An internist brought his wife in for psychotherapy and stated that he wished to give her history in her presence since he was certain that she would be unable to do so. As a preliminary, he stated that he had used hypnosis in his practice, had found it useful, but had abandoned it for no good reason except that he was more familiar with other methods. He hoped that this would not occasion offense to the author since he was certain his wife would require hypnotherapy.

In summary, the history was that his wife was exceedingly modest despite the fact that she was a registered nurse and that they had been married for 12 years. This modesty consisted of undressing for bed only after he was in bed. Then she would turn off all lights, go into the guest room in the dark, undress, put on pajamas and then a nightgown over them, and come into the bedroom in the dark:

> Our sex life was terrible the first few months, and then she became reasonable. When she finally got pregnant, I had to force her to see an obstetrician, but she wouldn't go until the seventh month. She made him give her ether and he had a hard time. Now our little girl is five years old and she is beginning to notice her mother, and I don't want her to grow up and give her husband the hard time I had.
>
> Then two years ago I demanded a showdown on this nonsense, which was a horrible mistake, only I didn't realize it. I ripped her nightie and pajamas off and made her come to bed and I wish to God I hadn't. She just went into a panic, developed tachycardia, became apneic, then had dyspnea. This was followed by a lot of hysterical behavior, and I had to sedate her. The next day she was phobic and had a compulsion to run out of the house. She would get clear to the end of the backyard before she could get control of herself. This got so bad that she couldn't do her housework. She trembled, she cried, she felt choked up, she had constant difficulty with her breathing, and all my apologies and promises

Unpublished manuscript, circa 1950s.

did no good. She just got worse and I took her to your colleague, Dr. X [a psychiatrist]. He hospitalized her for two months for an extensive work-up. I think every consultant in town saw her for everything. She received endocrine therapy, tranquilizers, and everything went well until suggestion of returning home was made. Then there would be more tachycardia, even snycope, and apnea and dyspnea.

Finally he transferred her to the private mental hospital, and he psychoanalyzed her six hours a week for six months. Since this led nowhere, he gave her twelve electric shock treatments. She has been home a year now. At first she was just quiet and subdued. She didn't have much to say and kept on coming to bed in the same old way. I felt like hell. During the last three months she has been getting progressively worse. I asked Dr. X what to do, and he offered to do more shock treatment. I don't like the results of that. Then I decided to consult you about hypnosis for her. Will you take her as a patient?

Throughout this narration his wife sat rigidly on her chair, now and then glancing from her husband to the author. She was obviously in a tense emotional state; she appeared badly frightened and embarrassed but in good contact with her surroundings.

Instead of answering her husband, the author asked her if he had given a correct history. She nodded her head and uttered a tremulous "Yes." In reply the author added, "That is, as correct as possible, since he could not really tell how scared you were and still are." To this she nodded her head affirmatively with vigor.

She was immediately asked, "Do you want to be my patient? Remember, I don't use electric shock and I might use hypnosis if I felt it would help."

Resolutely she answered, "Yes, I want help from you—no electric shock, no hormone shots. Just help me stop being so scared."

The rest of the interview was spent in securing additional details of history, indirectly confirming the fact that they were in love with each other, and also in endeavoring to encourage the patient to speak more freely. Any questions directed toward the original excessive modesty elicited profound embarrassment and apparently a hysterical apnea. A tentative diagnosis was reached—psychoneurosis of a mixed hysterical and conversion type. This diagnosis satisfied the husband and pleased the patient, who obviously feared, as she later confirmed, that she might be suffering from schizophrenia, a diagnosis that had been more or less broadly hinted at in the private mental hospital.

At the next interview, with her husband in the office with her, she tearfully pleaded that she be hypnotized at once. Both she and her husband stated that he had worked with her as a subject when he was developing his knowledge of techniques, but that, at best, she had been a light trance subject.

TRANCE INDUCTION UTILIZING RHYTHMIC EXPERIENCE

The intensity of her pleas and the pleading look upon her husband's face suggested the possibility of a *corrective emotional experience* (Erickson & Rossi, 1979) by means of hypnosis. As a possible clue to a method of approach she was asked, among other things, if she had ever done any painting or sketching, and had she ever seen or done any ballet dancing. Her answers were puzzled affirmations, and it was also learned that she was a fair pianist. She had also practiced ballet, had done much landscape sketching, and had painted portraits from memory, but all of this was previous to the birth of her child, her one and only pregnancy.

She was then asked to keep in mind some rhythms that she liked and to demonstrate one of them by beating time to it with her upraised hand. At the same time she was to recall her husband's most successful trance induction with her and, as she recalled it, to develop a comparable and then a progressively deeper trance until she could actually hear the music to which she had danced. She responded cooperatively, and shortly gave evidence of a deep trance, beating time with her feet and rocking back and forth in her chair in a childishly pleased and happy fashion.

UTILIZING OBSESSIVE COMPULSIVE PERSONALITY TRENDS FOR FACILITATING HYPNOTIC SUGGESTION

She was asked to listen to the examiner, and she was reminded that she came to receive therapy. Immediately a look of mingled despair and hope came over her face, and she asked, "Can you help me?"

"Only so much as you let me" was the reply, to which was added, "Very slowly I want you, still remaining in a deep trance, to feel completely unable to arouse from the trance, completely unable to do anything except what I tell you, and unable to forget that your husband is here all the time even though you cannot see him. Now there are many things I want you to do, and every one you must do without fail. You won't like to do those things, but such refusal will make it necessary for you to do something you will dislike much more.

"You will have no choice. You came for therapy, you want therapy, you will be offered therapy, and if you try to refuse it and to turn away, you will be confronted with therapy you will like even less. No matter where you turn, you will be confronted on all sides. I suggest that you endure helplessly the therapy that will be presented, because the therapy will be presented as gently as possible. I will only get rough if you try to avoid it." The purpose of this wording was to utilize the possible compulsive and obsessional elements in her behavior and to capitalize upon her long-established method of reacting as if she were behaving under duress.

In elaborating a therapeutic plan for her, the author kept fully in mind the utter childishness of her neurotic behavior that had persisted after a successful pregnancy and despite a reasonably good sexual adjustment. Reflection on the behavior she manifested suggested the possibility of an approach based upon some measure that would be equally childish and absurd, that would relate to her behavior in some contradictory fashion by being uncensored and uninhibited, and would contain in some reverse form the very behavior she had manifested over the years. In this approach there would have to be elements of impulsiveness and compulsive-obsessional coloring of a rather simple, childish, somewhat morbid character. A rather thinly disguised sexual theme seemed appropriate. A fortunate, highly neurotic sexual fantasy of another patient, along with cognizance of the capacity of the average person to be extremely childish, untrammeled, and unguarded in fantasies, finally permitted the formulation of a suitable fantasy for this patient. This could then be imposed upon her in the trance state and play upon the patient's own patterns of impulsive, and perhaps actually compulsive and obsessional, somewhat morbid patterns that had become habitual for her.

Not much time or effort was required by the author to organize the plan of procedure mentally while he watched the patient continue in the trance and to beat time to the hallucinatory music. Within a relatively brief time, which served to let the patient become more deeply absorbed in the hypnotic state, the author was ready. Accordingly, in a rather authoritative fashion he addressed her:

HALLUCINATORY EXPERIENCE TO REHEARSE THERAPEUTIC CHANGE

Now listen to me. These are the things you must do. Do them you must, and without fail. Item No. 1 is to open your eyes very slowly, to look at me, to see only me, to know that your husband is here, but you are to be unable to see him. Item No. 2 is that you are to see whatever I tell you to see and to know that you *do not* know where you are, only that you are sitting somewhere in a room seeing nothing but me, hearing nothing but me.

Now, perform these two tasks. [Slowly her eyes opened, her pupils were widely dilated, and she stared unblinkingly at the author.] Look slowly about you, seeing nothing, hearing nothing except me and an empty room. [Slowly she turned her head from side to side, then looked at the author.]

Item No. 3 is very nice. With your eyes wide open, experience a feeling of profound relaxation and restfulness, a feeling as if you could not move or tense a muscle or breathe faster no matter how hard you tried otherwise. Just feel hopelessly, completely caught in a state of utterly profound, restful relaxation, completely unable to change your restful physical state *no matter how much you try.* And enjoy that feeling of *utterly helpless comfort as long as you can,* because something will happen that will make you mentally want desperately to shake off that warm, comfortable, relaxed feeling. But you will be so completely helpless and comfortable physically and utterly unable to do anything physically, and you will be so horrified mentally that you can derive comfort only from knowing mentally that your husband is here, even though you can't see him. You will be desperately glad he is here. Do you understand?" [She slowly nodded affirmatively with a pleased but puzzled look on her face and a somewhat hesitant character to the nodding of her head.]

Item No. 4 is to see before you a large mirror in which you can see both of us. Right? Now that you see it plainly, I am turning it until you see nothing in it except a small part of a vacant room and a door that looks vaguely familiar in a most peculiar way— just how, you can't imagine. From now on you will breathe deeply, comfortably, with slow regularity, 12 to 14 times a minute, and there is nothing you can do about that except to continue the same slow, deep respiration comfortably. You cannot move, you cannot close your eyes, you will just look and look and look!

Now you can lean gently, comfortably forward, but that is all, with a peculiar feeling that you know that door, that that door is going to open, that you don't want it to open, but it opens slowly, wide and wider—you can see your face—your own face—Look at that unexpected mischievous smile on your face—on your face— you wonder—you wonder—you have a peculiar impending feeling that something, something, is going to happen, that mischievous smile is getting broader and plainer—Why?—Now you see it fully, you just can't take your eyes off it, you can't close your eyes—you have a grateful feeling for some peculiar reason that the mirror is turned so I can't look in it because—because—look—look behind your face until you see your whole head, and now you can't believe it—you just can't—your neck and shoulders are bare, your chest is uncovered, your body is naked, you are standing there horribly in the nude, you feel so paralyzed in such a peculiar, comfortable way, it's so horrible mentally—you can't stop looking—looking! And watch—watch carefully—you are beginning to dance—ballet dancing—with a wild wild rhythm of joyous abandonment. And what is that? Kicking high, you stand frozen there on one foot, slowly turning your head to see—to see what—somebody is coming—somebody is coming—you can't move—you cannot even stop that mischievous smile—it's frozen—someone coming—sounds like a man. Slowly the mirror turns—slowly the man comes into view—it is your husband and he is laughing—he is clapping his hands—he likes your dance—you become unfrozen and you dance and dance with wilder abandon until you collapse in utter exhaustion and your husband picks you up—for what—the mirror vanishes—just the room is left. Now watch—watch—watch! Watch it all happening just as I described. You can hear my words as each thing happens. See it again—completely.

The patient sat rigidly immobile; only the rapid movement of her eyeballs and the shallow, irregular breathing of an intensely excited person betrayed what she might be visualizing. Suddenly she closed her eyes, slumped in the chair, and smiled, saying as if to herself, "I'm so tired."

She was instructed to rest fully, and that shortly, fully rested, she would sit up and indicate her willingness to listen. Within three minutes she straightened up in the chair, slowly opened her eyes, and stared unblinkingly at the author.

A rapid summary was given of what had occurred, and she was asked if she had watched fully, completely the whole time and had seen everything—everything." With a burning blush she nodded her head to indicate that she had obeyed.

Carefully, in a manner of utter authority, she was told, "You have done well. Now you will repeat that whole task until you have done it five times from beginning to end—see every single part of the entire tableau, collapsing so comfortably at each termination, resting fully for what seems a long time, then going on to the next repetition until all five times have been completed. You know now that you must do as I say because you can only guess what I would have you see if you tried to refuse to do this task." Slowly she nodded her head and proceeded to behave as if obeying. Thereupon she was told:

> There remains now a most important thing that you are surely going to do, are you not? Item No. 5 is that after you awaken, you will have a total amnesia for all of this that has occurred today in your trance. Today is Tuesday. Then comes Wednesday and Thursday with no memories at all, but you will have some peculiar, indescribable feelings. A feeling that you are going to do something! You will catch a glimpse of yourself in the hall mirror [penciled notes to the husband elicited special items of information], in the sideboard mirror. You will catch a glimpse of a haunting, mischievous smile, but you won't know what it is. You will feel like a tantalized, happy little girl, but horribly thrilled, vaguely certain, awful certain that *something is going to happen that you don't want to happen because you want it to happen.* But what? It will be so tantalizingly close to your mind that you will almost feel that you can reach out and grab it. And everytime you walk past a mirror, just as you stop looking in it, you will get a tantalizing half-glimpse of a mischievous smile, only you won't be able to recognize it. You will just half-see it.
>
> And Friday afternoon you won't understand why you are letting your little girl go to visit and stay overnight with the children of your friend. But no sooner has she left than you draw every shade in the house, you draw all the drapes. You will wonder why, why, why!
>
> You will prepare, for no good reason, the best meal you ever cooked, but you will know there is no special occasion, or is there? There will be so many odd, unexpected, intriguing little things happen—interesting, yet they won't seem to have any meaning. The nearer the time comes for your husband's return from the office the more happily alert you will get. And yet such feelings!
>
> You will eat dinner—you will enjoy it—dishwashing will be so easy—so different—never like that before. Why? What next?
>
> All evening you will be happily up and down—you will look in every mirror—just a hint of a glimpse. Oh, I just don't know all the simple little ordinary good things you will do, every one of which will seem to bring closer something fascinating, horribly, laughably devilish. You will almost itch all over with wonderment. [The use of the *itch* was entirely fortuituous, an item of fact that will be clarified in its pertinence later.]
>
> Your husband will go to bed early. Subdued, slowly, confused, dully, hopelessly puzzled, you will get ready for bed in the same

old way. Something will seem bewilderingly wrong! You will turn on the light. That's not really your regular nightgown—it's ready for the rag bag—those pajamas—an old cast-off pair of your husband's. Appalled, you stand—a sudden impulse—an awful impulse—with a giggle you tear them off—you bound out into the hallway, you snap on the light, you dash into the bedroom, you turn on the light, and you do a rapturous dance in the nude while your husband sits helplessly in bed and watches until—until——. Now that is what will happen and you won't even guess what happened to make you do all that until I think you should know. And now, you know you will do it, do you not?—She nodded her head slowly, perseveratively.

THE RESULTS

The following Monday her husband reported to the author, "As I listened to you last Tuesday, I didn't know whether to be shocked, horrified, appalled, pleased, or just plain mad at you. What you were saying to her seemed like a crazy, madcap, childish daydream, and I didn't know whether I ought to take my wife home and get another psychiatrist or what. But all of a sudden I kept feeling that I could see that mirror, and that jarred my eyeteeth. Then again I tried to look in it, and when I caught myself straining to do that, I thought I better leave matters in your hands. I knew I couldn't understand.

"We got back home all right. She was silent, sort of wrapped up in her thoughts. One thing that made me sit up and listen was that every time she got near the piano, she'd play a few snatches of dance tunes. Then she played a piece of classical music for me to hear that evening as she often does, and she threw in scattered bits of dance music. It was weird. I'll swear she didn't know it. Bedtime, same old thing. I said nothing, as you indicated to me.

"Wednesday morning, Thursday morning, I saw her ducking her head at first one mirror and then another. I don't know what happened during the day, but I guess she was too busy to have symptoms. She said she was trying to clean out the storeroom, but I noticed a lot of sheet music that we brought from her home when we were first married. And every time she passed the piano, she would ripple her fingers down the keys. And she kept having a puzzled look. There was more classical music, some of her favorites with a lot of little pieces of dance music dropped in. Bedtime, the same.

"Friday noon she called me to tell me Jenny could go to visit with Martha's kids overnight.

"That dinner was wonderful, drapes drawn, candlelight, romantic as could be. She kept turning her head from side to side as if she had heard someone or expected someone. It was funny the way she kept looking at her reflection in the silverware. Half the time she had the most entrancing smile on her face, but every time she looked in a mirror, it would vanish. I could scarcely control myself. She didn't talk much at all. Just silent and absorbed.

"Bedtime, I looked in the guest room. Where she dug them up I don't know, but she hoards dust rags. Then I sneaked into our bedroom.

"Everything happened on schedule. It was literally a honeymoon. Saturday morning I called Martha and told her to keep Jenny until Monday morning. Enough said.

"No symptoms yet. Where do we go from here?"

"Come in tomorrow; that is Tuesday. I'll take over then."

The next day, as reported by the husband, the patient rebelled at the proposal that she accompany her husband to the author's office. However, after much insistent persuasion she came in exceedingly embarrassed. Her opening remark was, "I am too embarrassed even to look at you, Dr. Erickson [she had her hands over her face and was hanging her head]. I know everything that has happened to me. I've got a full memory of what you had me do in a trance in the office—if I just close my eyes, I can see the whole thing just as vividly now as I did then. I'm embarrassed. What will you think of me? I remember all the things I did Tuesday, Wednesday, Thursday—and please don't make me tell about Friday. You would be proud of me, but it's so embarrassing that I don't want my husband to tell you even. Will it be all right if I just say I did everything that you or my husband could want? Oh, I mean that differently! Everything that my husband could want and that you would think I should do. Is that enough to tell you, please?"

She was reassured but told, "All I want to know is about your so-called phobia."

She dropped her hands and declared angrily, "I'm glad you asked about that. I could kill Dr. X for giving me shock treatment for that and psychoanalyzing me and putting me in the hospital for months and giving me all kinds of hormones until I was a human pincushion!"

There was much more said in this same angry vein, but after expressing herself freely, the patient continued: "I just don't see why I couldn't have had just simple common-sense therapy. If I ever see that man again, I'll slap his face! That isn't very ladylike, and I hope you will forgive me, but my husband is a doctor and I'm a nurse, and we all know that there are some awfully stupid doctors. I even asked him about hypnosis and he sneered and——." Here she was told, "Quiet down, that's in the past; now tell me about your phobia."

Her reply was, "That's in the past, and I just can't understand how I ever got into that awful way of behaving, but I couldn't stop. I was just a scared little girl, too scared to think, and I just followed the path of least resistance, only it kept getting worse and worse.

"Then when you made me do those things, it was just like my phobia—compulsive I mean. I felt exactly like a little child—a frightened little child with some kind of a horrible, morbid curiosity. And the more I looked, the more I wanted to, and the stranger it got. Honest, I don't believe I know half of all the weird things I did Tuesday night and all day Wednesday, Thursday, Friday." With a flaming-red face she added, "And don't you dare ask me about Friday night or Saturday or Sunday. You can just be proud of me as a patient. But why did I have to be such a silly child? I wonder if it was because I would think I was too grown up to do something silly like that. I don't know, but anyway, I'm glad."

Her husband added a comment here to the effect, "The more I think about it, and the more I think about neurotic behavior in my patients, the more I wonder if they have grown up emotionally. It looks to me, and I'm no expert, as if some of these neurotics ought to be handled on a simple childish level so you can get their understanding." Here his wife interrupted with, "You can say that for me."

SUBSEQUENT COURSE

Over a period of five years the patient has been seen at regular intervals for a seasonal dermatitis from which she has suffered since about the age of five years. Previous treatment by various allergists had always been only mildly successful. With the close of certain pollen seasons, her dermatitis would vanish. The season following her hypnotherapy she sought hypnotic relief and amelioration of her skin condition.

This was attempted and proved much more successful than the treatment by the allergist. She reported to him what she had done, and he advised her to continue with the author stating that she was, at least for that season, securing much more relief than he could give her. Hence, each year she reports for her hypnotic symptom relief, and the allergist has continued to check her condition each year because of his curiosity about her much greater response to purely psychological measures than to his method.

40. Sterility: A Therapeutic Reorientation to Sexual Satisfaction

Milton H. Erickson

A college professor and his wife, happily married for five years and ardently in love, abhorred the thought of children. Both were absorbed in their careers and their home life together. They enjoyed sex relations frequently and intensely and gladly practiced contraception, finding it no significant annoyance. By chance the man was asked by a friend doing research on spermatazoa to furnish a specimen, which he did willingly. Since the friend knew the attitude of the professor and his wife toward children, he did not hesitate to inform the professor that the specimen disclosed complete absence of sperm cells. Interested at once, the professor asked for recheck examinations, and these confirmed the original finding.

Delighted with this news, the professor and his wife abandoned contraceptive measures. During the ensuing year both the professor and his wife became increasingly irritable with each other, and their sexual ardor decreased greatly. Finally they began to discontinue sex relations and to absorb themselves unhappily in their individual activities.Because of continued increasing disharmony for six months, the professor sought psychiatric aid from the writer.

The above history was elicited, and he was then asked to comment on how he felt about the absence of spermatazoa in relationship to himself. He declared that it should be a comforting fact to him, since it did not interfere with him sexually and it removed a possibility that was appalling to both himself and his wife—namely, an undesired pregnancy. Nevertheless, after his first rejoicing, some unrecognized emotional element of a disturbing character had crept into his total affect. What it was, he could not state, but gradually he had begun feeling that he was lacking seriously in those things inherently necessary to himself as a man. Sexual activity had become increasingly meaningless to him, and he had experienced a feeling that his wife was reacting the same way. This had resulted in ever-increasing friction between them until the now-desperate situation had developed.

No attempt was made to discuss his problem with him immediately.

Unpublished manuscript, circa 1950s.

Instead, he was asked to send his wife to the writer for a consultation. She was found to be remarkably frank and clear-thinking. She related a similar story with comparable significances.

At first she had been delighted at the opportunity to discontinue contraception. After some time—at first vaguely and finally with distressing clarity—she had realized that as a sexual mate her husband was biologically deficient—that is, that he could not constitute a biological masculine complement to her biological femininity. It was not that she wanted to be pregnant; it was merely that she, as a biologically female creature, needed to feel that her mate could, really could, impregnate her. She had reacted to this understanding by trying to force herself to look upon the situation as a fortunate happenstance. Failing in this, she had suppressed her ideas forcibly, with the result that the marital situation had grown increasingly more difficult. Their last sex relations had been more than four months ago and had amounted to no more than a labored, futile, unpleasant effort.

No attempt was made to do anything other than to elicit the above story in clear detail. Then a joint appointment was made for both of them. They entered the office rather diffidently and hopefully, seeming to be eager for help. They were assured most earnestly that their problem could be solved if they could attend to and understand the ideas that would be presented to them. They were told that the discussion about to be offered would be based upon medical concepts that were pragmatically valid and that could reasonably be applied to them. Much of the preliminary discussion would seem irrelevant, they were told, and it would appear to have no relation to their problem. However, it would constitute the essential and elementary foundation upon which they could base an understanding of the correction of their problem.

INDIRECT TRANCE INDUCTION WITH AN ABSORBING ASSOCIATIVE NETWORK

Thereupon, in the most hypnotically persuasive way possible, they were presented with a systematic discussion of concepts of psychosomatic medicine, and numerous case histories and examples were cited to illustrate the effects of psychological forces upon somatic functioning.

When they seemed to have sufficient understanding, a long, specious* argument was presented that:

---

*In this writer's opinion a patient kept awake by severe pain but who sleeps restfully and well as a result of a hypodermic injection of distilled water benefits more than he would from an injection of morphine.

1. Their joint desire, so strong, to have no children quite possibly could alter their procreative functioning.
2. Their use of contraceptive measures quite possibly could reinforce the psychosomatic effect upon their procreative functioning.
3. The continuance of contraception kept alive and active the psychosomatic forces militating against procreative power.
4. The discovery of aspermatazoa had resulted in the assumption that it signified biological failure with no realization that it was quite possibly a psychosomatic development protective of their actual needs.
5. The mere assumption that the aspermatazoa was biological and not psychosomatically functional led to an altered psychological state in them in which an essential element of their lovemaking was absent—namely, the protection of the other from procreation.
6. With the discontinuance of contraception, there could result a change in gonadal functioning, but since there was a profound psychological need to avoid procreation, another type of protection would be provided psychosomatically.
7. This new psychosomatic protection against procreation would be the progressive and finally complete loss of sexual interest in each other, a loss that would be distressing and troublesome.
8. Therefore, with these new understandings of possible psychosomatic functioning, it might be well for them to return to their original pattern of happy sex relationships. Thereby, any alteration in gonadal functioning that might have resulted from their abstention and their disturbed emotional states could be corrected by the reestablishment of the original behavioral pattern, and thus they could again have a sense of completeness in their sexual relationships.

They listened to this exposition of ideas* with intense interest and seemed to comprehend adequately. A few general questions were answered, and they were given an appointment in another month. At that appointment they reported happily that the understandings they had received had resolved their problem and that their marriage was back on

---

*Not only is the writer aware of the superficiality and speciousness of the ideas presented to these patients, but he is also aware of the utter absurdity of their problem and of the appalling readiness with which people can seize upon some inconsequential idea and elaborate it into an overwhelming catastrophe. Furthermore, the writer recognizes that complete awareness of absolute truth is much less available than happy adjustments based upon those partial understandings acceptable to individuals and available and suitable to their own unique limitations.

its original status. The professor summarized the entire matter by ruefully commenting upon the human tendency of people, however intelligent, to draw far-reaching conclusions from insufficient data from another field of understanding and to make extensive unwarranted applications of it. Several years later they were still adjusting happily.

41. The Abortion Issue: Facilitating Unconscious Dynamics Permitting Real Choice

Milton H. Erickson

This report concerns a problem of brief duration, decidedly acute in character, and marked by terrified, obsessional, insistent demands.

The patients were a young couple in their early twenties. Both were attending college, and they had been engaging in sex relations regularly for nearly a year. They had just discovered that there existed a pregnancy of about two months' duration. Both sets of parents were furious and unforgiving and asserted emphatically that "it better be gotten rid of, or no more college" (one more year of college for each remained). Extreme and unreasoning emphasis had been placed upon the shame entailed for all relatives and friends. The young couple had planned to marry but not until after graduation from college.

The couple were seriously distraught by their situation and by the parental attitudes which had developed to include "no college and no marriage unless you spare us this shame." The father of the young man furnished him sufficient money and advice on where to go to secure the abortion. A friend of the young man, knowing about the situation and aware of the highly disturbed emotional state of the couple, suggested that they see the author and get "tranquilized" before undertaking the risks of an illegal abortion.

Their distress was greatly augmented when the author uncompromisingly discountenanced an abortion. Nor would they listen to the author's suggestions of other, more reasonable possibilities. For two long hours they insistently repeated demands that the author approve the abortion and that he undertake the task himself by using hypnosis to induce physiological activity, thereby making it "legal," and that he prescribe tranquilizing drugs to "calm" both of them. They expressed fear that their overwrought emotional state, in view of the author's lack of cooperation, might cause an abortionist to reject them as too much of a risk, since neither could keep from bursting into hysterical sobs at frequent intervals.

Scattered items of information disclosed that each was an only child,

---

Unpublished manuscript, circa 1950s.

highly protected by rigid and domineering parents, and that they were completely dependent on their parents for everything, including even their opinions in general. They were genuinely in love and were expecting to be married with parental blessings upon being graduated from college. Among the planned wedding presents were a secure position in the firm of the father-in-law-to-be for the young man and a beautiful home from the young man's parents. Now all of this, their entire planned and desired future, was at stake unless they abided by parental commands and secured the abortion.

Two full hours of desperate endeavor failed to make the slightest impression upon their insistent, hysterical, highly obsessional, repetitive demands.

TRANCE INDUCTION BY UTILIZING OBSESSIVE BEHAVIOR, QUESTIONS, NOT KNOWING, AND A REVERSE SET OF SURPRISING IDEAS

Finally the author decided to capitalize upon the obsessional, fearful behavior they both manifested by using that very behavior itself. As everybody knows, it is impossible to hold a stopwatch to time one's self and to avoid thinking about an elephant for one whole minute. This simple childish challenge seemed to present a method of dealing effectively with the problem they presented. Accordingly, the author emphatically demanded:

> All right, all right, quiet now, quiet, if you want the help you ask. Be quiet and let me tell you how to ensure getting the abortion you are desperately trying to prove to me that you want. You have told me you want the abortion. You have told me that there is no other choice. You have told me that, regardless of everything, you are going to go ahead with the abortion. You declare most emphatically and resolutely that nothing can stop you. *Now let me warn you about one thing that can stop you, that will surely stop you, against which you will be totally helpless if you are not warned about it in advance. Quiet now! Listen attentively because you need to know this if you really want the abortion, if you really intend to get the abortion.* Now listen quietly and attentively. Are you listening? Both nodded their heads silently, expectantly.*

* Editor's Note: This attitude of heightened expectation and probably unconscious head nodding is characteristic of Erickson's patients when they are in a state of therapeutic trance without being aware of it.

You do not know an important thing, a vitally important thing. That essential information is this: You do not know whether that baby is a boy or a girl. You do not see, cannot see, the vital connection between that question and the abortion you have told me that you want. *Yet that question will prevent you from getting the abortion since you don't know the answer.* Your personalities, your psychological makeups make that question important. You do not know why, but who expects you to know? Let me explain! If that baby were going to be kept by you, you, not knowing if it were a boy or a girl, would have to think of a name for it that would fit either sex, such as Pat, which could be either Patrick or Patricia, or Frances for a girl or Francis for a boy. *Now that is the very thing you must avoid at all costs.* Under no circumstances, not even once, after you leave this office, are you to think of a possible name for that baby, a name that would fit either sex. *To do so and to keep on doing so would compel you pyschologically to keep the baby,* not to get an abortion. Hence, under no circumstances are you to dare to think of a name for that baby. Please, please don't, because then you won't get an abortion. Every time you think of a name, that thinking will definitely deter you from getting an abortion. You will be forced into taking the money you have and seeing a justice of the peace and getting married. You want an abortion, and you can't have it if you think of a name, so don't, just don't don't don't think of a name, any name for the baby *after you leave this office, because if you do, you will keep it, so don't don't don't think of a name, any name.* Now without another word, *not one word, not a single word, especially not a baby's name,* leave this office at once.

Thereupon the author took them by hand and led them quickly to the door to hasten their departure.

Several days later they returned, smiling in an abashed fashion, stating, "After we got married *because we just couldn't help thinking of dozens of names, and every name made the baby more precious to us,* we realized that all you did was bring us to our senses before we did something awful foolish and awful wrong. We had just lost our heads, and our parents didn't help either—that's why we acted like such awful fools in your office."

Inquiry disclosed that both sets of parents accepted the elopement instead of an abortion with a profound sense of relief. The original plans for setting-up the young couple were carried out when the husband was graduated.

The young mother had to delay her graduation for some time. Then the grandmothers alternately baby-sat so that the young mother could complete her college work. At the present time little Leslie has several younger siblings.

From the very beginning of the interview with this distraught couple the extreme obsessional character of their behavior, thought, and emotions was most marked. They seemed, as persons, to be basically sound yet caught in a situation they could not handle. Hypnosis was obviously not a suitable procedure, but it was realized, as observation of them continued, that a hypnotic technique of suggestion, seemingly worded to favor undesirable results, could effect positive results and that a specious psychological contingency could be so emphatically suggested to them that their own hysterical obsessional behavior would make it effective in securing a desirable end result. The emphatic presentation of the problem of not thinking of a name befitting either sex *outside of the office,* only incidentally mentioning marriage by a justice of the peace without actually suggesting that they resort to it, precluded any tendency for them to rebel because they had been "told what to do." This created a favorable climate for their voluntary marriage by a justice of the peace, since they were not recognizably so instructed. Fundamental to this evolution of results was their own sense of guilt, their own desire for marriage, their need to do something, the unexpressed and unrecognized anger at their hiterto loving, permissive parents, their outraged feelings at the parental rage and demands that they obey parental commands, and the suggestion of the friend that they seek "tranquilization." All this had so disturbed their emotions that they were left in an essentially irrational state. The author then simply and deliberately employed their own state of irrational thinking to effect a favorable outcome by the use of a hypnotic technique—the presentation of ideas in a fashion conducive to acceptance despite their overwrought emotional state. Additionally, that technique of suggestion, unwittingly to them, subtly transformed the problem from "we must get an abortion" to "we must not think of a name for the [our] baby." This could only be a losing battle, and the very desperateness of their efforts not to think of a suitable name could only serve to bring them closer and closer to marriage—as, indeed, it did.

42. Impotence: Facilitating Unconscious Reconditioning

Milton H. Erickson

THE PROBLEM

The patient was a 42-year-old physician, actively and successfully engaged in the general practice of medicine. With much embarrassment he doggedly gave the history of his complaint. It was, he declared, "psychogenic impotence," and he knew that this was the correct diagnosis since he could and did masturbate with ease and he could maintain a state of full tumescence up to the moment when sexual relations became an immediate possibility. Detumescence, but without ejaculation, resulted at once if any effort were made at vaginal insertion or even at intercrural placement. He could be masturbated successfully by a woman if it were done manually. Enfoldment of his erect phallus between a woman's breasts as a masturbatory measure led to immediate detumescence, even as did the mere suggestion of fellatio.

This problem, he stated, began in his first year in college. Together with friends he had visited a bawdy-house, but without success, although he had told his friends otherwise. Thereafter, he had secretly visited the same and other bawdy-houses, "always with the same humiliating failure. I could walk a mile with a full erection, choose the girl I wanted, go to the room with her O.K., undress, and start to get into bed with her, and then, kerplop, just like dropping a baseball bat, I'd lose my erection. That, literally, is the story of my life."

He continued his account by relating extensively his efforts at self-therapy. He had visited innumerable professional and clandestine prostitutes and had offered them large rewards all to no avail. He had engaged in campaigns of seduction of girls he had been informed were permissive, but however successful his campaign the desired result was not achieved. He had sought out women of the other races without achieving his goal. He had ventured "to try community stuff," which meant several men and

Unpublished manuscript, 1953.

several women all engaged at the same time in the same room in various forms of sexual activity with a repeated interchange of partners. All that he had achieved was successful manual masturbation of his partner, while she successfully masturbated him manually. He had once attempted to approach a "swish homosexual," but this had been so offensive an idea that he could not bring himself to make even a verbal approach. He had served overseas in the armed forces, but "I was in combat service repeatedly with casualties all around me without ever getting wounded, but sexually I was a total casualty before every engagement overseas."

He had tried alcohol in various amounts to overcome his difficulty, and before graduating from medical school he had sought out "hopheads and got hopped up with everything they recommended, but it was all no good."

After graduation from medical school and the completion of his internship he had searched the medical literature extensively and had experimented with every drug preparation that seemed to offer even the slightest hope, but all to no avail.

He had tried two other measures: stage hypnotists, whom he soon came to regard as patently fraudulent because of their extensive claims unsubstantiated by any scientific knowledge or results, and "bedmates," attractive, willing women he paid to sleep regularly with him over a period of many weeks, in the hope that "sooner or later," he might awaken with an erection during the night and succeed in having relations. This measure also was a failure.

His reason for seeing the author was twofold. In the first place he had been aware that ever since World War I medical interest in hypnosis as a scientific modality had been growing, and he was aware of the author's interest in medical hypnosis. Secondly, six months previously he had fallen "desperately in love" with a 32-year-old woman who had responded to him as intensely as he had to her, with mutual declarations impulsively made by the end of three months of their acquaintanceship. This had forced him into a full confession of his sexual incompetency, although not of the extensive "therapeutic" measures to which he had ineffectually resorted.

She was appalled by his difficulty, but she was convinced that their intense emotional regard for each other would constitute an effective cure. He was doubtful of this, but after several weeks of persuasion by her he agreed reluctantly (since he feared the outcome) to let her discard her moral standards and sleep with him. Approximately a half-dozen futile attempts were made to effect his "cure" by her proposed method.

They then discussed the possibility of a happy marriage with only sexual play and affectionate embraces; but, despite her belief in such a possibility, he felt that the frustrations entailed would inevitably result in marital discord. They finally decided "to date regularly without any attempt at sex, but this was frustrating too."

Then one day he happened to read an article on the surgical use of hypnosis, and this led him to secure an appointment with the author.

Having listened carefully to his story while making adequate notations, the author told the patient that his problem would require at least two weeks of thoughtful study before any opinion could be reached, and that he might then request another appointment.

TRANCE INDUCTION WITH THE CONSCIOUS-UNCONSCIOUS DOUBLE BIND

For the next two weeks much time was spent mulling over the nature and character of the patient's circumscribed, rigid, fixed neurotic behavior and the measures by which that distorted pattern of sexual behavior might be reordered constructively. At the end of this time the patient was seen and informed that therapy would be undertaken, that hypnosis would be employed, but that in no conceivable way would he have any comprehension of what was being done or of how it was being done. Instead of his having any intelligent appreciation of his therapy, he was to be blindly, stupidly obedient to every instruction given to him by the author.

He looked puzzled but nodded his head affirmatively while sitting quietly and expectantly in his chair. Then he was then told:

> As you sit there, close your eyes; listen intently to everything I have to say. Ask no questions; you have nothing to say. You are to develop whatever degree of trance is necessary, and that is what you are to do all the time you are listening to me. The only thing that is important is what I have to say, so listen intently with both your conscious and unconscious mind, especially with your unconscious mind, letting your unconscious mind take over more and more completely as you listen intently. It is not necessary for you to remember consciously, because your unconscious mind will remember what I say and what is means, and that is what is necessary. I shall tell you things you are to do, and do them you will, doing them as certainly as you are hearing me and being bound to do them as much as you are bound to hear them, and hear them you will, and do them you will.
>
> So listen intently, ever more intently, going into that necessary trance to hear me the better by your unconscious mind, which can alone assure that you will listen, hear, understand, and then act. And that you will.

First of all there is to be no discussion, not even with M——. I and only I will discuss with M——.

Next, you must and will arrange with your colleagues and the medical society and your answering service that you will take no night calls for the period of three long long months. [Many times in his story he had made mention of two three-month periods.] Nor will you take calls before eight in the morning.

If necessary, simply take a three-month vacation from your medical practice just to do what you must do. But do it you will.

Now listen with continuing intensity. Each morning you will note the calendar date, and each morning as you note the calendar date you will realize that day will end at midnight, and at midnight, every one of those midnights, for exactly three, three long intolerable months at the stroke of midnight up to the very end of those three long long months, you will know exactly what you are to do, and do it you must, and do it you will, up to the very end of those three intolerable long long months.

Now listen yet more intently. At the stroke of midnight for three long months, and only three long months, and for exactly and precisely only three long months, you will drop into sound physiological sleep at the stroke of midnight for each night of those three long months. And do it you will, for each night of those three long months, each night, no more, no less, for three long months.

Still listening intently, obediently, mindfully, and well. Each day you will dine with M—— at exactly 8:30 P.M. Following this you may converse with M——, listen to music, or watch television—whatever you wish so long as you engage in no sexual activity whatsoever. Then, exactly at 11:00 P.M. you are to be in bed and the light turned off at exactly 11 o'clock. Not one minute before, not one minute later, but at exactly 11 o'clock the lights are to be turned out.

There you will be, lying quietly on your back in the dark, saying nothing, doing nothing but lying there waiting for the stroke of midnight so that you may fall asleep in sound, restful, physiological sleep. And as you wait, tumescence will develop fully, and you will know, know thoroughly and well that you can do nothing at all about it, that you will not even try or even hope to do anything about it. All you can do is to lie there with full tumescence, waiting to fall asleep at the stroke of midnight, and this you will do for three long months; exactly at the stroke of midnight you will fall sound asleep in physiological sleep. Then, when sound asleep, and only then, can detumescence occur. Only then can detumescence occur, only then.

Now, once more, maybe twice more, I shall repeat instructions as you continue listening intently in your trance, and then when I open the door, you will gently arouse and quietly leave. One final understanding that is to be achieved by you and you alone is that three long months is intolerably long, even as would two months be intolerably long, even as one month would be intolerably long, and all you need to know or to understand is intolerably long, whatever that means to you, so now listen while I repeat my instructions.

The instructions were then repeated verbatim, altering only the emphasis to effect, if possible, better unconscious understandings by the patient.

POSTHYPNOTIC BEHAVIOR INDICATING TRANCE DEPTH

At the expiration of the session the patient departed alone in a state of self-absorption. He apparently did not recall that Miss M——had accompanied him to the office at the author's request. Nothing had been said to him about seeing her also. It was for this reason that the author preceded the patient out of the office so that she might be signaled not to attract his attention. The author had hoped for such posthypnotic behavior on the patient's part, but considered it unwise to suggest it. Its spontaneous appearance indicated the depth and effectiveness of the patient's trance. Had such behavior not appeared, the experimental procedure would have been repeated immediately to secure more intense hypnotic responses.

TRANCE INDUCTION AS "DEEP SLEEP"

After the patient left, Miss M——was called into the office. To take advantage of her bewilderment at being so obviously forgotten by Dr. B., an explanation was offered: "I have just been working hypnotically with Dr. B. in relation to the problem that concerns the two of you so much. So just be seated there in that chair, close your eyes gently, and go deeply asleep in a deep hypnotic trance."

Within a few minutes she was obviously in a deep hypnotic trance, and a presentation of instructions to her was easily made for which she developed a subsequent posthypnotic amnesia and full obedience.

Her instructions were rather simple but very explicit. She was told to avoid quietly and unobtrusively any form of sexual behavior with Dr. B., to avoid even any form of affectionate physical contact with him, to be unquestioning of all of his behavior, to have dinner ready to 8:30 P.M. without fail, and to be in bed ready to go to sleep at 11 o'clock sharp, since Dr. B. would unquestionably turn out the light at that exact moment. Then in the dark she was to go to sleep quietly, comfortably, and in an expectantly happy state of mind that would be continuously present whether she were awake or asleep. All conversations were to be on topics unrelated to Dr. B.'s problem. Even if he should mention it, there was to be no discussion on her part. Since they had been living in the same apartment for some time, this was to be continued on literally a sister-brother relationship, so that she would lie quietly on her side of the double bed, contrary to her previous practice.

She was assured that all of this was utterly vital to the correction of Dr. B.'s problem.

She seemed to accept all instructions readily and to be quite passive in her attitudes. She left the office manifesting an apparent amnesia for the events of the office visit and for the manner of her arrival at the office. She accepted as a matter of fact the calling of a cab to take her home.

The results

Just 30 days later, after office hours, both Dr. B. and M——appeared unexpectedly in the office. His opening statement was simply, "I would like to introduce you to my wife."

There then followed a somewhat disordered account, which was noted in full by the author and subsequently put into a more coherent form for this presentation.

> You know the problem I came to you for and explained in such great detail. Then I came again about two weeks later, bringing M——with me. I really don't remember much about that visit except that you began talking to me. M——tells me I forgot to take her home. But I do remember what I did. There was a young resident I liked very much who had just completed his residency. I asked him to take over my practice completely, because I had to be unavailable for about three months. I told him all income was to be his, and that if it wasn't sufficient, I would make up any additional reasonable amount. Everything turned out O.K. for him.
>
> Then I took a leave of absence from the office, but M——and I continued to live in the apartment. We went water-skiing, swimming, dancing—but not much of that because our evenings were so funny. Even when we dined out, we always sat down at

the table at 8:30 and ate, even if it was no more than a sandwich or some fruit. Neither of us said a thing about this. It just seemed to be a way of life, no matter where we had been that day. Since we are hi-fi addicts, we usually played records. I've got a large collection, and we enjoyed them a lot. Once in a while we would watch television. I even had my telephone disconnected.

But the funny thing was that we both had a compulsion to be in bed ready to sleep at 11 o'clock. We never kissed good night. We didn't even say good night. Sometimes we were in bed a few minutes before 11, and I would watch the clock, and when it was exactly 11, I would snap off the light. We were like a couple of dummies. We were living a queer sort of way without even thinking about asking why.

And every night after I turned off the light I'd get a full erection, but I would just lie there not doing anything about it, just waiting until it was midnight, because I knew that I could fall asleep then and that I wouldn't lose my erection until after I fell asleep. I was just a zombie. I just didn't do any thinking. I just acted like an idiot.

Then the other night [inquiry disclosed it to be the 27th night of the suggested three-month period] after I had turned off the light and developed an erection, I suddenly realized that I was unusually wide awake and that I just couldn't go to sleep. Then while I was trying to fall asleep and couldn't, it dawned on me that I couldn't lose my erection until I did fall asleep. While I was wondering about this and still trying to fall asleep, I suddenly realized what it meant that I could not lose my erection until I fell asleep, and I suddenly exploded and I began making love to my wife.—Yes, we went to Mexico the next morning and got married, honeymooned the next day and night at a motel near Tucson, and today came in to see you.—Well, we just kept on making love until we both fell asleep. When we woke up, we were too excited to think about anything except getting married in Mexico right away. Then we honeymooned, as I said, but today on the way back to Phoenix to get an Arizona license to marry, we got to discussing what really had happened. But M—— can't give much information, and what I know mostly is that I was hypnotized in your office and you told me what to do from day to day. But the important thing seems to be something that I'm confused about. It's that three months is just as intolerable as two months and two months are just as intolerable as one month, and there's something about understanding what intolerable really means. I don't suppose I need to know since I know I'm over my problem, but I am curious and so is M——. Both of us are completely satisfied, but we both feel that even if we don't know nothin' from nothin', it won't upset the applecart if you let us in on what happened.

They were asked if they wanted all the details or if they would be content to know that hypnosis had been employed to set up certain psychological patterns of behavior that would resolve the entire problem. To this was added, "To ask me to explain is like a surgical patient asking the surgeon to explain a gastric resection." To this Dr. B. replied, "You may add that your patients are progressing postoperatively in a most favorable fashion."

More than five years have passed. The marriage has been a happy one. There are no children, but children were not wanted by either. From time to time Dr. B. refers a patient to the author or telephones the author to give special information about a referred patient and then to converse casually about matters in general.

DISCUSSION: HYPNOTHERAPY VIA PSYCHOPHYSIOLOGICAL CONDITIONING

To discuss what was done for this patient requires oversimplification and general interpretations. The patient had experienced an unfortunate mishap in a situation of mixed, varied, and guilty emotions, which resulted in a distressing and embarrassing frustration. He sought to correct his mishap by returning to the scene of his misfortune, only to repeat the same unfortunate behavior again. Why it happened in the first instance can be attributed to mixed emotions and inexperience. Why he returned to the place of misfortune can be attributed also to lack of experience and to a misdirected effort at self-help. The second recurrence of his mishap was simply a repetition of his first learning, believing naively that his difficulty could be corrected only by more repetitions of self-help. At some one point in all those 22 years of frustration he reached the conclusion that an unhappy, meaningless detumescence constituted an absolute certainty for him, and he maintained that conclusion. For him detumescence must follow upon tumescence without intervening experience. He became practiced in this sequence of events and learned no way of altering it. To state the situation concisely, he found himself caught in a psychophysiological bind that led only to hopeless frustration, a learning he endlessly reinforced.

Now what was done therapeutically? The nature of his problem was assumed to be a frustration deriving from what, for convenience's sake, was regarded as a psychophysiological conditioning that would not lend itself to any recognizable therapeutic endeavor. He had had too much unfortunate experience to accept a contrary belief. Therefore, it was decided that therapy might be accomplished by setting up a second psychophysiological conditioning contradictory to his traumatic conditioning. This would have to be done with the patient's full cooperation but without his understanding of what was occurring. Thus, a pattern of behavior was suggested hypnotically (hypnotically because "no one in his right mind would accept such silly suggestions in the waking state," where too often the needy listener sets himself up as a final judge despite any degree of ignorance). This proposed pattern of behavior permitted tumescence and conditioned any detumescence to the development of full physiological sleep. Conversely—and this could not be recognized—tumescence was conditioned to the wakeful state. Only by falling asleep could he lose his erection; conversely while he was awake after 11:00 P.M. tumescence had to persist.

Then came the task of working out the details of behavior that would permit this reconditioning, then the task of obscuring the reconditioning to protect it from destructive recognition. At the same time provision had to be made to ensure, within a reasonable time (what was reasonable the author did not know), that the patient would find himself inexplicably confronted by the new state of affairs with no comprehensible way of resolving or understanding the bewildering turn of events except by "doing what comes naturally." So strong was the reconditioning that "doing what comes naturally" was terminated by complete satisfaction and restful physiological sleep, exactly as he had been intentionally reconditioned in this regard.

Once his goal had been so happily and well achieved, his problem could no longer exist. This the author knew before he undertook the case. The only problem was how to facilitate human behavior in a manner to lead to certain goals, to guard against interference by awareness of what was being done, and to create a slow, progressive development of emotional tensions (understanding what "intolerable really means") that would result in a state of uncomprehending awareness of a reality that could only be met adequately by activity favored by the state of passivity so thoroughly instilled in Miss M——. Thus, they achieved their actual goal. Just how that suggested behavior led to the final result is, at best, merely speculative. The discussion offered above seems to be a fair account of the author's understandings.

43. Latent Homosexuality: Identity Exploration in Hypnosis

Milton H. Erickson

A social service worker, Miss X, who had been supervised by the writer in her work and who had, at various times, acted as a demonstration hypnotic subject, decided to be psychoanalyzed because of personality problems. What these were she could not state, other than to declare that she was hostile, antagonistic, exceedingly aggressive, unable to adjust socially, and most unhappy because of periodic depressive reactions.

After a year of "classical" psychoanalysis, five hours weekly, she sought an interview with the writer on a Saturday morning. Her reason was that she had "wasted" the year of analysis in "stupid resistance." For the past three months she had spent each session either in silence or in giving accounts of her daily reading of current books and magazines, and she had not discussed anything pertinent to herself. She asked that the writer put her in a trance and "force" her to "get down to business." Otherwise, since her funds were being rapidly dissipated, she would have to discontinue analysis. In fact, she had twice discontinued analysis but had returned after a week's absence, each time in the hope of doing something other than "showing resistance." On this occasion, however, she had informed the analyst that, unless results were forthcoming within the next three sessions, she was terminating therapy.

She was informed that the writer could do nothing about her request, since she was under the care of another physician. She was rather angered by "such ethics," but accepted the refusal. She declared that she felt entitled to ask such a favor from the writer because of her services as a hypnotic subject in the past. This led to the writer's request, that, as a favor, she would again act as a demonstration hypnotic subject for a lecture before a medical group to be given that afternoon. She consented, commenting that it was apparently all right for the writer to ask a favor but that it was "unethical" for her to do so.

Unpublished manuscript, 1935.

TRANCE INDUCTION AND HYPNOTIC ROLE-PLAYING

Since the writer knew her well, he had formed a private clinical judgment about her personal problem. Also, he was thoroughly acquainted with her officemate, Miss Y, a most feminine girl. Accordingly, at the lecture she was deeply hypnotized and, among other things, depersonalized, then induced to assume the identity of Miss Y. She did this in a startlingly accurate and impressive fashion. As Miss Y, she expressed an intense dislike for Miss X, but could give no reason for this attitude. When the demonstration of this and other hypnotic phenomena had been completed, she was awakened, thanked and dismissed with a posthypnotic amnesia for the trance experiences.

She was seen a week later, very happy and excited. Her story was that she had kept her Monday appointment with the analyst and spent the first half-hour in sullen silence. Then, suddenly, the thought of Miss Y came to her mind, and this had loosed a whole flood of free associations. For the first time in her analysis she became communicative. Each session thereafter had been most productive. She stated that she was now making progress and that, when her analysis was completed, she would inform the writer of the nature of her conflicts.

Three months later she was discharged as requiring no further therapy. Shortly thereafter she sought an interview with the writer, explaining that she attributed the success of her analysis more to the writer than to the analyst. Also, for some reason, Miss Y should be credited in part, although she had disliked Miss Y until recently. However, therapy had corrected her dislike. She continued by explaining that her personality conflict had centered around "strong latent homosexual tendencies," which she had not recognized and which she had repressed with "every ounce of my strength." Because of those tendencies she had reacted with bitter hostility to men and to women in general, especially attractive, highly feminine girls such as Miss Y. Once this material came forth in free association in analysis, she made remarkably fast strides in her adjustments.

She concluded her account with the statement that she was confident that the writer and Miss Y, in some unusual way, had made it possible for her to recognize her problem and to free her of the repressions. Beyond this statement she could explain no further. She asked if any explanation could be given to her.

She was hypnotized and asked if she still wanted an explanation of her conscious belief. She confirmed her desire. Accordingly, she was instructed to remember all of the events of that Saturday-afternoon demonstration. She did so easily in chronological order, reporting her recovered memories readily until she reached the point at which she had been depersonalized and induced to assume the identity of Miss Y. Then she paused and, after much thinking, declared, "So you knew what my problem was all the time. And you made me become a feminine woman. And you made me enjoy it. And I did enjoy it. It was wonderful. I felt so good and so relaxed and so comfortable. And when you changed me back to myself and awakened me, I woke up so mad that I wanted to slap you. I was so glad when you told me I could leave because I was afraid I was going to slap you. I didn't know why. I couldn't sleep that night, and all day Sunday and Sunday night I was horribly depressed and angry. Monday afternoon at my hour session I was just mad at everything, nothing in particular. Then I happened to think of Miss Y, and that opened the floodgates. My analyst was so pleased that I had broken through the resistances. Now I can see that you recognized my problem, that you deliberately forced me into a position where, when I was Miss Y, I could think about myself as a stranger. I told you then I didn't like me, even though I didn't know it was me I was talking about. But I really saw me and it wasn't pleasant—all those repressed homosexual fears and conflicts."

"Then in that hour when I started to free associate, I really could do it! My analyst was so pleased, too. Any time you want to use me as a subject, you can, I owe you so much."

She has since married happily and is enjoying a career other than social service work, combining it with rearing a family. Subsequently she explained her reason to the writer for abandoning social service work, which was her realization that her original interest in such work was primarily a search indirectly for therapy and, at the same time, a denial to herself that she needed therapy.

44. Vasectomy: A Detailed Illustration of a Therapeutic Reorientation

Milton H. Erickson

A college graduate in her early thirties, with three children, was married to a professional man. She sought psychotherapy because of what her husband described as "sexual obsessions" that had come to dominate their daily life during the past two years. These centered around an insatiable curiosity about the love affairs of people she knew and those she read about in the newspapers. The husband could not understand her "incessant talk" on the subject, since they were well-adjusted and active sexually. Nor did she have any doubts about his fidelity, since he had confessed his premarital experiences and had had no desire for extramarital experiences since marriage. Neither did she have any suspicions regarding him. However, she was convinced, and this was confirmed by her husband, that several permissive women had undue interest in him. One of them had actually suggested a liaison, should he be interested.

In discussing their sexual adjustments both husband and wife disclaimed any disharmony. After the birth of the third child they agreed on vasectomy as the most convenient method of birth control. The operation had been done four years previously when the youngest child was five years old. There had never been any feelings of regret experienced so far as either knew. They were entirely satisfied by the size of their family and relieved by no further concern about precautions for birth control.

The first part of therapy for Mrs. A was devoted to her explanation of her curiosity. Newspaper stories, neighborhood gossip, and general speculations constituted her communications. Next she began offering an extensive, well-organized, elaborate discourse upon the significance of sexuality in adult daily marital and family life in establishing emotional bonds and a sense of personal fulfillment. After several hours of this she declared that obviously she was making no progress and that she had decided that there was much in her unconscious that she was repressing and concealing by an avid interest in external matters. Therefore, she felt that hypnosis should be employed and that her unconscious should be encouraged to give free rein to expression.

Unpublished manuscript, circa 1950s.

THERAPEUTIC TRANCE AND POSTHYPNOTIC SUGGESTION

She proved to be a fair subject and readily accepted posthypnotic suggestions that she talk freely and without attempting to give orderly ideas. Upon awakening, she announced a full recollection of what had been said to her in the trance, declaring that she would not act as had been suggested. Instead, she had decided to speculate freely upon how a woman would think, feel, and act in considering how to establish a liaison.* She then described various men she knew, speculated upon their attributes, general attractiveness, sexual prowess, capacity to establish emotional relationships, possible attitudes toward liaisons, and numerous other considerations. Next were considered places, times, physical settings, social settings, and the general atmosphere in which a liaison could be culminated.

This was followed by an extensive consideration of the emotional effects and results of a single extramarital experience and the results of a continued affair. She discussed well and comprehensively the effect of liaisons upon the individual lives of the participants, their family relationships if they were married, their individual emotional lives, the influence of past training and conditioning, and the immediate and subsequent developments. This was followed by a consideration of guilt feelings, their impingement upon the individual aspects of life, upon the liaison itself, and the separate family lives.

Thereupon she began discussing in detail how she would react in establishing a liaison, how active and how passive a part she would take, and what she felt would be the ultimate outcome. Her conclusion was that she was certain she could adjust happily either to one single sexual experience with a highly desirable, respectable man, or to a discreetly conducted affair of at least a year's duration with a similar man. Usually an hour or two, sometimes more, was necessary to complete her discussion of these various topics. During them she was remarkably objective and serious in all of her remarks.

The next development was her declaration that she had only been "stalling for time without knowing it." She explained that all of the previous discussion had been but a slow introduction to the really important things she had to say. Thereupon she lapsed into a troubled

---

*Editor's Note: The reader should recognize that a statement about not carrying out a posthypnotic suggestion is frequently followed by actually carrying it out in a rationalized or semidisguised form. The patient can thus resist and yield at the same time: She can have her cake and eat it too.

silence, after explaining that she knew what her trouble was but did not have the courage to state it. The next hour was also spent in silent emotional distress.

At the next appointment she began with the assertion that she might as well begin to disclose her problem, which she had not previously recognized until she had remarked about "stalling for time." She then asked permission to speak frankly and freely. When this was granted, a torrent of words poured forth in the language of the street. In essence she declared that she was an adult woman, a married woman, a woman who had borne children, that she was a sexualized female, and that, as a healthy normal living creature, she was entitled to have her biological needs and hungers completely satisfied. Therefore, as a living healthy normal female, with healthy normal appetites, she was entitled to be satisfied by a male who was completely a male and not one who was "expurgated" or "bowdlerized." He did not have to have two legs or even one, nor two arms, nor even two testicles. All that he had to have was enough penis and testicular tissue to be able to ejaculate semen—live, potent semen—upon or in her genitals. Thus, and only thus, could she have the biological satisfaction of being a sexualized female. She did not want more children, she had no desire to become pregnant, but when she had intercourse, she wanted to have it with a man capable of impregnating a female and not capable of only simulating such an act. In fact, she had never objected to contraceptives because the capacity to impregnate existed, and therefore a biological potency existed.

She had not realized that a vasectomy would constitute so serious a deprivation for her. In fact, she had not even been aware of such a possibility. She had first looked upon vasectomy as a simple solution to a minor nuisance, but after a year a growing unrest and dissatisfaction had developed. She had met this by increased sexual activity and ardor, to her husband's great satisfaction and the seeming happiness of their sexual adjustments. As her vague unrest developed, she had first reacted by dropping some old friends and replacing them with new acquaintances. As she looked back, she realized that the rejected friends were either unmarried or childless couples and the replacements were couples with children. Additionally, she had developed a predilection for people who were grandparents, particularly those whose sons had borne children, thereby signifying a continuance of masculine biological potency.

Also, as she reviewed the men she had considered as possible lovers, every one, whether married or divorced, had fathered children. The only single man in the list had been involved in a bastardy case. In her obsessional interest in love affairs, rumored or published in the news, the only ones that had interested her were those of men, married or divorced, who had fathered children. She went on to declare, in direct Anglo-Saxon terms, that the essence of her problem was a compelling desire, once more, to have sex relations with a biologically complete man, even at the risk of an illegitimate pregnancy. This last assertion was taken as a point of departure in summarizing her problem for her. Accordingly, the following discussion was offered:

1. What she wanted was an emotional experience, an emotional satisfaction, a satisfaction related entirely to her inner needs.
2. The question of risks involved, of times, places, physical setting, social atmosphere, etc., were all unimportant, since the problem was one of her emotional satisfaction.
3. The man himself would be no more than an instrument, that it was not a part of her need to establish an emotional bond, such as marriage and a home, that all she desired was her own response to a specific stimulation that could effect a satisfaction of her emotional needs.
4. Therefore, her problem did not center around the giving of sexual satisfaction, but the gaining of complete sexual satisfaction at an emotional level in relationship to a man.
5. Hence, it would not be necessary for the man to do anything or to provide anything actually material to her sense of complete sexual satisfaction other than to be a potent male. His potency as a procreator would be the only important consideration.

The patient was most attentive to these ideas, and care was taken to prevent her from analyzing them too closely. The suggestion was offered that they ought to be presented in detail to her unconscious mind to permit an even more adequate understanding of them. She agreed and developed a definitely better trance than before and listened attentively to the discussion offered her a second time of the above ideas. Thereupon the suggestion was offered that her needs could be met in a remarkably adequate fashion and in a manner that would please and intrigue her without emotional repercussions of any sort. She was urged to accept this idea of this possibility, even though she did not know exactly what was meant. She asserted that she would do whatever was asked.

POSTHYPNOTIC SUGGESTIONS FOR THERAPEUTIC DREAMS AND FANTASY

The explanation was then offered that that night she was to sleep most soundly and, during her sleep, she was to dream vividly of the past. This dream was to center around a period of time just previous to the conception of any one of her children (they were all "planned children").

The dream was to be most vivid and active, and it could be as erotic as she wished. Upon awakening the next morning, she could, if she wished, remember the dream. On the second, third, and subsequent nights she would continue to have similar and even more vivid dreams.

At her next appointment she reported that her dreams had been as suggested and that in them she had relived previous satisfying experiences with her husband. As a result of her dreams her sexual appetite had increased greatly, but nevertheless she still had her compelling drive. A new series of posthypnotic suggestions was given her. This time, in addition to her nocturnal dreams, she would, upon awakening, recall them and engage in a fantasy about them. Thus, she would suddenly discover, during the fantasy, that sexual excitement was developing, culminating spontaneously in an intense orgasm.

When seen four days later, she related this new development. Her first fantasy had been a recollection of her courtship days. She had been suddenly overwhelmed with excitement and embarrassment upon recalling a specific instance in which the question of premarital sex relations had been discussed, and she had reacted by experiencing a violent orgasm.

The next morning, while recalling her dream, she chanced to see her husband's photograph on her dresser. This had been taken just shortly before the conception of the second child. Upon looking at it she developed sexual excitement, which culminated in an orgasm. Later that day she had taken out an old photo album to look over her collection of snapshots of her courtship days. In so doing, she came across the picture of a former admirer, now married and the father of several children. To her amazement she became sexually excited and had an orgasm. This had astonished her so much that she "did not know what to think," and she remained preoccupied and self-absorbed throughout the rest of the day.

That night, after satisfying sex relations with her husband, she fell asleep comfortably and began a series of dreams. In each dream she saw, spoke to, or merely thought of various men, and as well as she could remember the dreams, she had in each instance experienced an orgasm. Then in the morning, when wide awake and reviewing her dream behavior, she had deliberately chosen to fantasize about one of the men she had previously named, and had been delighted to experience an orgasm as a result. That afternoon she picked up her husband at his office. While waiting for him, she had greeted his business associate, a married man with a large family, and had quietly and immediately had an orgasm. That evening she had insisted that she and her husband call on a married couple she admired greatly. While playing cards with the host as her partner, she had an orgasm.

Since then she had been thinking things over, and she felt that she now had no problem of any sort. She had, she explained, a feeling of inner conviction that she was truly a biological female, capable of responding adequately to any biologically competent male at any time she chose and in a way that met her needs adequately without creating problems. In the two years that have elapsed since the termination of therapy, she has been seen on occasion for advice concerning her children. As for her problem, it no longer troubles her. She feels free to have her own sexual response in her own way, but usually she resorts to a dream, almost invariably about her husband and in relationship to the time of planning for a pregnancy.

VIII. Self-Exploration in the Hypnotic State: Facilitating Unconscious Processes and Objective Thinking

The papers of this section all illustrate the facilitation and utilization of the patient's own inner resources for solving personal problems. In a number of these illustrations, Erickson did not even know the nature of the problem that the patients solved within the privacy of their own trance experience. In some cases it is evident that even the patient does not consciously understand the entire nature of the problem, or exactly how it was solved. It always delights Erickson when the patient has a trance experience that leads to the resolution of a problem on a more-or-less unconscious level. This approach to problem-solving that takes place on an unconscious or preverbal level may involve right-hemispheric processes that are not always available to the self-reflective understanding of the left hemisphere (Rossi, 1977; Watzlawick, 1978).

The apparent reversal of this process of unconscious problem-solving occurs when Erickson utilizes therapeutic trance to facilitate "objective thinking"; that is, a concentrated period of thinking about a problem without any interference from emotional sources (see Chapter Eight, Emotional Coping, in Erickson & Rossi, 1979). This process of "objective thinking" usually involves a hypnotic dissociation between the process of experiencing and an observational modality that watches the process of experiencing. The therapeutic relationship between experiencing and observing is discussed in the following dialogue that took place in the early 1970s, when Erickson and the editor first met.

E: When you are aware of hypnotic dissociation and know how to use it, you can then take up other physical problems of the patient: The patient who has the pain of cancer, the patient who has sexual problems, the patient who is afraid of intercourse or being kissed. You can watch how that person might behave if he were to be kissed by some appropriate person. The patient can take his eyes away [be an

393

objective observer watching himself] and watch those lips being kissed by a father or mother or brother or sister or cousin or aunt, grandma or grandpa. You can ask a woman who complains of frigidity to watch for the possible responses of her body to intercourse and discover that perhaps there might be a nice feeling. A pregnant woman who fears delivery can be induced to watch it [in her own mind].

R: To *watch* it but not *experience* it.

E: Just *watch* it! She can watch the growth of the pregnancy. She can speculate about her abdominal size and the process of childbirth and remain free and unconcerned because it's interesting to watch.

R: So you emphasize the observer modality to help a person get through whatever is bothering him or her. What does that do, putting the patient into the observer modality?

E: It removes the questionable aspects of the experience from the patient's awareness. It allows him to objectify that thing, and then he can be curious about it as an objective phenomenon.

R: You arouse the patient's curiosity now.

E: Because now the feared experience is only an objective thing.

R: Before, the person's sense of distaste was warding off the experience.

E: Yes, because of subjective values. *What you're doing is taking something which is a personal experience and rendering it into an objective matter.* The patient can now be free to observe the objective.

R: He is now free from his former biases of distaste.

E: All the subjective fears and biases.

R: That freedom from former biases later helps him get into the subjective experience with a more desirable frame of reference?

E: Yes, when the body of a woman can be rendered an object to be viewed undergoing an experience, then an appraisal can be made by that woman, apart from any fearful associations to the experience. You remove the subjective and let the objective work.

R: Yes, I describe this process of interaction between the objective and experiential levels in my book *Dreams and the Growth of Personality* [Rossi, 1972a; see also Rossi, 1972b]. This is why I originally became so interested in your work. You described, from the perspective of your work in hypnosis, exactly what I thought I had discovered as a healing process in dreams. When I wrote my book, I was not aware that anyone else was systematically utilizing the observer modality as it interacts with the experiential as a form of psychotherapy. All my work to date has led up to exactly this point you are now discussing: How can we utilize these two modalities in order to facilitate the process of psychotherapy? In traditional Jungian analysis the observer modality is emphasized, I believe, at the expense of the experiential. In Gestalt therapy, on the other hand, it appears as if the "here and now" experience is emphasized at the expense of the observer modality and the value of its perspective.

In dreams, however, I found that the observer and experiential modalities interacted spontaneously and naturally to effect personality growth and behavioral change in a manner that was, to some extent, unrestricted by the programming and learned biases of the conscious mind. In your hypnotherapeutic work, I now find a systematic use of this interaction between the observer and experiential modalities that appears similar to the naturally occurring process of change and growth which I observed in the dreams of my patients.

E: I have found it an extremely valuable approach.

R: Some hypnotherapists try to effect cure by having the patient *reexperience* a trauma or problem. But you do something different. You have the patient just watch objectively and dispassionately from a perspective outside of the original emotional experience. Other therapists say that the problem of neurosis is that the person is just an observer in life; cure is effected by having people experience. So they try to plunge their patients into experience and experiencing.

E: But that's just what a lot of people are trying to avoid.

R: That's right! The patient became an observer to escape unpleasant aspects of experience that he is either unwilling or unable to face on an emotional level. But sometimes the patient gets stuck in the observer modality and feels himself increasingly estranged and separated from life's experience. (In the extreme, this can result in psychosis.) The patient is in this dilemma because he jumped to the observer modality as the first step in solving an experiential problem. But once he removed himself to the observer level he either forgot, or lost his courage, to deal with his essential task: To use his observations toward solving an emotional problem.

E: [Dr. Erickson draws the analogy of first testing the temperature of a pool with a toe before plunging in.] Having tested the water temperature, the person is now going to experience it in a much more complete way.

R: Yes, since the individual has gotten through his fears and blocks by utilizing the observer modality, he can effectively test and predict parameters for a safe experience. Maybe that's why the observer modality evolved in nature: It had survival value for the extraordinarily complex and sensitive entity that is man [Rossi, 1972b].

This is a regular therapeutic technique you use. You put a person in the observer modality while in the trance state, have him observe whatever is traumatic or distasteful, and then when he comes out of the trance, he is more likely to resolve the observed experience in a subjective and satisfactory manner.

E: The patient knows it now. He has observed it, he has it. You can also
   have a patient hallucinate a protective shield or an opaque cloth, and
   you can have that shield or cloth get thinner and thinner and more and
   more transparent in order to view the area of anxiety. You can stop the
   transparency at any stage you choose. You have such a total freedom
   for exploring and solving problems when you put the patient in the
   observer modality.

45. Pseudo-Orientation in Time as a Hypnotherapeutic Procedure

Milton H. Erickson

In every attempt at psychotherapy there is always the need to utilize the common experiences and understandings that permeate the pattern of daily living, and to adapt such utilization to the unique needs of the individual patient. Hence, to a significant degree psychotherapy must necessarily be experimental in character, since there can be no foreknowledge of the procedures exactly applicable to any one patient. Furthermore, the entire field of psychotherapy, in itself, is still in the course of early development, thereby enhancing the need for continued experimental studies.

For these reasons the following case histories are reported to illustrate an experimental therapeutic technique employed by this writer from time to time for the past 15 years. This technique was formulated by a utilization of those common experiences and understandings embraced in the general appreciation that practice leads to perfection, that action once initiated tends to continue, and that deeds are the offspring of hope and expectancy. These ideas are utilized to create a therapy situation in which the patient could respond effectively psychologically to desired therapeutic goals as actualities already achieved.

This was done by employing hypnosis and using, conversely to age regression, a technique of orientation into the future, or "time projection." Thus, the patient was enabled to achieve a detached, dissociated, objective, and yet subjective view of what he believed at the moment he had already accomplished, without awareness that those accomplishments were the expression in fantasy of his hopes and desires.

PATIENT A

The first of these case histories is that of a 30-year-old divorced man who held a minor clerical position, lived in a wretched rooming-house, and had no friends of either sex. He did no reading, did not attend church or the theater, ate all his meals in one cheap restaurant, and limited his recreation to aimless driving about the countryside.

For three years he had been under the care of a general medical man because of innumerable somatic complaints involving all parts of his body. At one time he had been hospitalized as a possible candidate for abdominal surgery. He had reacted traumatically to his admission to the surgical ward by developing extreme terror, sobbing, screaming, and complaining of agonizing abdominal pain. An exploratory laparotomy disclosed no pathological condition, but a routine appendectomy was performed. His convalescence was prolonged for a month and marked by even more complaints than he had expressed previously. Additionally, he was periodically depressed, cried a great deal, and was most reluctant to leave the hospital. The operation and his related behavior convinced him that he was a "coward," that he was "no good," "worthless" and "incapable of being a man."

Thereafter he had functioned at an even lower level personally and economically. He visited his physician two to four times a week, plaintively seeking help for his weakness, backache, headaches, gastric pains, etc. Efforts to refer him to psychiatrists proved futile. They "did not understand" him. In turn, the psychiatrists variously reported him as a "character defect," an "inadequate personality," a "profound hypochondriac," and a "psychopathic personality of the constitutional inferior type." All agreed that he was not amenable to therapy. However, the writer's clinical impression was much more favorable.

Approximately 18 months after his laparotomy, he was referred to the writer for hypnotherapy, and the extensive case history which his physician had taken was made available.

Rapport was easily established with the patient. He was pitifully eager to be hypnotized, and he proved to be a remarkably fine subject. For a month he was seen weekly for a three- to four-hour session. During this time all efforts were devoted to training him to develop readily every hypnotic phenomenon of which he was capable. For all of these sessions a profound amnesia was induced. No therapy was attempted other than establishment of good rapport and a general feeling of trust and confidence.

The next two sessions were spent having him hallucinate a whole series of crystal balls.* In them he was induced to see a great array of the outstanding emotional and traumatic experiences of his life. These hallucinated portrayals were "fixed"—that is, he could look from one scene to another and back again without having to rehallucinate. Thus, he

---

*The idea of crystal balls lends itself readily to popular understanding, and hallucinated crystal balls are convenient, easily manipulated, and remarkably economical.

could see himself depicted in various situations and at different times in his life. Thereby he could observe his behavior and reactions, make comparisons and contrasts, and note the thread of continuity in his reaction patterns from one age level to the next.

A most extensive and elaborate series of events was thus viewed by the patient. His reaction to the total experience was one of hopeless resignation, "Anybody that has had all that happen to him ain't got much chance." Even after being awakened with an amnesia for each session, his mood was one of discouragement and general depression.

The next session was spent by having him discuss in the waking state all the things he wished for himself, the hopes he had, and all the ideas he had of what might be possible for him. This session was not satisfactory since much of the time was spent emphasizing his complaints as insuperable barriers to anything he could want. At the close of the session he was most discouraged.

At the next session he was hypnotized deeply and instructed to repeat the task of the preceding session. His wistful, plaintive hopes for the future can be summarized as follows:

1. The enjoyment of "just fair" physical health.
2. An economic adjustment "about average."
3. Personal adjustment sufficient so that he could "get along" in relation to recreation, personal habits, social activities, and personal interests and friendships.
4. "Not too much" fear, anxiety, and feelings of compulsion.
5. "Enough guts to be a man" if he ever had to have an operation, or, if he had to defend his rights, "to take a licking like a man."
6. A desire to be able to "take in my stride a little better" all the bad things that had happened to him or might happen in the future.
7. A wish that he could achieve "maybe enough" emotional maturity so that he could marry for love and not "because someone pitied me."

He was awakened with an amnesia and departed in a general depressed mood.

In the two preceding sessions, as in the previous sessions, no effort was made to do more than to elicit his responses. At the next session, with the patient in the waking state, a vague general discussion was elaborately offered of what he could expect in the future. This, it was explained, *would be the opportunity to look back over the past, to review his complaints and difficulties, and to recall the developments of therapy. Then, most importantly, he could examine all those accomplishments, resulting from therapy, that represented his achievement of those things signifying normal adjustments. However, this latter could be done only after a lapse of time, probably several months, following the termination of therapy.*

He was then hypnotized deeply, and the same discussion was repeated in similar general terms. Still in the deep somnambulistic trance, he was then disoriented for time and then oriented or projected in time * to some future date.†

The projection into the future that this patient achieved was approximately five months, and the setting was an office visit. The purpose of his visit—since, for him, enough time had elapsed since terminating therapy—was to give an account of what had really happened since then.

The suggestion was offered, to which he readily assented, that he might like to begin with a brief but comprehensive review of the past as depicted in crystal-ball scenes. Some 10 minutes were spent by the patient in this hallucinatory review. During it his emotional manifestations were those of sympathetic interest rather than the intense fear, anxiety, and concern he had frequently shown in previous similar situations.

Then the suggestion was made that he might be aided in giving his report on the therapeutic developments he had achieved by visualizing the significant incidents in another series of crystal balls. Thus, he could enjoy watching the progressive unfolding of each event as it had occurred.

He agreed enthusiastically, and as he viewed the various hallucinatory scenes in the crystal balls, his enthusiasm and pleasure increased. Frequently he would either comment excitedly or demand that the writer observe what was happening.

Some of the reports he gave may be summarized briefly as follows:

---

* Essentially, this is a simple though detailed technique of suggestions by which the deeply hypnotized subject is reminded of the current date; told that the seconds, minutes, and hours are passing; that tomorrow is approaching, is here, and now is yesterday; and that as the days pass, this week will soon be over and then all too soon next month will be this month. Particular attention must be given, in using this technique, to be most accurate in verbalizing the transition from the future to the present to the past, and to do it easily and gradually without rushing the subject.

† The date for the patient, as a consequence of preceding waking and trance discussions, would necessarily be several months in the future. Such future dates are best selected by the subject, since the hypnotist might choose one inauspicious for the situation. Also, the selected period of time should not be too exactly defined. For example, if an actual future date, such as the next birthday, is desired, the orientation should be to "some days before your next birthday." Then it becomes a simple matter to let the subject define the date progressively more exactly. When the actual future date is unknown, having the subject glance out of the window and describe what he sees may indirectly reveal the time of day, the season of the year, and the location. Thus, one subject described the noonday Christmas shopping rush in a distant city.

1. I'm walking down the street. I'm turning. I'm going to see Dr. X (his physician). No, I'm walking past. I'm thinking, "Thank God, I don't have to go there again."
2. I'm swimming and—watch me, I'm going to do a high dive.
3. Look, I'm asking the boss for a raise. He's going to give it to me. Damn it, I couldn't hear how much. I don't understand that. (His attention was hastily distracted.*)
4. My goodness! Did you see that? That was that great big lug who always parked his car just to be mean so I couldn't get my car out until he came out half an hour later. Now I'm telling him off and thinking what a sap I was to keep parking my car where he could pull that dirty trick.
5. I'm in the theater. (He was asked what the picture was.) Who's looking at the picture? I'm necking my girl.
6. That's a different girl and I'm taking her to the art gallery and then we are going out to dinner. She's pretty.
7. I'm giving a speech to a group of men. I wonder which one that is because I gave another speech, too, but I can't see plainly.
8. My car has been painted and I got a new suit. Looks good. I even wear it to work.

He was unwilling to discontinue his crystal-gazing, expressing much pleasure in his accomplishments and a desire to describe more of them.

However, he was reoriented to the current time and given extensive posthypnotic instructions to have a complete amnesia for every possible thing that might have occurred during the session. Additionally, he was to make no response of any kind to any of the things that might have happened during the session except a full obedience to the instructions just given.

He took his departure, complaining of extreme fatigue.

He was seen the next day, and the same routine was employed. He was carefully oriented about seven months in the future, and he made a similar initial response to this projection in time.

He was addressed as follows:

> As I remember, I saw you last about two months ago. You came in to report upon your progress. I put you in a trance and had you visualize yourself in crystal balls so that you could give me full accounts.
>
> Now, suppose you remember tonight all the things you said and

---

*Constant alertness must be exercised to prevent any undue thinking that might break down the established psychological orientation.

saw that night about two months ago. Never mind anything I saw or did; remember only the things you said and saw and did while you were giving me the report. [This was to prevent him from recalling anything about preliminary or subsequent hypnotic instructions, particularly in relation to time projection.]

Now review all those things. Some of them go way back to our first meeting and even way back to the beginning of the problem you brought to me. Think them over carefully, clearly, extensively, and then discuss things for me.

The essential content of his discussion follows:

> I was really a sorry mess when I met you. A whining crybaby. I don't see how you could have stood me. Dr. X deserves a gold medal for what he put up with. It embarrasses me to think about it.
>
> I don't really know what happened. It was like a dream, but it wasn't a dream. Whatever you said to be became true. I was a little boy, I was older, I was still older, sometimes all at the same time. Some way you made me live my life all over so I could see it. I really lived it, too.
>
> Then you made me see it in moving pictures in crystal balls. I was in the crystal balls. And I was outside watching. Some of the things I saw were pretty darn sad. But I was a sad sack myself.
>
> But the thing I really liked but didn't have any hope about was when you made me tell you all the things I wanted to do. Then somehow I began doing those things. I can't understand that because I must have been in this room and I wasn't. [He was immediately interrupted, and extensive hypnotic instructions were given that he report only on what he himself saw and did and that he was not to try to understand the situation.]
>
> Well, I did every one of those things. Surprised myself! Boy, I really felt good about it. I enjoyed doing them. I sure was surprised when I asked that waitress for a date. She's a nice girl. And that raise was $10.00. And when I told off that lug about blocking me in with his car, he took it like a man. And I felt like one! I've got to look up Dr. X some day because he was really interested in me. I guess he believed in me, even if he didn't help me.

He continued to review extensively, with confidence, assurance, and pleasure, a further wealth of fantasied accomplishments, all in keeping with a suitable reality situation for him. They all had, apparently, the significance of absolute realities for him.

When he had apparently finished, he was told that he was to be hypnotized. By this approach it became possible to reorient him to current time. Again, as in the previous session, he was given extensive posthypnotic suggestions to induce a comprehensive amnesia for trance events of all sorts.

Still in the trance state, he was instructed ambiguously that his next appointment was possibly for next week but that it might or might not be kept; that various events would develop which would determine both the time and the manner in which he would keep the appointment. However, he would certainly be seen again, if not next week, quite possibly in two months' time.

He was awakened with posthypnotic instructions for amnesia and dismissed with no mention of a future appointment. He appeared exhausted and self-absorbed.

He was not seen until eight weeks later. He arrived in a new suit, and his car was newly painted and had new seat covers. An attractive young girl, a secretary, accompanied him. His opening statement was that he felt that he would like to give the writer an account of the recent events that had occurred. His report may be summarized as follows:

> For about a week after the last session he had felt confused and bewildered, but at the same time he had a "feeling" that "something good was happening" to him. Then one day he had wondered about his next appointment while at work, but before he could clarify his thinking, he had impulsively asked his employer for a salary increase. Not only had this been granted, but he had been transferred to another and better position. This had given him a tremendous feeling of elation and self-confidence.
>
> Upon leaving work that night, instead of waiting in his car and raging helplessly, because he was boxed in, he hailed the man and invited him to have a beer. During the drinking he had told the man in a simple, matter-of-fact tone of voice, "I think you have been blocking my car regularly because I've been such a damn sissy. From now on, you damn bastard, cut it out and have another beer on me." This had ended that petty persecution.
>
> Much elated by this, he dined at a different restaurant that night, fell into conversation with a waitress, and asked her for a date. She refused but, unperturbed, he went to the theater alone.
>
> Subsequently he had moved to another and better residential section. In the process of moving, he "went through all the trash I've been saving for years. I threw out all the junk, I really cleaned house."
>
> He had joined a Young Businessmen's Club and had maneu-

vered himself into a position on the weekly program. He felt that he had acquitted himself creditably.

From then on, "I began living a normal respectable life and enjoying things like an average man. I just suddenly got out of all my bad habits and feelings. It was easy once I got started. I just never tried that before. But one thing just naturally led to another and instead of feeling bad like I used to, I just get out and do something I ought to.

I met my girl at a dance, and we're going steady. But we are going to wait awhile to see if we're really interested.

My health is good. I don't pay attention to every little ache or pain the way I used to. You got to put up with a cold or something like that instead of getting scared to death. Some day I'm going to see Dr. X and let him see me the way I really am. He was a good scout with me."

After still further discussion, during which no effort was made by him to inquire into what had occurred in relation to the writer, he departed.

He was seen casually from time to time thereafter in a social way. Two years later he was still adjusting satisfactorily, and he and the secretary were completing their plans for marriage.

PATIENT B

This case history concerns a long-continued, highly circumscribed form of compulsive behavior.

The patient's mother had died when he was 12 years old. His father insisted that the son visit the mother's grave and place flowers on it every Saturday, Sunday, and holiday regardless of anything except absolute physical incapacitation. On several occasions the boy had played truant and had been brutally beaten by the father, who had reacted to the mother's death by becoming a severe alcoholic.

When the patient reached the age of 15, the father, first giving the boy a most brutal beating to make him remember to visit the grave, had deserted him. For a year the boy had lived in the home of a distant, unfriendly relative before striking out on his own.

For 15 years, summer or winter, rain, shine, or snow, he made his pilgrimages to the grave, sometimes having to make regularly a round trip of 20 to 40 miles. Even during his courtship he regularly took his fiancee on the Sunday pilgrimage.

During the years physical illness had confined him to bed on several occasions and made him miss his regular trips. He had reacted by making extra visits during the week. The result had been a compulsion to make a daily trip. At the time of seeking therapy he was making a daily round-trip of 20 miles.

He had attempted to break the compulsion by placing bouquets of dandelions or wild chicory blooms from the roadside on the grave, even limiting the offering to a single bloom and then to none at all. However, the compulsion proved to be that of a visit only. Then he tried to break it by merely driving past the cemetery and hurrying home. A dozen such attempts had caused him such extreme anxiety, insomnia, panic, gastric symptoms, and diarrhea that each time he had been forced to make a midnight trip to fulfill his "obligation."

His reason for seeking therapy was that he had recently been offered a most advantageous position in a distant city and the deadline for his acceptance was approaching. While both he and his wife were most eager to make the change, the thought of being unable to make the daily trip to the grave caused him to suffer intense panics.

Because time was short and his problem was circumscribed in character, intensive hypnotherapy was employed. He proved to be an excellent somnambulistic subject and was easily taught to manifest hypnotic phenomena.

In a deep trance he was asked to review his innumerable pilgrimages, his memories of his mother, and the nature and character of his feelings, particularly his resentments, toward his father. He found this a most difficult task and possible only if he did it silently. Hence, this approach was abandoned.

Accordingly, he was disoriented for time and systematically oriented by projection into time *two weeks in the future*. Essentially, a technique comparable to that used for Patient A was employed. During the process of orienting him in the future, elaborate instruction was given to him to ensure a calm, comfortable feeling and to induce an overwhelming interest in whatever the writer might have to say.

As soon as the new orientation had been secured, a casual conversation was begun with him and carefully guided to the subject of his remarkably good muscular development, of which he was exceedingly proud. This led to an extolling of the patient's adherence to his principles in not smoking or drinking and of living a good, clean, industrious, hard-working life.

When these ideas had been built up sufficiently, he was challengingly asked, apparently in a spirit of camaraderie, if he had the strength to stand up like a man under a shock. He replied that he could "stand up under anything that any man could dish out." This led to the writer's declaration that he could easily "floor" the patient "with a good wallop." Entering readily into the spirit of the verbal exchange, the patient declared that the writer did not have "enough beef." After still further similar persiflage, he was warned, "Pick a spot on the floor to take a tumble, because I'm going to hit you hard and unexpectedly. Listen, here it comes. Now listen! You are a beautiful physical specimen, you live right, you work hard, you are a strong man, you are feeling good. Now here's the punch. Listen! *For two whole weeks you have not visited your mother's grave—not once for two whole weeks.* Are you alive, are you strong, or are you a weakling that I can lay out with my little finger?"

His startled response was, "Good God, how did I stop?"

Before he could elaborate that question, he was emphatically admonished that it was not the how, *but the fact that he had stopped that was of significance, and that he could now feel happy and relieved that it had been done.* Without pause the writer continued with a rapid, general discussion of all the problems involved in packing, moving, finding a new home, and getting settled. The patient was admonished emphatically to work out these matters to the last detail, since it was a problem that would require every possible bit of energy.

Very rapidly, then, he was reoriented to the current time and awakened with extensive posthypnotic suggestions for a continued amnesia of all trance events. He was given an appointment in two weeks' time and dismissed. (Since it was known that his grave visits were a sore topic at home and never mentioned, no special precautions had to be taken.)

He reported promptly for his next interview and was cheerful and enthusiastic. He had accepted the new job; arrangements for moving were practically complete, and would be accomplished within the next week.

Special inquiry had been made secretly of his wife, who reported that, while he had worked regularly, he had been home each night approximately an hour earlier. Also, he had worked busily at packing the full day both Sundays as well as during all spare time during the two weeks.

Accordingly, his enthusiastic account of his new preparations was suddenly interrupted by the inquiry, "How does it feel to be happy, content, enthusiastic, and really interested in the new job and *free from having to visit your mother's grave?*"

In startled amazement he declared, "Good God, I haven't done that for two weeks. I've been so busy."

Immediately, by means of a posthypnotic cue to which he had been trained to respond, a deep trance was induced.

As if there had been no alteration in his level of awareness, the writer replied, "Yes, now that you are asleep, you now know that you were too busy. More than that, *you know now by actual experience that you don't need to visit the grave anymore.* But, of course, if a legitimate occasion ever arises, you can do so in a normal way. Thus, on Mother's Day you could, or some such occasion."

After some silent thought he asked, "Is my father alive?" Reply was made, "Neither you nor I know if he is dead and gone; we know only that he is gone and that you are a man."

Return was made to the question of the new job, and after some further discussion he was awakened. At once he returned to the moment preceding the posthypnotic cue by remarking, "Two whole weeks! I don't understand it, but it's sure O.K. with me. Maybe taking that new job did something for me."*

Return was at once made to discussion of the new position, and shortly he was dismissed.

In the 10 years that have followed only on those rare occasions when he visited the hometown would he visit the grave, and then only if it were convenient. Also, there have been no other neurotic manifestations developed to replace the original compulsion.

PATIENT C

This next case history also concerns a circumscribed problem but of another type. Psychiatric help had been repeatedly sought and always rejected on the specious grounds that cooperation was impossible.

The patient was a 20-year-old student nurse. When she was less than a year old, her mother had secured a divorce, broken off all ties with everyone she knew, moved to another state, and had destroyed every possible evidence of the father that she could.

As the patient grew older and inquired about her father, the mother simply stated that she had divorced him, that she knew nothing about what had happened to him since then. Additionally, the mother firmly refused to give any description of him or even to reveal the location of her former home.

Upon reaching the age of 18, the patient made a determined effort to learn something about her father. The mother's marriage certificate and divorce decree were locked, she was informed, in a safety deposit box and would remain there. As for the patient's birth certificate, it disclosed only that she had been born in Chicago. Her mother explained that her birth had been unexpectedly early and had occurred while she and the father were visiting some of the father's relatives in Chicago. As for the mother's maiden name, that, like the father's surname, was utterly commonplace and there would be no possible way of tracing identities.

Thoroughly frustrated by this, the patient had sought out psychiatrists who used hypnosis. She would demand that they hypnotize her and thereby compel her to remember something about her father. However, she would immediately establish an impasse by declaring that such a procedure would be ridiculous, since she had no memories of him. Hence,

---

*Therapeutically there was no reason for the patient to think otherwise. In final analysis the outcome did derive from the opportunity for a new job.

all that would be secured would be her "imaginations" and she did not want to have them passed off as genuine. She invariably refused to cooperate and at no time was she ever hypnotized.

When she came to the writer with the above story, her request was refused on the grounds that a search for memories before the age of one would be futile. (Actually, of course, she represented an interesting problem if her cooperation could be secured by a judicious use of negativism on the writer's part.) She was reassured by this refusal of her request, but before the interview was terminated, she had become interested in hypnosis simply as a personal experience.

Accordingly, arrangements were made to train her for "experimental work." She readily became an excellent hypnotic subject except for the one procedure of age regression. This she would not permit, and when indirect efforts were made, she invariably awakened to protest that "things seem to be going wrong."

Therefore, the measure of projecting her into the future was decided upon as a possible approach to her problem.

Consequently, while she was in a profound somnambulistic state, an "experiment" was outlined for which she was to do some learning tasks. Then, it was explained, she was to be projected into the future, and she would report upon that learning. Thus, the nature and character of her forgetting could be studied. However, as a "preliminary" bit of training she would first be projected in time and induced to have fantasies of activities during the period of time between the current date and the future date.

Following these explanations (actually disguised instructions for her guidance), she was disoriented and then oriented to the future. No effort was made to ascertain the approximate date, but various remarks permitted the deduction that the time projection was about two months.

She was asked to give a full account of that "remarkably interesting patient" she had cared for since that "last interview with me quite a few weeks ago." She executed this fantasy and several others of a comparable character. During the narration of them mention was made repeatedly that she had probably forgotten a lot of the details, to which statement she was induced to agree.

She was then reminded that "quite a long while ago" arrangements had been made to study her rate of forgetting and that the time had now come. Speaking rapidly to ensure her full attention and to preclude her analyzing the statements made, she was told:

1. I am positive you have forgotten completely a task I had you do a while back.
2. I want you to work on the full assumption that you did it, even though you can't remember doing it.

3. I want you to recover as systematically as you can the memories of what you did.
4. It was an unexpected task for which you could make no plans to remember. Hence, you forgot it.
5. This task was done between the time of the last interview you remember and this present moment. (Projected time.)

The task was then described to her as regressing in age and recovering a variety of memories about her father, all of which she had now forgotten.

The proposal was offered that she now try to recall what she might have discovered in that age regression by whatever means she chose, crystal-gazing, automatic writing, flashes of memory, or any other means she wished.

She hesitatingly suggested crystal-gazing. Immediately the suggestion was offered that in a series of crystal balls she would see herself at descending age levels until she saw herself as an infant-in-arms. (As for Patient A, these crystal balls were "fixed.") She was to study these portrayals carefully, until she felt certain that she had "rediscovered" the forgotten memories.

For half an hour she sat silently, absorbed in this task. Finally she turned to the writer and indicated that she was through. Instructing her to keep the memories and to report them in any way she wished, the crystal balls were removed by suggestion. (The reason for this was to prevent her from developing tangential interests by observing again the crystal balls.)

She was asked what she thought about the experience. Her reply was the startling request that the writer examine the back of her right knee.

That examination revealed an old, small, jagged scar. Told about this, she explained, "I saw myself as a little girl. I was six years old. I was playing. I was running backward. I tripped over the root of a tree. My leg hurt. I got up crying. Then a lot of blood ran down my leg. I was scared. Then the crystal ball disappeared."

After some moments of silent thought, she continued, "I'm all mixed up. I think different ways about time. I don't like it. I think you better straighten my mind out and tell me to remember everything. I think I'm in a mixed-up trance. Wake me up."

She was reoriented and awakened with instructions for full recollection of memories.

Soberly she began, "I saw me fall. I've got the scar. You found it. I don't remember it. I just saw it in the crystal ball. Maybe the other things are true, too."

"First I'll tell you and then I'll tell my mother. Then I'll know. This is what I saw: I could say 'Daddy.' My father was holding me. He seemed to be awful tall. He was smiling. He had a funny looking tooth, a front tooth.

His eyes were blue. His hair was curly. And it looked yellowish. Now I'm going home and tell my mother."

The next day she reported, "They were real memories. It shocked Mother. When I got home, I told her, 'I've found out what my father looked like. He was tall, blue-eyed (she and her mother were brown-eyed and five feet three inches tall), and curly-haired. It was almost yellow and he had a gold front tooth.' Mother was frightened. She wanted to know how I found him. So I told her about what we did. After awhile she said, 'Yes, your father was six feet tall, blue-eyed, yellowish-red curly hair, and he had a gold tooth. He left me when you were 11 months old. I'll tell you anything else you want to know now, and then let's not talk about it anymore. I know nothing about him at the present.'"

However, the patient's curiosity was satisfied. She was used subsequently for experimental work. Although she was given opportunities over a year's time to manifest further concern about her original problem, she seemed to have lost all interest in it.

PATIENT D

This case history centers around an impasse reached during therapy and the utilization of a fantasy about the future to secure an effective resumption of therapeutic progress.

The patient suffered from a profound anxiety neurosis with severe depressive and withdrawal reactions and marked dependency patterns. A great deal of hypnotherapy had been done and her early response was good. However, as therapy continued, she became increasingly negative and resistive.

Finally, the situation became one in which she limited herself, during the therapeutic hour, to an intellectual appraisal of her problems and her needs, while rigidly maintaining the status quo at all other times.

A few examples will suffice to illustrate her behavior. For cogent reasons she could not tolerate her parental home situation, but she persisted in remaining in it despite actual difficulties and in the face of favorable opportunities to leave. She resented her employment situation bitterly, but she refused to accept a promotion actually available. She recognized fully her need for social activities, but she avoided, often with difficulty, all opportunities. She discussed at length her interest in reading and the long hours she spent in her room futilely wishing for something to read, but she refused to enter the library she passed twice daily, despite numerous promises to herself.

Additionally, she became increasingly demanding that the writer must, perforce, take definitive action to compel her to do those things she recognized as necessary and proper but which she could not bring herself to do.

After many futile hours she finally centered her wishful thinking upon the idea that, if she could achieve even one of the desired things, she would then have the impetus and firmness of intention to achieve the others.

After she had emphasized and reemphasized this statement, it was accepted at face value.

She was then immediately hypnotized deeply and, in the somnambulistic state, instructed to see a whole series of crystal balls. In each of these would be depicted a significant experience in her life. These she was to study, making comparisons, drawing contrasts, and noting the continuity of various elements from one age level to another. Out of this study would slowly emerge a constellation of ideas which would be formulated without her awareness. This formulation would become manifest to her through another and larger crystal ball in which she would see herself depicted pleasantly, happily, and desirably in some future activity.

She spent approximately an hour absorbedly studying the various hallucinatory scenes, now and then glancing about the office as if looking for the other crystal ball. Finally she located it and thereupon gave all of her attention to it, describing the hallucinated scene to the writer with avid interest.

It was the depiction of a wedding scene, that of a lifelong family friend, which in actuality was not to take place for more than three months. She saw frequent "close-ups" of herself and of the others. She described the wedding ceremony, the reception, and the dance that followed. She was particularly interested in the dress her image was wearing but could only describe it as "beautiful." She watched the dancing, identified some of the men with whom she danced, and named the one who asked her for a date. Over and over she commented on how happy she looked, and what a contrast there was between her appearance now and her appearance at the wedding.

It was difficult to get her to cease watching the scene of the wedding party, since she was so interested in it and because she was so pleased by her behavior in it.

Finally, she was instructed to keep all that she had seen in her unconscious and to have a waking amnesia for the trance experiences. Furthermore, it was explained, it would constitute a tremendous motivating force by which all of her understandings could be utilized constructively. She was then awakened and dismissed with a posthypnotic suggestion for continuance of the amnesia.

There were only two more therapeutic interviews, and both of these were limited in scope by the patient. Each time she stated that she had nothing to say until she had been hypnotized. Once this was done, she stated both times that she wanted instructions to remember in her unconscious very clearly all that she had seen and thought and felt as she watched the wedding scene. The desired instructions were given each time, and after about half an hour of silent thoughtfulness in the trance state she asked to be awakened and dismissed. At the second visit she terminated therapy.

She was not seen until several days after the wedding, three months later.

Then she entered the office without an appointment and explained, "I've come to tell you about Nadine's wedding. I have an odd feeling that you know all about it and yet don't know a thing. But I do know that I have to give you an explanation for some reason."

Her explanation was that she and Nadine and the bridegroom had been lifelong friends and that their families were intimate friends. Some three months ago, following a therapeutic session, she had felt impelled to discontinue therapy and to devote her energies to getting ready for that wedding. When she was asked to be a bridesmaid, she decided to make her own dress. This had made it necessary to get promoted at work so that she would have better hours. Additionally, she had taken an apartment in town so that she would not lose a total of three hours going back and forth from work. She had gone on shopping tours with various friends to help select wedding presents, and she had arranged for "showers" for the bride-to-be. All in all she had been exceedingly and happily busy.

She described the wedding scene, the reception, and the dance. She was decidedly startled when the writer asked if she had danced with Ed and if he were the one who asked her for a date. She answered in considerable bewilderment that she could not understand, since she had not mentioned his name, how the writer could ask such a specific question. However, she had danced with Ed but had forestalled his request for a date since she considered him not to be up to her standard. However, she had accepted a date from another dancing partner.

Finally, she was reminded of her original purpose in seeing the writer. Her reply was simply, "I was a pretty sick girl when I first came to see you; I was horribly mixed up, and I'm grateful to you for getting me straightened out in time so that I could get ready for the wedding." She had no awareness that her preparations for the wedding constituted her recovery.

She has been seen occasionally since then on a casual basis. She is happily married and the mother of three children.

PATIENT E

In this case history the patient was not interested in therapy and did not know that she needed therapy, but she was interested in hypnosis as a personal experience that might be enjoyed. Very early in hypnotizing her the realization was reached that, despite her seemingly good adjustment, therapy was seriously indicated.

She was a 19-year-old student nurse of good intelligence, pretty, vivacious, likable, but annoyingly flippant in her general attitudes. She proved to be an excellent somnambulistic subject and interested in experimental hypnotic work. However, it was soon discovered that she had a mild avoidance phobia for water fountains and flower vases. Hypnotic exploration of this rapidly disclosed other items of psychopathology, which she confirmed in the waking state. Among these were the following:

1. She had learned to swim well when she was about 10 years old. However, for some unknown reason she had not been able to swim for at least the last five years. Yet, each season she would go to the lake to swim, don her bathing suit, and walk expectantly down to the shore. As her feet touched the water, she would turn and run away screaming, as a result of a sudden, unexpected impulse. Several hundred feet away she would gain control of herself and embarrassedly walk back to the shore, fully expecting to swim, but only repeating her previous uncontrollable impulsive behavior. Yet each time it occurred, she did not believe it would happen again.

2. She would accept an invitation to go to the theater with some young man. Once inside, she would slip away from her escort and then leave by a side entrance and go home alone. Or if she went to dinner, she would, at the close of the meal, excuse herself to go to the rest room and either wait it out there until her escort left in disgust or she would depart by a back door.

3. Her attitude toward marriage as a possibility for herself was one of bitter intolerance. So intense was her hostility on this topic that she would not discuss it except to declare that this was her "normal" feeling and that she had no particular reason for disparaging marriage so completely.

4. There were a number of other items of psychopathology, but these were not discovered until after therapy had been accomplished.

When the question of therapy was raised with her, she agreed to it provided the therapy were limited to the correction of her swimming problem. She did not realize that therapy in that regard might correct other maladjustments.

Treatment was initiated by training her fully as a hypnotic subject. This she enjoyed, but she was really interested in therapy.

Age regression was employed extensively with her, and a series of traumatic, deeply repressed memories were recovered and the experiences relived by her.

Some of these were as follows:

1. When she was about five years old, she and her two-year-old sister were playing about a washtub full of water, while the mother was out of the room. The sister fell into the tub, and the patient struggled to pull her out while screaming for her mother. When the mother came, she rescued the baby, who had "turned blue," and finally spanked the patient most severely "for pushing sister in the water."

2. At about the same period the sister, while sitting in the high chair at the table, managed to tip herself over. The patient rushed across the room with arms outstretched to rescue her. She arrived too late and just as her mother entered to see the patient's outstretched arms and the toppling chair. Again she was severely punished.

3. When she was about six years old, a neighbor volunteered to teach her to swim. This neighbor believed that a child's fear of water is best cured by complete immersion. The patient became extremely frightened, fought, screamed, and bit. Her "misbehavior" resulted in another spanking.

4. At about this same age a neighbor died and the patient was sent to the grandmother's house while the mother attended the funeral. That night the patient returned home and was awakened by her father's coughing (he was bedridden and slowly dying of pulmonary tuberculosis). Distressed by the coughing, she aroused her mother and explained that she wished her father would die. Without seeking the patient's reasons for this wish (when people die, you go to Grandmother's and get cookies and candy, and Daddy likes cookies and candy, so why can't he die and go to Grandma's?), the mother punished her severely.

5. When she was about eight years old, contrary to her mother's orders, she tried to cross a creek on a fallen log used as a footbridge. She slipped, fell, and saved herself by embracing the log. After much screaming on her part, she was finally rescued by

her older brother, who subsequently intimidated her by threats of reporting the escapade.

6. When she was about 12 years old, she and her sister, both having learned to swim well two years previously, went swimming. The water was cold and the sister became cyanotic but refused to leave the water despite the patient's frantic pleading and crying.

7. Because of the above experience, she had later refused to go swimming with her sister and brother. He had forcibly dragged her into the water. She fought him so furiously that they "both nearly drowned." She could not remember ever again swimming.

Although the patient relived these various experiences with vivid emotional intensity in the trance state, she protested that they had been forgotten events. Therefore, they ought to remain forgotten, and she declared emphatically that she would not remember them when she awakened.

Furthermore, she demanded that the writer begin therapy on her swimming problem immediately, doing this in a "subtle" way so that she would not suffer any more emotional stress. Efforts to correct her attitude while she was still in the trance were futile, as proved to be the case when she was awakened.

At the next interview the patient was definitely hostile. She declared that she had lost her interest in experimental hypnosis; she was interested in prompt and immediate correction of her "swimming problem and nothing more." In the trance state she confirmed this attitude but was much less hostile. She also declared that she did not want to remember consciously any of the memories previously recovered in hypnosis, since they had "once been forgotten and might as well stay that way."

Accordingly, her demand was accepted, and she was assured that all efforts would now be directed as she wished.

She was then disoriented for time and reoriented approximately three weeks into the future. Immediately she was told that, since therapy had been terminated the first part of June and it was now the latter part, one thing remained to be done. This task was that of "putting into effect the therapy that had been done." The opportunity to do this, in fact, was rapidly approaching. Her vacation would occur in the latter part of July and the first part of August. Therefore, it would be well to plan how to utilize that vacation to establish her therapeutic gains on a reality basis.

Thereupon, collaboratively, she and the writer devised the following plan. She would spend the vacation at a summer home on a lake well known to her. She was to purchase a new bathing suit and a small waterproof silk bag large enough to hold a package of cigarettes and matches. This bag would be carefully attached to her bathing suit for the first two days, if necessary, but would probably be dispensed with in much less time.

The cigarettes and matches would now be presented to her, a package of Lucky Strikes* on which the writer would, in her presence, inscribe, "This really is a lucky strike." These she would now put into her handbag with the matches slipped into the cellophane wrapper, and she would keep them hidden from her conscious mind until the time came to use them.

At the lake, and in the form of posthypnotic behavior, she would attach the waterproof bag containing the cigarettes and matches to her bathing suit. Then, consciously, she was to stroll down to the beach, speculating about sitting on the raft and wondering whether she would sit facing out over the lake or facing the shore.

Once on the raft she would experience an overwhelming desire for a cigarette. While wishing for one and dangling her feet in the water, she would "accidentally" discover the waterproof bag and explore the contents. She would be so delighted that she would immediately light a cigarette and only while puffing it would she begin to wonder where they came from. Examination of the package would lead to the discovery of the writing on it. While she pondered its meaning, she would finish the cigarette, toss the butt into the water, and strike out for shore, still puzzled about the inscription.

Upon reaching shore, she would realize that she had left the cigarettes on the raft, and she would turn and strike out for the raft again. Upon arriving at the raft, she would be hungry for another cigarette and would smoke again.

As she smoked, she would suddenly remember completely everything that had happened since she had donned her bathing suit.

The patient listened attentively to these elaborate instructions and comprehended readily what she was to do. Then, while she was still in the trance state, she was "disoriented" for "the latter part of June" and projected in time to September in the situation of entering the office.

She was asked, "Well, what really happened on your vacation?"

Her narrative was essentially as follows:

> When I started to get undressed to put on my suit, I had an awful time. I was so absentminded. Then, when I went down to the beach, I was wondering why nobody was on the raft, and I decided to sit on it. The next thing I was ravenous for a cigarette. Then everything happened just as you said last June. I smoked a cigarette and struck out for shore, but then I had to go back and get my cigarettes. And then I started to remember everything

---

*Ordinarily she refused to smoke other than her own particular brand of cigarettes.

about undressing and getting that silk bag fastened to my suit and thinking about the raft and swimming out there twice. And then I knew I was over my swimming problem and I really enjoyed swimming every day.

Now I'm back at work and everything is swell.

She was reoriented to the current time and emphatically instructed to obey, to the last detail, all instructions that she had ever, at any time, been given when in a trance state. With equal emphasis she was instructed to keep all unconscious knowledge from her conscious mind. This must absolutely be done until such time, if it ever did occur, that both she and the writer independently would approve of her conscious awareness of things unconscious. This instruction, in accord with her previously expressed attitude, she accepted most readily.

She was awakened and dismissed. The cigarettes and matches had been carefully wrapped in tissue and concealed in her handbag.

She was seen again in September. She entered the office with a merry laugh and declared:

Well, you already know everything that happened on my vacation. It all happened just as you said. By the end of my vacation I got so puzzled by everything that I sat down one day and deliberately remembered everything. It was so confusing because I started with the appointment I had with you in the first part of June. I really had a lot of trouble getting straight about "the last part of June," and then "September," and making them both fit into the real time. Puzzling that out was a job, but I got it straight. You ought to try to think a thing out like that. At first, the last part of June and September were just as real as any other memories. I knew they couldn't be so, but they were real and it was a terrific job, but exciting and interesting.

But when I got them straightened out, I could see them as ideas that I had for the future, and then I was straight in my mind.

That's when the real merry-go-round started. That's when I started to remember everything that happened since you began to work with me—all those things you dug out of me. If you had as much fun digging them out as I had remembering them and putting them together to make sense, I won't have to apologize for being so stubborn.

The whole thing went pretty fast. I puzzled all morning one day, and then after lunch I really sat down and started my think-trap going, and by dinnertime I had everything straight.

That first September report wasn't right in some things. What really happened started in June, after that trance that really started things. I started getting ready for my vacation, and the first thing I had to do was to get a bathing suit. I was looking for a special suit, but I didn't realize it then. I didn't know it was blue.

Then I had a job finding a waterproof silk bag to send overseas to someone—I hadn't really made up my mind who, so I couldn't send it after I got it. Then I misplaced my handbag. Every time I found it again, it got misplaced again. The last place I found it was in the suitcase I took to the lake. I can remember now all the tricks my unconscious played on me to keep those cigarettes hidden from my conscious mind.

Well, the rest at the lake was like you said, except that when I was hanging my feet in the water on the raft, I kept worrying about the toenail polish coming off. But the rest was like you said. But I kept wondering what happened to me because I was enjoying the swimming.

But that isn't all. After I remembered all those other things you dug out, I knew I could handle them, but I didn't know what I was going to do. I had to wait till I got home.

I'll tell you them now, all except one. I'll tell you that next time.

She continued:

For years and years I have wanted to take a hot soak in the bathtub. I always filled the tub full and then I would step in, pull out the plug, and take a shower. It always made me so mad, but I did it every time. And if there wasn't a shower, I'd just stand in the tub and sponge myself. Now I can take a tub bath.

Another thing! I can drive a car now. I had to give it up because I got in the habit of shutting my eyes and speeding up, sometimes in the city, sometimes in the country. Remember the footbridge— well, I always did that to cross bridges, but I just realized that up at the lake. Now I don't shut my eyes to drive over a bridge.

Those poor guys that dated me and took me out! That neighbor that took me out in the water and wouldn't let me come back and ducked me. Well, I let those poor fellows take me out and I made sure I got back.

And Sis and the high chair! You couldn't hire me to stay in a place where there was a baby in a high chair. Some of the nurses invited me to their homes for dinner, and after I got in the house I just walked out. I didn't know why then. Now I can visit people who have babies in high chairs.

And Sis getting blue when she was a baby and then when we went swimming that time. I've never worn anything blue because of that, and it's becoming to me. First the blue bathing suit and now this new outfit I've got on.

And I've joined the church. I always wanted to go but couldn't stand being in a church. I even took my training in a Catholic hospital because I'm a Protestant and I wanted to be sure to keep away from church. But just because they have funerals in church doesn't stop me. There are a lot of other little things, but you get the general idea. What I don't understand is how I kept all this in my unconscious and made everything so tough for me. How can a person be so stupid and so stubborn? But I suppose you're going to call me stubborn now because I'm not going to tell you the most important thing that happened. But I'm not really stubborn because I've got a good reason this time, and I'm going to tell you the next time I see you.

She was not seen again until mid-October. As she entered the office, she said:

I'm ready to tell you, but first I've got to explain a little. Mother had it awful hard when we were kids—looking after us, taking care of Father, earning a living for us. I thought that marriage was horrible, just trouble and work and heartache, and that husbands were always sick. I just never straightened out that idea. So last month I visited Mother and had a long talk with her. I didn't tell her those things you dug up out of my unconscious; we just talked about when the kids were little and my father was sick. She really loved Father, and she doesn't think she had it so hard. I wish I'd had enough sense to get her ideas before, instead of keeping my kid ideas in my unconscious. So I told her about Joe, how we're going steady since I got back from vacation. She was very pleased when I told her I was going to get married some time next year. She never did like nursing for me, and now I wonder why I took it up—my father, I suppose. But now I want a home and kids and a husband. So now I'll introduce you to Joe—he's waiting outside.

The young people were seen casually on several occasions before their marriage. When their first child was about a year old, a visit was made to them, and at this time the mother was met.

During the course of that visit the mother, who knew that her daughter had been the writer's patient and had been hypnotized, expressed an interest in being hypnotized also. Immediately the daughter was asked if she had ever given any account of her hypnotic experiences to the mother. This was disclaimed.

The mother proved to be an unusually good subject and responded readily to age regression. She was regressed to the time, "when your daughter was between four and a half and six years old, at which time something may have occurred that frightened you and her very much."

Among the things elicited was a similar account of the washtub episode. The patient's age was given "as almost two months past her birthday." Similarly, a comparable account was obtained of the high chair episode. The patient was then about five years and nine months old.

The swimming lesson by the neighbor and the funeral episode were both adequately confirmed, including the midnight spanking for the "death wish."

The fallen log footbridge episode apparently was not known to the mother, but she did relive an episode, when asked to be sure to speak to her daughter about something on the west side of the house, of anxiously cautioning the patient "never, never walk on that tree that fell across the creek in that bad windstorm."

The mother was awakened with instructions to remember fully what had happened in the trance. She was tremendously startled by the recovery of these memories, and she, her daughter, and the writer spent a considerable period of time discussing those past experiences. The mother showed good capacity to understand, and she was relieved to know that the "death wish" was something entirely different.

Some months later the mother was seen again. The purpose of her visit was to find out if there were any other things that she had done that she ought to talk over with her daughter. She was hypnotized and told that she could remember freely and comfortably and discuss anything of actual interest to her daughter whenever the occasion arose.

A social telephone call from the daughter some months later disclosed that the two of them had been reminiscing happily and contentedly and that she had a very pleasing recollection of her childhood.

The patient's adjustments have remained good. Her relationship with her mother has continued to be happy, and she is very much interested and contented with the raising of her two children.

GENERAL COMMENT

Perhaps the first discussion of these therapeutic experimental procedures should concern how fantasied accomplishments could have proved such effective measures of therapy. We all know, from common experience, how easy it is to fantasy great deeds, and how far short fall the endeavors in reality. The fantasied story is such a masterpiece until it is set on paper, and the beautiful painting, so clearly visualized in the mind's eye, becomes a daub when the brush is applied to the canvas. However, it must be borne in mind that *such fantasies as these are conscious fantasies.* Thus, they represent accomplishments apart from reality, complete in themselves, and expressive, recognizedly so to the person, of no more than conscious, hopeful, wishful thinking.

Unconscious fantasies, however, belong to another category of psychological functioning. They are not accomplishments complete in themselves, nor are they apart from reality. Rather, they are psychological constructs in various degrees of formulation, for which the unconscious stands ready, or is actually awaiting an opportunity, to make a part of reality. They are not significant merely of *wishful desire* but rather of *actual intention* at the opportune time. Thus, one can endeavor to record a fantasied story on paper, but its merit may derive from the "sudden flashes of inspiration that come unbidden to the mind." Or an author may consciously endeavor to write a novel and find that his characters "do not behave but run away" with him.

In these case histories extensive emphasis was placed upon fantasies concerning the future, and every effort was made to keep them unconscious by prohibitive and inhibitive suggestions. By so doing, each patient's unconscious was provided with a wealth of formulated ideas unknown to the conscious mind. Then, in response to the innate needs and desires of the total personality, the unconscious could utilize those ideas by translating them into realities of daily life as spontaneous responsive behavior in opportune situations.

An experimental illustration of this may be cited. A normal hypnotic subject who disliked ostentatious display of learning and who spoke only English was taught in a deep trance to recite "Die Lorelei." This was done as a seeming part of an experiment on memory that was being completed and without informing him that he was learning a poem or that it was in German. A posthypnotic amnesia for this task was then suggested.

About two weeks later at a social gathering, through prearrangement, a colleague of the writer's offered to entertain the group by singing and reciting variously in Polish, Austrian, Italian, French, and Spanish. After listening with increasing displeasure, the subject remarked, "I can talk in nonsense syllables, too," and proceeded to recite "Die Lorelei." To his full conscious understanding, the subject's utterances were no more than nonsense syllables spontaneously offered in the immediate situation. Rehypnosis was necessary to convince him otherwise.

This experiment differs from the case histories in that future possibilities in a life situation were not a part of the experimental situation. Rather, the subject's unconscious was provided with special learning, and then, later, an opportunity was created in which that special learning could become manifest in response to inner personal needs.

For the patients, special understandings for the future were developed in their unconscious minds, and their actual life situations presented the reality opportunities to utilize those ideas in responsive behavior in accord with their inner needs and desires.

The fashion in which the patients made their fantasies a part of their reality life was in keeping with the ordinary natural evolution of spontaneous behavior responses to reality. It was not in compliance with therapeutic suggestions, nor did it seem to derive even indirectly from anything other than the patients' responses to their realities. Furthermore, their behavior was experienced by them as arising within them and in relation to their needs in their immediate life situation.

Thus, Patient A vaguely wondered about his next appointment with the writer and acted on a sudden impulse to ask for a raise in salary, which, in turn, led to a series of events. Patient D did not leave the parental home for the cogent reasons she had discussed with the writer but because she wanted to make a dress she wished to wear. And Patient E responded to her fantasies by searching blindly for a bathing suit that met unconscious needs related to her distant past. So it was with the other two patients.

The kind of fantasies by which the patients achieved their goals is of marked interest and significance. They were not of the elaborate, grandiose type that one commonly has when fantasying consciously about one's wishes. They were fantasies in keeping with their understandings of actually attainable goals. For example, Patient A was pitifully modest in wishing for "just fair" health. Nor did he think of winning a fight, but hoped to be able to "take a licking like a man." Patient B's thinking did not center around visions of receiving one promotion after another but dealt with the humdrum realities of packing and moving. Patient C validated her fantasies in terms of a reality scar, and her father was just a man with a "funny-looking tooth." And Patient D saw herself in her fantasy not as a star in the entertainment world but as a happy guest at a friend's wedding.

So it was with all the fantasies about the future experienced by these patients. There was no running away of the imagination, but a serious appraisal in fantasy form of reality possibilities in keeping with their understandings of themselves.

To speculate upon the question of why and how "time projection" proved to be an effective therapeutic measure for these patients is difficult. One can hardly do more than to draw parallels with experiences common in everyday life. For example, advertising and salesmanship extensively utilize appeals that stimulate fantasies of the future. An example more closely comparable to the above case reports is that of writing, after much indecision, a letter accepting a new position. Once it has been written, even though not yet mailed, there develops immediately a profound feeling that the die has been irrevocably cast. There results then a new psychological orientation of compelling force, effecting a new organization of thinking and planning. The writing of the letter constituted an initiation of action, and, as was mentioned earlier, an action once initiated tends to continue.

For these patients, apparently, the establishment of a dissociated state, in which they could feel and believe that they had achieved certain things of benefit to them, gave to them a profound feeling of accomplished realities which, in turn, resulted in the desired therapeutic reorientation.

46. Facilitating Objective Thinking and New Frames of Reference with Pseudo-Orientation in Time

Milton H. Erickson

A common, repetitious learning of everyday life is the frequent, marked discrepancy between anticipation and realization. The value and significance of hopes and wishes, upon becoming realized, so often prove to be quite different from what was originally expected. This is particularly true in situations centering around emotional problems. There is a natural tendency to overemphasize the importance of immediate understandings and subjective attitudes in preference to a thoughtful, objective consideration of eventual probabilities and possibilities.

This common experience of daily life has been utilized extensively by this author for many years as the basis for a special therapeutic technique in the handling of a wide variety of emotional problems that have been experienced by the patient as too difficult to evaluate satisfactorily. In essence, this technique is not new—the author has published previously on experimental therapeutic methods employing basically similar principles. Its central feature is the instruction of the patient, hypnotized and pseudo-oriented in time, to view the problem for which therapy is being sought as one deriving from the remote, recent, or immediate past, the current situation, or the impending near or remote future. In this way the pressing emotional urgency of the actual current situation can be altered by the interjection or interpolation of a sense of perspective in time, thereby creating an opportunity conducive to more comprehensive and objective thinking. In this regard, one need only call to mind such familiar plaintive utterances as: "I knew all the facts even then, and I should have foreseen this outcome; if only I could do it all over, I'd do the same things but for entirely different reasons and with such different results." And, "If only I could have known for sure, or just had the feeling that it was going to happen, I could have changed my feeling so easily."

This comprehensive, objective viewing of stressful matters is thus carried out against suggested backgrounds of various possible understandings. Ideally, objective thinking is possible in the ordinary waking state,

Unpublished manuscript, circa 1940s.

but emotional stress is likely to constitute a serious interference, if not an actual barrier. In contrast to the functioning of the ordinary state of conscious awareness, hypnosis permits a dissociation of ideas and attitudes in one relationship and a vivification and intensification of others in another relationship, thereby facilitating a much more effective examination, identification, and evaluation of wishes, fears, beliefs, and understandings. In this way clear comparison of intrinsic values, a resolution of conflicts, and an integration of understandings can be more readily effectuated.

This technique was in part developed from an experimental therapeutic study conducted in the early 1930s and published under the title "Unconscious Insights."* It is also essentially a narration of the technique described in "Pseudo-orientation in time as a hypnotherapeutic procedure" (Erickson, 1954). The actual procedure is rather simple. Upon inducing a medium or deep trance, suggestions are offered to effect a dissociation from the immediate environment and then to emphasize the unimportance of the identity of the day of the week and then of the month, culminating in an amnesia for time, place, and situation, but with an awareness of the general identity of the self.

Clinical Data (Fragmentary Notes)

Edward and Jean: A childless couple, content to be childless. His mother lived with them, dominating the household completely. Jean finally rebelled and gave Edward his choice between kicking his mother out or divorce. Edward sought counsel.

Techniques of unconscious insights employed in both directions. His discovery of a desire for paternity. The ejection of his mother. Reconciliation. Two children.

Walter and Willa: Incessant quarreling for six years, with threats and counterthreats of divorce. Weekly visits by her parents. Weekly dinners at her parents' home. Walter finally rebelled and "laid it on the line." Willa seen as patient. Solution: Weaning from the parents and several additional pregnancies.

Howard and Margaret: Children grown. No desire for further family. She was only 35. Both decided on a vasectomy and both came for counseling. Her unconscious fears of his infidelity. His unconscious fears of infidelity. Consideration of salpingectomy is rejected. Decision for contraception.

---

*Editor's Note: This study was never published, but the fragmentary notes on the cases presented at the end of this paper are part of the clinical data MHE was collecting for it. "Unconscious Insights" is indicative of MHE's interests and initial hypnotherapeutic orientation at that time.

Marie and Ralph: His infidelity. Guilt and confession. Her desire for revenge. Her request for counsel and her own discovery of a profound sense of guilt.

Dr. B: Sought counsel concerning vasectomy. He and his wife were content with one child. They wanted no more. In the trance state he recognized his definite, though unformulated, ideas of infidelity. Also, he discovered serious fears of the consequences and a feeling that a divorce would result.

Without disclosing his fears to his wife, he raised the question of vasectomy vs. salpingectomy. He rejected her offer, rejected his trance learnings, underwent vasectomy, was eventually divorced for the reasons originally feared.

James and Joyce: Ages 23 and 22. Married when she was 16. Four children by the age of 22. Much debate between them regarding vasectomy vs. salpingectomy. Salpingectomy rejected. Vasectomy accepted and counsel sought by both. Both rejected unconscious insights. Divorced three years later.

Charles and Carol: Both aged 25. Both only children. Both resolved to have no children. Both rejected contraception. Sought counsel regarding vasectomy or salpingectomy. Unconscious insights confirmed five years later by several pregnancies.

Albert and Janice: History of 11 miscarriages. Majority between the second and third month. Much bitterness and resentment and depression. Salpingectomy proposed. Consistent rejection in the trance state. Five successful subsequent pregnancies.

Leon: Aged 38. Chronic alcoholism. Wanted to know his future. Unconscious discovery of homicidal attitudes. Twelve years of sobriety.

Joe and Ann: Ann, university graduate. Joe, grade school education. Counsel requested concerning advisability of marriage. Unconscious insights approved.

Jack and Jill: December and May situation. The man's unconscious insights objected.

James and Patricia: The prospective bride requested counsel regarding a premarital sex relationship. Invariably rejected premarital relationships in the trance state.

Phil and Nancy: Marriage counseling for mixed racial marriages and mixed religions.

47. Self-Exploration in the Hypnotic State

Milton H. Erickson

INTRODUCTION

This brief study is reported in detail for a number of reasons. It is an account of a classroom experiment proposed and executed by a medical student as an intellectual project for classroom purposes. Actually, it was an unconscious seeking by the student for specific psychotherapy in the guise of an intellectual effort.

The fashion in which the proposed task was to be done, apparently to illuminate the intellectual aspects, served in reality to define the manner in which the student wished unknowingly to achieve his therapy.

While every effort was made to avoid giving the student assistance, other than that of creating a favorable situation, various suggestions were nevertheless seized upon by him to develop his task.

The results obtained by the student serve to illustrate with remarkable clarity:

1. The obvious but unrecognized unconscious motivations and needs served;
2. The separateness of unconscious and conscious memories;
3. The actual possibility of dissociating the affective and the cognitive elements of a traumatic experience;
4. The process of the transfer of memories from the unconscious to the conscious mind;
5. The extensive effects of a single, deeply repressed traumatic experience upon the personality and the comprehensive changes achieved upon its reintegration into the experiential life of the person; and
6. The numerous minor clues, given during the task performance, highly informative of the significances involved.

Quoted from the *Journal of Clinical and Experimental Hypnosis*, 1955, *3*, 49–57. Copyright by the Society for Clinical and Experimental Hypnosis, 1955.

STATEMENT OF EXPERIMENTAL PROBLEM

One of a group of medical students being trained in hypnosis had shown an almost compulsive-obsessional interest in psychiatry and had studied avidly on the subject. He early volunteered to be a hypnotic subject for the group but had placed a restriction on his role as a subject by declaring that no intimate or personal questions be put to him. He proved to be easily trained and most capable of developing complex hypnotic phenomena.

After some weeks work with the group, at the beginning of one session this student announced his wish to raise a special question for the evening's work and discussion. This question he explained as follows: People normally forget many things and hence do not know that they have forgotten them. These things may be only of past significance, or they may be of actual present but unknown and unrecognized significance. They may be of a minor or a major character and importance. And they may be of a traumatic or a nontraumatic nature.

Therefore, would it be possible for a person to set himself the task of remembering some definite but actually long-forgotten event and to recall it vividly and comprehensively?

The reply was made that this question was worth investigation and that he could retire to the next room for half an hour and really work on recovering some completely forgotten memory of his own. He replied that he had been thinking about the question off and on for the past week without formulating any ideas, but he would be glad to devote an intensive half-hour to the subject.

During his absence the question was discussed with the other students. At the expiration of half an hour he was summoned. He explained sheepishly that the task of attempting to remember something that was completely forgotten and that had occurred at a time and in a situation that could not be recalled was as futile a task as trying to describe some totally unknown place. He had, however, recalled many things, but these were not forgotten things, but merely things he had not thought about for varying lengths of time.

The suggestion was offered that he might spend the next half-hour endeavoring to recover a forgotten memory of something that had occurred previous to his tenth year and about which he had not even thought for at least 15 years.*

---

* All emphasis in this suggestion was placed upon the word *might,* thereby rendering it a permissive suggestion, offering only a general concept of possible time periods.

Half an hour later he reported that the task was even more hopeless than ever. He had recalled innumerable things, but they were memories about which he had had no occasion to think, and they did not constitute recoveries of forgotten things. He then raised the question of whether or not he could be given the same task in a hypnotic trance. He was answered that he could be given the task, but he would have to discover for himself whether or not he could perform it. He agreed to that stipulation.

He was hypnotized deeply and instructed to review mentally his question and his two half-hour efforts and to spend at least 10 minutes considering the feasibility of the task.

After 10 minutes he stated that the entire problem still looked hopeless to him.

Still maintained in the trance state, he was asked if he wanted any help or guidance, and he replied that any assistance would vitiate the purpose of the effort, since such assistance would direct and aid in memory recovery, and it was his desire to see if such a memory recovery could be effected by a person in either the waking or the trance state and accomplished solely by personal efforts in mental searching.

He was told that he would be given no aid but that certain general remarks could be made to him which would give him more opportunity to do the task. Hesitantly he agreed to hear the remarks, but upon hearing them, he accepted them readily. These remarks were offered to explain the following matters. Since he was in a somnambulistic trance and usually manifested catalepsy, it would serve no purpose either to maintain or abolish catalepsy, which was only an incidental part of his trance state and not an integral part of the proposed task.

Therefore, in performing his task, no incidental item of behavior such as catalepsy should be permitted to interfere with his efforts. Also, since he usually kept his eyes open in the trance state, that behavior item should be regarded in the same manner as the catalepsy.

Since he would be doing his task in the presence of the group, he should recognize it as solely his task in which nobody else had a part; it would be well to limit himself to his task without including any member of the group by any response of any sort. In other words, he was essentially to isolate himself from the group.

Inasmuch as the forgotten memory belonged to him, it should not be shared in any way until he had an opportunity to consider that sharing as a distinctly separate problem. Hence, his task should be a mental performance occurring within himself. Additionally, it would be necessary for him to keep in mind that, for example, when the task was done, it would be desirable for him to establish contact with the writer to give instructions about awakening him, or for any other contingency that might arise. Then, too, he might want instructions about what to do with whatever results he secured. Therefore, he could, at any needful time, address inquiries or remarks to the writer.

After these remarks had been repeated to him to enable him to think them over thoroughly, he asked, "How do I start?"

The reply was cautiously given, "It is your task. You will start by waiting until I announce the time and as soon as I do, you will begin in your own way."

While waiting for the time announcement, he stated, "I'm going to look for a forgotten thing just as I said before. It should be something like you said that maybe happened before I was 10, and it should be something I haven't even thought about for at least 15 years. I think that is a reasonable problem."

THE EXPERIMENTAL PROCEDURE AND RESULTS

The time of 7:30 P.M. was announced. He settled himself in a chair, still in a deep trance, bowed his head, and closed his eyes.

At 7:50 P.M. he called, "Dr. Erickson, I have a feeling that I am getting something, but I don't know what it is. But I am curious." Reply was made, "Thank you for telling me."

About 10 minutes later he asked if it were warm or cold. Reply was made, "I find the temperature comfortable."

About five minutes later he announced, "I am getting scared, awful scared, but I can't think of anything." No reply was made.

Within a few minutes he presented a distressing picture of indescribable terror that seriously alarmed the medical students. Falteringly he gasped, "I'm scared, awful, awful scared. I'm going to get sick. But I don't know why. Tell me to rest."

He was told, "Stay just where you are in your mind, but rest a few minutes."

Immediately he relaxed and declared, "I am terribly scared, but I can't remember anything. It is the awfullest feeling. I think I am going to get sick. Don't let me get sick."

He was told, "I do not know what you are doing. Getting sick might be part of it. I will not tell you how to do your task."

To this was added, "Do you want to wake up and rest or just rest in the trance with your gears in neutral, the engine just idling, neither going ahead nor backing up?"

He answered, "Just as I am."

A few minutes later he asked the time, and as it was stated, the look of intense terror reappeared; retching but no vomiting developed. His breathing was labored and spasmodic, his hands clasped and unclasped convulsively, and he seemed about ready to collapse.

Suddenly he gasped, "Rest."

Immediately he was told, "Hang on but rest."

Again he relaxed and declared, "It's too big, I can't do it. Tell me how." He was told, "I can't tell you how, but I can offer a suggestion. You say it's too big. Why not do it a part here, a part there, instead of the whole thing at once, and then put the parts together into the whole big thing?"

He nodded his head, asked the time, and again manifested, as the time was stated, intense emotions of varied types. *Rage, terror, grief, fear, hatred, hysteria, sickness, despair, bravado, shock, horror, agony* were the words written down by the students as they watched him and recorded their interpretations of what they saw manifested by him, and the writer was willing to agree with them.

Finally, a state of what appeared to be stark terror developed. His face was contorted, his hands were tightly clasped, his jaws were clenched, his breathing was labored, his neck muscles were taut, and his body was rigid.

After about two minutes he shuddered, relaxed, sighed, and said, "Rest."

Asked how he wished to rest, he answered, "I've got started. I've got the feelings. I don't know what the memory is. Wake me up and let me rest, and then hypnotize me and just tell me to finish the job. I still got the whole thing to do yet. But I got to rest."

He was awakened with instructions to rest and to have a comprehensive amnesia for what had happened in the trance. He awakened, wiped the perspiration from his face, remarked that he must have eaten something that disagreed with him because he felt sick to his stomach, wandered about the room opening windows, remarking about the heat, and added that he hoped to learn something if the writer would start discussing the question he had propounded. Thereupon he returned to his chair, sat down, but jumped up and asked one of his classmates what the assignment was in dermatology. Without waiting for an answer, he started a casual conversation with another student.

After about 10 minutes he returned to his chair, sat down, looked expectantly at the writer, and developed a deep somnambulistic trance.

He was told, "You said just before you took your rest, 'I still got the whole thing to do.' The time is now nine o'clock."

He closed his eyes, a look of interest appeared on his face, then one of amusement. Many head movements were made, as if he were looking from side to side. This lasted for a few minutes, and then his head movements became jerky and his hands and arms moved slightly in a jerky fashion. Suddenly a look of anger appeared on his face, followed by a short jerk of his body. Then he stiffened in his chair, his face contorted, his hands clenched, and his biceps contracted. There followed then a tremendous variety of facial expressions as described above, with much jerking of the head from side to side and twisting of his body.

After about 10 minutes of this he slumped exhausted in the chair and gasped, "Rest."

Immediately he was told, "Stay where you are in your mind and rest."

He relaxed and declared, "I'm through. I did it. But I don't know what to do now. You got to tell me or I'll forget it all over."

He was answered, "I can give you some suggestions. Listen carefully. I think you have recovered a long-forgotten traumatic memory. [He nodded affirmatively.] You know it now in your unconscious mind. You do not know it in your conscious mind. Keep it fully remembered in your unconscious mind. I will awaken you and let you find out for yourself if you want to know it consciously. Is that all right?"

Since he nodded his head affirmatively, he was told to awaken with only a conscious amnesia and to rest awhile. Then the writer would discuss matters.

He awakened, complained of feeling "horribly washed out," "sick," "tired," and "like I just took an awful beating."

He added, "I'd swear that someone had just been kicking me around and punching me. My gluteals feel like they've been kicked. And my ribs hurt. I feel as if Joe Louis had given me a workover."

He went out to the water fountain, took a drink, returned, asked the same student about the dermatology assignment, and again did not wait for an answer. He wandered about the room, began and interrupted conversations, and was exceedingly restless.

Finally he sat down and remarked that it was getting very late, that the writer ought to discuss the question he had propounded at the beginning of the evening.

The writer began by summarizing the question he had raised and then went on to state that such a forgotten memory as he proposed to discover would probably be a rather deeply repressed memory. Hence, there was a good probability that the repression would derive from a traumatic character of the memory. Therefore, recovery of such repressed memory would entail a lot of distress, pain, and actual misery. Furthermore, self-protective tendencies would make such recovery slow and difficult.

With hypnosis there could be a more rapid recovery of the memory, and the self-protective tendencies would be greatly minimized. However, such recovery would first be limited to the unconscious mind. Then there would arise the question of whether or not the unconscious knowledge could or would be shared with the conscious mind. If it should be, then the person would have to experience mentally the original trauma with all the personal pain that would accompany the recovery of the repressed material.

In his case there would be a number of questions he would have to consider. Would he be content to recover it and let it remain in his unconscious? Or would he want to know it consciously? Also, while his willingness to work on such a problem in the presence of his classmates implied his willingness to have them see his behavior in so doing, would he want them to see his conscious reactions to a conscious realization? Then, too, even if he were willing for that, would he want them to know the content of the repressed material?

As for the method of achieving a conscious understanding, there were certain considerations he should have in mind. Would he want the whole thing to irrupt into his conscious mind all at once? Or would he prefer to have it come piecemeal, one part at a time, with the possibility of halting the process and mustering his strength so that he could more easily endure the next development? Would he want to separate the affective from the cognitive elements and experience the one or the other first? Or would he like to have the recovery follow the same course of development, the same chronology, as the original experience?

He interrupted to declare that the latter sounded best and to ask when a beginning could be made.

Reply was made, "The other students are here."

Thoughtfully he answered, "I don't care what they see, but I don't want them to know until I know first. We're all medics, so I figure that they ought to be able to take it. But I want the first look. When can we start?"

He was told, "It is now after 10 o'clock. What do you think you have been doing? Why do you feel so tired, so beaten up?"

After a long pause he said, "You mean, I've done that job I talked about when I came, that I know it in my unconscious and that you are waiting for me to figure out if I want to know it consciously? I'm pretty sure that's right—I better think it over. I'm not just beginning the job. I'm on the homestretch and I'm sick. Give me a few minutes."

Shortly he declared, "I'm going to take it just like it really happened. What time is it?"

He was told 10:30.

He smiled and began, "That's funny. A scene just flashed into my mind. It's just as clear as if I were there looking on. I'm back in Oklahoma. Let's see. I'm almost eight years old. And there is that shirttail cousin of mine. I haven't seen him since I was eight years old. He moved away." Then, in the manner of one who is hallucinating visually a past experience, he continued, "Us kids are playing. We got short pants on and we are having fun." Then in a detached fashion he added, "Nothing traumatic about this. I can see us wrestling and pushing and kicking up in the straw. We are in the cowbarn. We are having a whale of a time. Hey, he pushed me. That hurt. I hit him. He hits back. What a fight. Slugging away. Oh no, no, no, no, don't, don't, don't."

At this point he stopped verbalizing, closed his eyes, and shuddered; there followed a duplication of his previous disturbed behavior, with one new addition. Repeatedly he seemed to be endeavoring to speak but unable to do so. For about 20 minutes he was absorbed in the throes of this experience, and finally he collapsed in his chair in exhaustion and said, "Thank God, he will live."

Slowly he straightened up in his chair and remarked, "Yes, he lived, and I forgot the whole thing. I haven't even remembered him. I never dared. I couldn't. I haven't remembered it for years and years—more than 15 years. I just put it out of my mind completely."

After further similar comments he suddenly remarked, "I might as well tell the rest of you what it's all about," and he proceeded to relate the story. In summary, his account was as follows:

One summer day before his eighth birthday he was playing in the cowbarn with a distantly related boy of his own age named Johnny. They were wrestling and tussling, and unintentionally they hurt each other. This led to an active fight, and Johnny, smaller than he, was getting the worst of the battle. To even the contest, Johnny grabbed a pitchfork and attempted to jab him. In turn, he seized a pitchfork used in cleaning the barn and unfortunately stabbed Johnny in the left calf. When Johnny screamed, he horrifiedly jerked the fork tine out and was even more horrified by the pulsing stream of blood.

Johnny ran screaming and limping to the house, while he turned and ran to the pump and began pumping water frantically into the horse trough.

As he learned later, his father applied a tourniquet and summoned a physician. While waiting for the doctor, the father came to the well and, seizing him, went to the horse trough, sat down, and proceeded to spank him thoroughly, as he lay across his father's knee, staring at the green scum of algae in the horse trough. Then his father roughly dragged him to the house and made him stand and look at Johnny.

The physician arrived and dressed the wound, then wanted to see the fork. His father cuffed him and sent him to get the fork, which he did in a turmoil of emotion.

After examining the fork, the doctor administered antitetanus serum, explaining the reason. Upon learning this the father beat his son again.

Just before the doctor left Johnny developed anaphylactic shock. His eyes swelled shut, his tongue enlarged and protruded from his mouth, and he became a "horrible greenish color."

He saw the doctor give another injection, which he thought was again antitetanus (afterwards he learned it was "medicine to help Johnny live"), saw the doctor insert a spoon in Johnny's mouth (to lessen respiratory embarrassment), and then take out a knife (scalpel) to cut Johnny's throat (do a tracheotomy). He was all the more terrified that Johnny was to be "butchered like a pig."

However, Johnny responded to the adrenalin injection and no tracheotomy was performed, but the doctor did explain the reason for considering a tracheotomy. However, to him, it still sounded like a plan to butcher Johnny.

After the doctor left, his father trounced him soundly again and forced him to stand for hours by Johnny's bedside and to watch and give the alarm if Johnny developed "breathing trouble so he would have to have his throat cut."

All that night he dreamed of Johnny's skin turning a "horrible green like the scum in the horse trough." The next day he was forced to watch the doctor redress the wound, the surrounding area of which was "all awful color, green and nasty." Furthermore, the doctor in examining the wound remarked that it was a most "nasty thing." Later that day he neglected to pump water for the horses, and was again thoroughly spanked by his father, while in the same position as the previous day.

Shortly thereafter Johnny's parents moved out of state, and all contact was lost. As far as he could determine, the entire matter then became a closed incident, and a year later his parents moved to a distant city, and farm life became a forgotten thing.

Tired, exhausted, self-absorbed, the student took his departure with the others, who had been instructed not to discuss the matter till later.

A week later the student visited the writer, stating that he had learned some amazing things about himself as a result of his recovered memory.

First of all, he doubted if he was as seriously interested in psychiatry as he had previously thought. Internal medicine was proving more interesting.

Secondly, his attitude toward dermatology had changed completely. Previously, he had been unable to study the textbook, despite repeated efforts. Either he went to sleep or immediately became distracted. Each time he went to the dermatology clinic, he became sick and had to leave. Also, despite frequent faculty warnings, he had consistently avoided the lectures given on the subject. Now he was studying dermatology with interest, and he enjoyed the clinics. (He eventually secured a good grade in that subject.)

He was seen regularly in class sessions for the rest of the year and also throughout his internship, during which time he discussed his future plans, which included a residency in internal medicine. However, he still retained a good, though secondary, interest in psychiatry.

He has since completed a residency in internal medicine and is now in private practice, utilizing his knowledge of psychiatry extensively in handling his patients.

CONCLUSION

Little need be said in summary about the informativeness of the student's performance. The directness, the economy of effort and time, the effectiveness with which he accomplished his task, and the significance of the results to him as a personality, together with the ease with which one can follow and understand what occurred, is most impressive.

It is difficult even to imagine such a task performance in the ordinary waking state, even as the student himself discovered. Yet, in the hypnotic state a seemingly impossible task became comprehensible, feasible, and ready of accomplishment in a recognizable fashion.

48. Self-Exploration in Trance Following a Surprise Handshake Induction

Milton H. Erickson

A medical man who had used hypnosis for many years suffered the tragic loss of his oldest son, who had been his first hypnotic subject. The man reacted to this by a severe depression, following which he abandoned hypnosis and practiced his profession at a minimal level. After approximately seven years he attempted to resume the use of hypnosis, but each time he found himself seriously blocked psychologically, stumbling for words, becoming confused, and reacting with a brief severe depression at each failure.

He sought therapy in a rather rigid, compulsive way, entering the office, placing a check on the desk, and explaining, "That will pay you for your time. All I want is to have you hypnotize me, remove my block against hypnosis, and send me on my way." Reluctantly, he gave the above information and insisted upon the therapist proceeding forthright with no other preliminaries. He sat rigidly upright in his chair, arms folded across his chest, and stared unblinkingly at the therapist, following every movement made. The suggestion that he lean back and relax elicited the answer, "I'm perfectly relaxed—just go ahead and try to hypnotize me. I've given you a check large enough to pay you for the next two hours of your time."

INITIAL FAILURE AT TRANCE INDUCTION TO DEPOTENTIATE RESISTANCE

Against this background of resolute, insightless resistance the therapist made a seemingly intense effort at hypnotic induction, employing first one and then another induction technique, taking care each time to force issues unduly or to fail to take advantage of any slight yielding to suggestion. Thus, failure of the effect to induce hypnosis was ensured. Now and then, as the therapist continued his efforts, the patient was observed to smile. At the end of two hours' intense effort absolute

---

Unpublished manuscript, 1952–1954. A detailed analysis of the dynamics of the handshake induction is provided in Erickson, Rossi, & Rossi, 1976.

inability to induce a trance was admitted. The patient smiled graciously, reassured the therapist that it did not matter, that he was merely on his way to the Grand Canyon and had stopped in only as an incidental visit to see if he could be hypnotized. Now that he knew this could not be, he would abandon his search for therapy.

A SURPRISE HANDSHAKE INDUCTION

After shaking hands with the patient and bidding him a pleasant trip, it was suggested that he might like to meet the therapist's wife (the office is in the home). He consented, the introduction was made in another room, casual remarks were made about his trip, and he was again bidden farewell. The therapist again shook hands with the patient in a normal, vigorous fashion. However, the hand was withdrawn in a slow, lingering, indefinite fashion that served to fixate the patient's attention completely, to induce a state of catalepsy and a profound somnambulistic trance.* He was immediately led into the office, assured that his purpose in seeking hypnosis had been achieved, and that he should spend the next hour primarily in thinking through and understanding his total life situation, using the therapist merely as a sounding board for ideas.

The patient sat quietly, now and then murmuring inaudibly to himself, now and then asking some simple question pertaining to the therapist's opinion about his future use of hypnosis and his reestablishment of his full practice. Simple reassurances were given.

At the end of the hour the patient was aroused from his trance state, congratulated on his competence as a subject, and asked to keep in touch with the therapist by mail should problems arise in his use of hypnosis in his practice. Then he was again bidden farewell.

Eight years have elapsed. The patient has a full and active practice, is enthusiastic in his use of hypnosis, and has encountered no further difficulties.

* Editor's Note: The effectiveness of this surprise handshake induction was due in part to the fact that his resistance had already been satisfied and thus depotentiated by the earlier ostensible failures at hypnotic induction. The patient was thus permitted to both refuse and accept trance.

49. The Reorganization of Unconscious Thinking without Conscious Awareness: Two Cases with Intellectualized Resistance against Hypnosis

Milton H. Erickson

CASE 1: THE REORGANIZATION OF UNCONSCIOUS THINKING WITHOUT AWARENESS

A 40-year old patient, suffering from a chronic respiratory disease of a progressively disabling character, sought hypnotherapy for long-continued excessive smoking, amounting to three to four packs of cigarettes daily. The explanation was offered by the patient that the smoking was entirely compulsive, that there was no possibility for self-control, and that hypnotherapy had been sought repeatedly without avail. Now, as a final endeavor, hypnotherapy was once more being sought as "a final despairing gesture." This phrase was explained as signifying the patient's absolute conviction that any attempt at hypnosis would fail.

TRANCE INDUCTION WITH AN ASSOCIATIVE NETWORK OF TRUISMS

The therapist silently agreed with the patient, who sat watching every move made with almost pathological intensity. However, the patient demanded that an effort at hypnosis be made and seemed both relieved and disappointed when he did not experience any recognizable hypnotic response after half an hour of systematic trance induction. The patient demanded further effort, but was dissuaded by the therapist, who suggested the following:

1. The patient was to fixate visually upon the corner of a desk clock—"to hold the eyes still."

Unpublished manuscript, 1956.

2. The soft ticking of the clock was to be attended assiduously—"to hold the ears still."

3. Random thoughts, orderly thoughts, systematized thoughts were to be free to wander through the mind freely and spontaneously or even to linger.

4. At all times the patient was to feel wide-awake, alert, and attentive to the adequate performance of the tasks assigned or to be assigned. At any hint of any hypnotic suggestion or attempt to induce a trance, the patient was to give full attention to the therapist and to disrupt thereby the assigned tasks.

5. Although paying attention to the ticking of the clock, there could be any degree of additional auditory awareness of sounds within the office, in the next room, outside the office, in the street, in the skies.

6. There was also to be a constant awareness of the physical self, with attention fluctuating from one part of the body to another, from the feet to the hands or the thighs, to the cloth around the neck, to the hair on the head, and back again with any variation desired.

7. At all times the patient was to feel free to listen consciously to whatever the therapist said, but this, it was explained, was actually unnecessary, since the constantly present unconscious mind would be within hearing distance of the therapist and could listen by itself while the conscious mind busied itself with the clock, with thoughts, with various sounds, and whatever else interested it, including the fluctuations in body awareness.

8. At the close of the interview the eyes and ears would slowly shift their attention from the clock to the therapist.

The patient was most cooperative, obeying instructions excellently. Within five minutes he presented the appearance of a deep trance state. This was tested, after 10 minutes, by laboriously searching the desktop for a manuscript, during the process of which the clock was apparently "thoughtlessly" removed from its position and obscured from the patient's view. This resulted in no visible response on the part of the patient, whose gaze remained fixed and unchanged at the spot where the clock had been. The pupils were noted to be widely dilated, as is frequently the finding in deep hypnosis. Neither was there any apparent awareness of the therapist leaving his seat and wandering aimlessly about the office. Nor did the patient seem aware of a sudden noisy flight of jet planes overhead.

Therapy was accomplished by discussing matter-of-factly the patient's physical needs to discontinue smoking and by raising the question variously of the relative values of smoking, physical health, freedom from compulsion, and peace of mind.

As this discussion was offered, the patient was admonished from time to time to continue fixating on the clock, both auditorily and visually, to entertain any variety of conscious thoughts of interest, to hear and to be aware of whatever was desired, but above all to know that conscious activity was relatively unimportant in the therapeutic situation, that *the only thing of paramount importance was the reorganization of unconscious thinking taking place without conscious awareness.*

The patient was seen for a total of 11 hours over six days in one month. About half that time was spent in futile attempts to "hypnotize me," at the patient's urgent request, and in social chitchat far afield from the problem in hand. The rest of the time was spent in actual therapy essentially as described above. The therapeutic result was the reduction to three postprandial cigarettes and one just before going to bed.

The next month the patient returned with the plea that the remaining cigarette smoking be abolished, since it constituted the "doorstep for the reentry of the old habit." At this time a hesitant request was made several times for the use of hypnosis, but on each occasion the patient was fully as resistant as originally. Each time an apology would be offered, and the suggestion would be made by the patient that resort be had to the clock fixation "because that way I listen better."

The same routine as before was instituted with one exception: the smoking, which had been excessive since puberty, was a secondary matter. Present-day problems pertaining to finances and family matters were brought up for discussion. A total of 16 hours over a period of eight days was spent, about one-fourth in directed chitchat to elicit information and attitudes and the rest of the time as described above, but this time discussing the immediate problems other than smoking, which in five days was discontinued.

Upon the closing of the case, the patient expressed regret at the failure to develop a trance state and wonderment at a marked inability to perceive the passage of time correctly during therapeutic sessions. No request of any sort was made for any explanation of this, although in discussing matters with the patient's "unconscious mind," suggestions were offered that the patient should feel free to request explanation of any item not fully understood.

CASE 2: TRANCE INDUCTION WITH A SURROGATE THERAPIST

Comparable to the foregoing case was that of another patient, also a physician, who telephoned long-distance demanding a specific appointment for hypnotherapy at a specific hour, suggesting that any conflicting appointments already made be canceled. After some discussion an appointment was finally scheduled, but the day before he again tele-phoned long-distance to inquire if the therapist were prepared to abide by the wishes and needs explained over the telephone. A placating answer was offered, and preparations were made for his arrival.

He appeared promptly on time, walked briskly into the office, intro-duced himself, stated that he was a physician, well aware of his own needs, and demanded that he "be hypnotized if you think you can do it" without further history-taking or delay. He sat himself comfortably in the chair, leaned back, cocked his head to one side, smiled in a superior fashion as he folded his arms, and said, "Go ahed."

With equal insistence the therapist demanded a minimum of vital information about him, and the patient reluctantly agreed that he himself would so demand of a patient. When this was completed, the patient commanded, "Now go ahead, and use a dominating technique because I am a dominant personality. Take about 15 mintues. That will tell the story."

For about 15 minutes a strongly authoritarian technique was carefully employed, while the patient smiled condescendingly. After glancing at the clock, the patient ordered, "You might as well keep on for another 15 minutes, even though you are not going to get anywhere."

As predicted, the patient made no response to this approach, nor was one expected. The patient made a few caustic comments and then asked if the therapist knew any method by which hypnosis could be induced.*

Answering affirmatively, the therapist immediately stepped out of the office and returned almost immediately with a young woman. Without further ado she was instructed to develop a somnambulistic trance, which she did promptly. She manifested spontaneously a negative hallucination for the patient, and this was corrected by having her become aware of his presence. She was then instructed to sit quietly in the therapist's chair and, usin a soft gentle technique, induce a profound somnambulistic trance in the patient while the therapist absented himself from the office. Upon his return in about 15 minutes she was to transfer rapport to the therapist and then to leave the office, arousing from the trance imme-diately after her exit.

The therapist returned in about 15 minutes. The patient and the young woman were both in somnambulistic trances. The young woman fulfilled her instructions and departed.

The question of therapy was then taken up with the patient, and in the

---

*Editor's Note: This is another example of how MHE allows a resistant patient to experience his resistance successfully and then allows the patient to respond with the other side of his ambivalence by being successful in experiencing a therapeutic trance. See Paper 48 of this volume.

trance state he was found to be receptive and cooperative; it was possible to arrange with him to let the therapist govern the course of the therapy. Despite the patient's disturbed condition extensive and effective therapy was accomplished, sometimes with and sometimes without the use of hypnosis, as the immediate situation indicated.

IX. Facilitating New Identity

The papers in this section deal with what we may regard as the highest and most complex function of the psychotherapist—facilitating the evolution of new identity and consciousness. The cases discussed herein span 50 years of Erickson's experience in exploring the delicate balances between polar opposites of different psychotherapeutic approaches: *Provoking* and *facilitating, directing* and *nondirecting,* the *authoritarian* and the *permissive.* His approaches range from the apparently gross and professionally questionable technique of having a patient get drunk in order to tell off his overprotective mother, to utilizing the most delicate sensitivities in perceiving the nuances of relationship involved in a case such as that in "The Identification of a Secure Reality" where a foundation is created for the total personality.

This section begins with a series of papers on psychological shock and creative moments as instrumental in precipitating the need for new identity. Psychological shocks can come naturally with the unexpected happenings of everyday life or from those normal developmental stages that are characteristic of the process of personality maturation. When a normal developmental process does not take place because the patient is too fixated at an earlier or less adequate stage, the hypnotherapist may feel the need to administer the shock that tends to break the old frame of reference and thus precipitate a search for new development and identity. Most therapists are wary of administering such shocks. So is Erickson. Because of this the first paper in this section was formulated by the editor to present some views on the safe administration of therapuetic shock leading to problem resolution and new identity.

The major Ericksonian principles of indirect approach and utilization are more or less apparent in all these case examples. More than technique or theoretical principles are involved here, however. Wisdom and a deep appreciation of life processes underlay and enrich the therapeutic principles. Erickson recognizes each case as unique in the creative interplay that emerges between the psyches of therapist and patient.

50. Psychological Shocks and Creative Moments in Psychotherapy

Ernest L. Rossi

During the summer of 1972 Milton H. Erickson was quietly reminiscing over his 50 years of creative experience with hypnosis while Rossi gently probed with a question or two as he maintained the adjustments on his cassette recorder. It soon became evident to our mutual surprise and delight that Erickson was now giving expression to a basic aspect of his work that he had never really emphasized before—psychological shock. Shock could be creatively utilized in psythotherapy (with or without hypnosis) to break up maladaptive attitudes and patterns of behavior so the therapist could help the patient realign his life learnings in a more constructive manner. As Erickson illustrated his views with many case histories from his clinical practice, Rossi gradually began to recognize the necessary relation between psychological shock and the development of creative moments which he recently described as the basic dynamic of change in psychotherapy (Rossi, 1972a). In this paper we will first present a number of cases where Erickson successfully utilized psychological shock; we will then make an effort to describe the psychotherapeutic circumstances necessary for the safe and successful use of psychological shock; we will then outline some of the theoretical issues dealing with psychological shock and creative moments in their relation to hypnotherapy.

CASE 1

A 30-year-old university professor attended a university dance and saw a 30-year-old single woman on the other side of the room. She saw him, and they rapidly gravitated toward each other. Within a month they had planned their future and were married. Three years later they appeared in

This paper was written by the editor who expresses his appreciation to Milton H. Erickson for providing the case material and inspiring the discussion of its theoretical issues. He and his wife, Elizabeth Erickson, have generously contributed time, effort and editorial experience in its preparation. Reprinted with permission from *The American Journal of Clinical Hypnosis* July, 1973, *16*, 9–22.

Erickson's office and told their sad story. In telling it they were extremely prudish and embarrassed, and they used a most stilted and formal wording. In essence their complaint was that even before marriage they had planned to have a family, and because of the fact that they were each 30 years old, they felt that there should be no delay of any sort. But after three years they were childless despite medical examinations and advice. They were both present in the office, and in telling the author their problems, the man said:

> In my thinking and that of my wife we have reached the conclusion that it is more proper that I give voice to our trouble in common and state it succinctly. Our problem is most distressing and destructive of our marriage. Because of our desire for children we have engaged in the marital union with full physiological concomitants each night and morning for procreative purposes. On Sundays and holidays we have engaged in the marital union with full physiological concomitants for procreative purposes as much as four times a day. We have not permitted physical disability to interfere. As a result of the frustration of our philoprogenitive desires, the marital union has become progressively unpleasant for us, but it has not interfered with our efforts at procreation; but it does distress both of us to discover our increasing impatience with each other. For this reason we are seeking your aid, since other medical aid has failed.

At this point Erickson interrupted and said to the man, "You have stated the problem. I would like to have you remain silent and have your wife state the opinion in her own words." In almost exactly the same way and with even greater embarrassment than her husband had shown, the wife voiced their complaint. Erickson said, "I can correct this for you but it will involve shock therapy. It will not be electric shock or physical shock, but it will be a matter of psychological shock. I will leave you alone in the office for 15 minutes so that the two of you can exchange views and opinions about your willingness to receive a rather severe psychological shock. At the end of 15 minutes I will come back into the office and ask your decision and abide by it."

Erickson left the office and returned 15 minutes later and said, "Give me your answer." The man said, "We have discussed the matter both objectively and subjectively, and we have reached the conclusion that we will endure anything that might possibly offer satisfaction for our philoprogenitive desires."

Erickson asked the wife, "Do you agree fully?" She answered, "I do, sir."

The author explained that the shock would be psychological, involve their emotions, and be a definite strain upon them.

> It will be rather simple to administer, but you will both be exceedingly shocked psychologically. I suggest that as you sit there in your chairs, you reach down under the sides of your chairs and hang tightly to the bottom of the chair and listen well to what I say. After I have said it, and as I am administering the shock, I want the two of you to maintain an absolute silence. Within a few minutes you will be able to leave the office and return to your home 40 miles from here. I want the two of you to maintain an absolute silence all the way home, and during that silence you will discover a multitude of thoughts rushing through your minds. Upon reaching home you will maintain silence until after you have entered the house and closed the door. You will then be free! Now hang tightly to the bottom of your chairs because I am now going to give you the psychological shock. It is this: For three long years you have engaged in the marital union with full physiological concomitants for procreative purposes at least twice a day and sometimes as much as four times in 24 hours, and you have met with defeat of your philoprogenitive drive. *Now why in hell don't you f—— for fun and pray to the devil that she isn't knocked up for at least three months. Now please leave.*

As was learned later, they maintained silence all the way home thinking, "many things." When they finally got inside the house with the door shut, it was explained, "We found we couldn't wait to get to the bedroom. We just dropped to the floor and we didn't engage in the marital union. We had fun, and now the three months are barely up and my wife is pregnant." Nine months later a baby girl was born. When Erickson called on them to see the baby, he learned that formal speech and polysyllabic words and highly proper phrases were no longer necessary in their conversations. They could even tell risque stories.

This case history was related in full to an audience of over 70 practicing psychiatrists at Columbia University at the request of Doctor Herbert Spiegel. Preliminary to narration of the case history, Doctor Spiegel and Erickson had been discussing the ingrained attitudes of inhibitions for what are so-called Anglo-Saxon words, and the audience was asked if they thought that they could endure listening to the author make use of such words in relation to a psychiatric problem. The audience and Doctor Spiegel were certain they could, and Erickson also felt that they could. However, to the utter astonishment of Erickson, at the utterance of the key word he noted that the entire audience actually froze into rigid immobility for a few moments. Doctor Spiegel was noted to catch his breath, and Erickson noted that his own tone of voice very definitely changed. This was most revealing about the long-continued effects of the learned inhibitions of childhood and their continuance into adult life.

In Erickson's opinion the 40-mile drive in absolute silence made possible, in accord with the suggestions given them, a great variety of much repressed thinking which ran riot in their minds. This resulted in their sexual activity immediately upon closing the door when they reached home. This was what Erickson had hoped. When the couple were questioned about this, they stated that they believed that there had been an increasingly greater build-up of erotic thinking the nearer they got to their home, but they stated that they had no specific memories.

CASE 2

Erickson: A soldier in Yuma courted a Spanish-American girl whose mother was widowed while the girl was still very young. She had been escorted to grade school and high school by two maiden aunts and then escorted home again every day. They went to every child's party, every school party, every high school outing, football game, what have you. They went with her when she applied for a job as secretary. They took her to work, called for her at noon, took her out to lunch, escorted her home in the evening. At some football game this soldier stationed in Yuma was attracted to the girl. The two old maids went on every date. Somehow or other he proposed to her, properly and in the presence of the old maids. She promised to marry him, and he was allowed to kiss her once. She promised to marry him in June. In June she promised to marry him in July. In July she promised to marry him in August. That went on for 48 months—continuous delays.

Then the family physician called me up and said "I can't do anything with this girl." The girl had been escorted to the family physician's office and was properly chaperoned when the physician examined her. He called me when they left, "Would you take her?" I said, "Yes." So her mother and the two maiden aunts came with her on the bus to my office. They were horrified when I wouldn't let them come into the office with her. The mother and two aunts were forced to sit outside the door so I could see the girl alone. The girl told me the situation. I asked her if she wanted to marry the boy. She did. That was in June. The first of July she got a letter from him saying, "We're going to be married this month or I'm going to get another girl." She was most tearful. So I asked her, "Are you sure you want to marry that boy? Are you really, really sure?" She was. I told her "I can help you, there's only one thing you have to do—come from your home to my office alone. I know you're afraid to ride on the bus alone, you're afraid to ride in a car without your aunts, you're afraid to ride on the train without your aunts, but you come from Yuma, alone.

"Now, I don't care where you do it. You can do it in Yuma or in Phoenix: you buy a pair of short, short pants and come into my office wearing them, and when you come into the office, you are going to do exactly what I tell you to do. Absolutely, exactly, without protest without question. You'll silently do what I tell you to do. You'll think it over for a long, long time, and do you know, you're going to do it, you'll say 'I will, I absolutely will.'"

On her next appointment I had Mrs. Erickson in the office. Mrs. Erickson didn't know what I was going to do. The girl came in and sat down in a chair, I introduced her to Mrs. Erickson. I told the girl to just stand there, facing me, hands to her sides. "Now look straight ahead . . . take off your left shoe . . . your right one . . . take off your left stocking . . . your right stocking . . . take off your shorts . . . take off your blouse . . . take off your bra . . . take off your panties . . . point to your right nipple . . . your right breast . . . your left nipple . . . your left breast . . . your belly button . . . your pubic genital area . . . turn around, point to your right buttock . . . your left buttock . . . turn around, face me, tell me if you have a beautiful body. . . . All right, you do have a beautiful body. You may dress. Before you marry that man you'll board the train and go back to Yuma alone. You will tell your mother that you are getting married, and you will tell your mother what kind of wedding cake you want. You will tell your mother who the guests will be and you will tell your mother that if she thinks otherwise, you are going to be married by a justice of the peace (a terrible threat since they were Catholics)."

That was the beginning of July. She married on July 17th. She sent me a Christmas card in December with a picture of herself and her husband. The next year, she sent me a picture of her first child and Christmas cards on the following years announcing her second and third child. A few years later she brought the family with three children in to see me.

Rossi: Okay, how did that case work? Was shock involved?

Erickson: Could there be anything worse than undressing before your doctor in the presence of his wife and pointing to your nipples and your breasts and your belly button?

Rossi: She was never in a trance?

Erickson: No.

Rossi: Except what the situation might have induced.

Erickson: That's right, except for what the situation induced.

Rossi: There might have been an altered state of awareness that arose spontaneously due to the shock situation she was in. So what you did was to break through tremendous inhibitions.

Erickson: Great inhibitions—nothing worse ever happened to her.

Rossi: Having forced those responses, you broke through the lifelong pattern of conditioned inhibition of having those aunts around and so forth.

Erickson: Yes, it disrupted the rigidity that governed her entire life. Just as the first break in the shell pecked by a newly emerging chick immediately shatters the whole shell, so her whole life opened up. I just gave her simple statements. You do this, do that, no questions, just do it silently.

Rossi: And those simple statements, that you point to your breasts, your genitalia and so forth, what were those statements designed to do?

Erickson: To break her inhibitions, really break them! Notice how I engineered that: first the left shoe, then the right, the left stocking, and then the right. I carefully built up a momentum of an affirmative character so she finally took off all her clothes and followed all my suggestions designed to shatter her lifelong inhibitions. I made her promise to do everything. Anyone like that who gives a promise. . . .

Rossi: Ah, that's how you had her caught in a double-bind, so to speak. I notice that before you do this shock type therapy, you demand a promise of obedience, do you not? And the patient has to have a mental structure, I suppose, where they are going to go along with you. They are the kind of people who will keep a promise, and you capitalize on that. A psychopath you could not do this with.

Erickson: I can't imagine doing it with a psychopath, I wouldn't even try.

Rossi: It would have to be some who had a lot of . . .

Erickson: . . . Innate honesty.

Rossi: It occurs to me, was this therapy a symbolic rape?

Erickson: It was a rape.

Rossi: Did you think of it that way when you were planning it, as a symbolic rape?

Erickson: I did, it was a psychological rape.

CASE 3

Erickson: A professional man and his wife consulted me. He began by saying that they have been married 12 years. "We have a daughter, but apparently we are not going to have another child. This is the way we go to bed. I have to go to the bedroom, shut the door, undress, put on my pajamas. Get into bed then call my wife. She comes, turns out the bedroom light, all of the lights. Then first she draws the shades, and then the drapes over every window. She checks the doors, to make certain they're locked, the windows are locked. She turns out all the lights. She goes into the guest room and she undresses there, in the dark. She puts on her nightgown. Then she comes through the darkened hall into the dark bedroom and she gets into bed with me. I can have sex relations with her, I can even take her nightgown off, but the lights cannot be turned on. She will not allow me to see her nude."

I then said to her, "You've had one child, the lights were on and your nude body was seen by your obstetrician and nurses, and you're still alive. Now your husband wants this corrected."

She said, "But I can't do what he asks, I just can't let him see my body."

I said, "Well, that's your statement, 'I can't do it.' Now your husband is six foot two, weighs 210 pounds, able-bodied. I have a bad limp. I'm five foot six, weight 150 pounds. There's no question that I'm outmatched physically by your husband. I want you to sit quietly in that chair. Your husband's going to make you sit there. I can tell you and I mean it, you sit there. Now I'm going to do something to you, and I want your husband to watch." At that time the style of the skirts was down to mid-calf length. "Now I'm going to start moving your skirt a little bit over your thighs, I'll stop moving them only when you are in a deep trance. And you'll listen to me. And you'll not say you can't." Half an inch at a time I slowly began lifting her skirt. This was an unendurable thing for her to be aware of consciously, therefore her only escape was to go into a trance. She was aware of my use of hypnosis, since I had treated a friend of hers.

Rossi: Now this was setting up a double-bind, going into a trance that way.

Erickson: Yes. I slowly lifted her skirt, up and up past the knee. She was just looking at her skirt and my face.

Rossi: Yes, she went into a trance.

Erickson: "Now you're in a deep trance. I don't know why you've been having this foolish undesirable behavior for 12 long years, more than 12 long years, actually 13 years, before your daughter was born. But I want you to understand that you're going to change things. You'll not do it all at once. I'm not going to ask you to do it in my presence or your husband's presence. Each day at home, after your daughter's gone to school, and you're alone in the house, I want you to look in every mirror in the house. [A house is a woman's castle, her own protected territory in which she could feel free to experiment.] And look at that woman and wonder what she looks like, and I want you to discover bit by bit what she looks like in the nude, completely in the nude. Take off her clothes bit by bit. First the shoes, then the stockings, then the dress and the slip. The bra, the pants. Then I want you to dance. You will dance as a child, a ballet dance. You did ballet dancing in college. You'll enjoy dancing. You must within six months, perhaps after three months, undress in the guest room, in the dark, then walk into the bedroom, turn on the lights, and do a ballet dance for your husband in the nude.

Rossi: This was all said while she was in that trance state and her husband was present?

Erickson: Her husband was present. She could effect the cure at the right time at her own speed.

Rossi: Yes, very important that you allowed her unconscious to do it at its own rate.

Erickson: Its own rate, its own fashion. First the shoes, then the stockings. Or she'd take off her slip first or she'd take off her bra and her dress first, it didn't make a bit of difference to me.

Rossi: Right, this is all the freedom that you gave her.

Erickson: I placed the limit of within six months, and I offered her a period of three months to experiment by herself. This establishes the illusion of freedom of choice.

Rossi: Setting these definite time parameters within which she could have all the freedom she needed.

Erickson: You can imagine her husband's delight when she pranced in her bedroom, switched on the light, did the ballet dance for him in the nude.

Rossi: He must have been happy. So with that happening, presumably she was over her inhibition.

Erickson: Yes, and how! Now there's one thing I had said to her, "If you don't do it, your husband will bring you back here and you will do a nude dance for me in your husband's presence."

Rossi: It was going to be worse if she didn't do it for her husband since she'd have to do it for you too. So again you set up a double-bind. It was going to be harder if she didn't do it alone for her husband, so you gave her the easy way out.

Erickson: A very easy way out.

Rossi: You use a carrot but you use a whip too, don't you?

Erickson: There's iron under my velvet gloves.

Rossi: I'm becoming more and more impressed with that.

Erickson: Now, why should I investigate her past? The parental influence on her, her father's, her mother's, her teachers'. Why should I do anything at all by way of going deeply into her personal history? Therapy is often a matter of tipping the first domino. All that was needed was the correction of one behavior, and if that one behavior was corrected . . .

Rossi: All the other inhibitions topple like dominoes.

Erickson: Yes, we have a domino situation.

Rossi: Yes, perhaps the early analyst had to go back into a patient's history to learn psychoanalysis, to learn how those inhibitions were built up. But since we know all that, you don't have to go into it with each patient.

Erickson: It's so ridiculous to pore over what you did when you were five years old because it belongs to the unchangeable past and any present understandings of that are different than that of the five-year-old. The adult level of understanding precludes any real understanding of the child's or adolescent's world.

CASE 4

Erickson: Another shock case. This is such a beautiful one. Mary and Eve had been grade school and high school friends. They both married high school friends, and the two men were also high school friends. They both told me they confided everything to each other, and they both confided that they had to get a divorce. Each said her husband was a pervert, but neither admitted, neither dared to tell the other just what the perversion was. So in separate interviews I asked each girl to describe her husband's perversion to me. Mary said when a man and a woman have intercourse, a man's legs are between the woman's legs. And her husband always wanted to keep his legs outside her legs. Now when I later interviewd Eve, she said the exact reverse. She felt it was normal for the man to have his legs outside the woman's, but her husband perversely wanted to keep his legs between hers. I saw both girls at four o'clock on successive days. I told them not to tell each other what I had said or what they told me. And then the third day I had them come together for a joint interview. By this time they both had time to build up a lot of inner turmoil and emotion. I told them, "When one of you speaks to me, the other just listens and says nothing (this silence was to build up even more emotion)." Then as one told her story, the other would just listen to her. First Eve told about her husband insisting on keeping his legs between her legs. And then Mary told the reverse story. Their mutual horror is imaginable. Then I summarized how they both told their story and listened to each other most attentively in silence. Now they were to drive home together maintaining their silence all the way. "Now when you get home you will both have the urge to ask the other, what the hell is wrong with you?"

Rossi: I see, they had to be silent on the way home, so it would build up within their minds. . . .

Erickson: It would build up: what in the hell is wrong with you! They both had to say that to the other. Then they could talk. Think of the horrible buildup!

Rossi: Again, building up that tension to be discharged in a new way.

Erickson: Each had intercourse that night both ways and both enjoyed it.

Rossi: Fantastic. So here's another shock therapy involving a sexual problem, a sexual inhibition.

Erickson: It was more than a sexual inhibition. It was based on an insufficient awareness of human behavior.

Rossi: I see. That was their inhibition—a lack of awareness of the broad range of human behavior.

Erickson: Yes, and a rigid idea.

Rossi: Yes, so that's what shock therapy does. It breaks through rigid ideas.

Erickson: Rigid ideas they couldn't break. And when I shattered that rigid idea, it shattered the hell out of them. It even led them to try other positions. I hadn't told them there were other positions, they started investigating other positions on their own.

Rossi: Once you broke their rigid idea of only one set position. . . .

Erickson: It altered the place they could go for pleasure. It was a breakdown of a narrow, limited, restricted life existence. You can't be rigid in one area alone; it always spreads.

Rossi: So again, it's not mere behavior you're changing, but a whole existence.

Erickson: And you pick whatever lock is presented to you.

Rossi: I see, so this is as much existential therapy as behavior therapy or hypnotherapy. It's the total existence that you. . . .

Erickson: It's an old thesis.

Rossi: You pick whatever lock is presented to you.

Erickson: And once one lock is picked, all the other locks become vulnerable. [Erickson now elaborates many examples in the history of science where great advances were made by one man breaking through the inhibiting preconceptions of others.] Throughout history there has been a lot of shock therapy.

Rossi: Perhaps the whole history of innovation is shock therapy. Every scientific innovation is a shock therapy.

CASE 5

Erickson: American Jews aren't always orthodox—in fact, many Jews aren't. But this is the case of a very orthodox Jewish girl who came from a European family that observed all the most elaborate rules about food. They left Germany because they realized that Hitler boded no good for the Jews. Her father had to sell out all his belongings at a great loss. So great a loss that it shattered their former life-style, and this shattering permitted them to change. They took on the break that Hitler forced upon them and made it their own by breaking former traditions. They thus gave up bitterness and gave themselves a chance for happiness in America. This allowed them to encourage their daughter to change. Her parents were older and knew they could not change, but they encouraged the girl to adopt more liberal views so she could marry an American doctor who had proposed to her. He had insisted on a more liberal home. She said, "I want to marry him but I'm kosher." I said to her, "You are no longer German Jews, you're going to be an American citizen, you've already applied for your first papers. You're in love with an American Jew. He's a doctor who knows his business. He's got my respect. But he likes bacon and ham and he doesn't believe in two sets of kitchen utensils. I want you to eat a ham sandwich right now."

Rossi: You said this directly to her just like that!

Erickson: I told her to go across the street and get a ham sandwich, have the man wrap it and bring it to my office. You'll slowly unwrap it, first bite, the second, the third. . . . You won't believe you can possibly eat it, but I've never seen a persson die so I'll be glad to watch you eat it and die while you are eating it. Now there is nothing colder and harder than watching a person die. The fact that she doesn't die even though I said I would watch her die forces her to face the complete absurdity of the idea. The inhibition was shattered by a reductio ad absurdum. Can you imagine how she ate that sandwich?

Rossi: You tell me—a lot of inhibition, I suppose, or could it possibly have been with relish?

Erickson: With tension and fear. I watched her closely with a straight face. When she was half through with the sandwich, I said, "Wouldn't it be pure hell if you found the sandwich tasty?" She is now happily married.

Rossi: Again the shock was used to shatter lifelong inhibitions by forcing her, right there in your presence . . .

Erickson: No. I'm not forcing her. I'm watching her die, but she is eating the sandwich. The burden is on her for eating the sandwich.

Rossi: Oh, I see. The burden for the critical behavior change is always on the patient. You know, this begins to sound a little like some of the behavioristic techniques of helping a person to overcome a phobia by accompanying them on a certain journey . . . to a height, for example. Do you see a relation?

Erickson: Well, Wolpe says its behavioristic. But I think its more experiential.

Rossi: I see, it's their experience that's the important thing.

Erickson: Yes, and I'm definitely on the outside.

Rossi: How do you mean, you're on the outside?

Erickson: I'm just watching her eat, and she is eating so I can watch her die.

Rossi: Yes, and it's not the mere behavior of eating, but the whole experience, all of her inhibitions, all her lifetime associations, these are the things that are being broken. It's not the mere behavioristic act of putting ham in her mouth.

Erickson: Yes, you have expressed that quite well; it's the total experience.

CONDITIONS FOR THE SAFE UTILIZATION OF PSYCHOLOGICAL SHOCK

So unusual and obviously risk-laden are these examples of psychological shock therapy that the average, responsible therapist may feel inclined to throw up his hands and silently decide to leave this approach to a few master therapists who somehow know how to handle it. A careful review of Erickson's work, however, does reveal a number of conditions that appear again and again in many different guises when he illustrates the successful use of psychological shock. They may be summarized as follows:

1. Psychologically Binding Conditions

The most important condition for the safe and effective use of shock is that patient and therapist are bound together in therapeutic encounter by powerful psychological forces. C. G. Jung (1953) has used the ancient concept of the *temenos* (sacred precinct) to describe the psychologically binding conditions that are necessary to contain a conflict in order to permit a safe personality transformation to take place without the person being shattered by internal chaos or extraneous external circumstances. On a cultural-anthropological level, for example, the psychological shock and pain that is a regular feature of many initiation rites designed to promote personality change is safely contained in the *temenos* of the belief-system adhered to by initiators and initiates. In modern psychotherapy it is the *transference* or the *prestige* of the therapist that binds patients to the conflict-laden task of change. In its simplist form Erickson actually sets up morally binding conditions where he demands obedience when he knows he can get it. This is most clearly illustrated in Case 2, when he demands of the virginal girl, "Absolutely, exactly, without protest, without question, you'll silently do what I tell you to do." In cases 1, 3, and 4 the *temenos* contained husband and wife or friends who were required to interact in such a manner that their rigidly maladaptive patterns were shattered so something new could happen.

2. Protecting the Patient

Implied in the above is that the patient must be protected at all times. In Case 2 Mrs. Erickson was present as a chaperone during a critically important nude encounter; in cases 1 and 3 a spouse was present. Far more subtle is the protection that must be provided for the deeper levels of personality. Although Erickson admits, "There's iron under my velvet gloves," he makes an obvious effort to be scrupulously circumspect in respecting the patient's dignity. Erickson has previously described this need to protect the subject in his discussion of deep hypnosis and its induction (1967a).

3. A Central, Strategic Issue Is Dealt With

In his discussion of the domino situation in Case 3, Erickson makes it clear that psychological shock is to be used to jolt the basic crux of the patient's problem. Once a crucial behavior is actualized (eating a ham sandwich in Case 5), a rigid belief shattered (the "perversions" of the girls in Case 4), it is *suddenly* possible for many behaviors, attitudes, and inner experiences to change. Erickson reiterates this view with his lock analogy in Case 4—"And once one lock is picked, all the other locks become vulnerable."

4. Tension Is Kept High

Tension is not a mere epiphenomenon in psychological shock therapy. Erickson frequently sets up circumstances where tension will build in the therapeutic situation so that energy can suddenly be discharged in more desired channels. The clearest example of this is in Case 1 where Erickson (a) gives a psychologically weighty forewarning to the couple that he is going to use "shock," (b) allows the tension of that forewarning to build as he deliberately leaves the therapy room so the couple can privately discuss whether they want to take the "risk" involved, (c) tells them to hold on to the seat of their chairs as he is about to deliver his shock, and (d) most importantly he demands that they remain silent all the way home after he delivers his shock, so it will not be dissipated by needless intellectual discussion. In particular this maneuver of demanding *silence* during certain crucial periods is a way of building and maintaining optimal therapeutic tension (as well as *fixing the patient's attention*) very frequently used by Erickson.

5. Changing Behavior by Setting Definite Time Limits

Therapy is obviously doing as well as understanding. A certain amount of therapeutic acumen is needed to determine whether a patient is ready for immediate behavior change (as in Case 5, where the Jewish girl's orthodox parents had already encouraged her toward more liberal attitudes, so Erickson recognized she was probably ripe for the immediate behavior change of eating a ham sandwich) or a more leisurely pace of inner growth and transformation. In Case 3, where Erickson recognized it was going to take more time to radically change a lifelong attitude of prudishness, he (a) carefully set time parameters (between three and six months) within which the desired change was to take place, (b) carefully protected the patient by allowing her to experiment with nudity by herself at first, and (c) helped her to make the desired change by associating the difficult problem of nudity with her skill and joy in dancing. The setting of definite time parameters for psychotherapeutic change may be something more than borrowing a leaf from Otto Rank's time-limited approach to therapy: Time is required for the actual process of psychotherapeutic transformation, to which we will now turn our attention.

PSYCHOLOGICAL SHOCK AND CREATIVE MOMENTS IN HYPNOTHERAPY

Rossi (1972a) recently described *creative moments* in therapy as follows:

> But what is a creative moment? Such moments have been celebrated as the exciting "hunch" by scientific workers and "inspiration" by people in the arts (Barron, 1969). *A creative moment occurs when a habitual pattern of association is interrupted;* there may be a "spontaneous" lapse or relaxation of one's habitual associative process; there may be a *psychic shock,* an overwhelming sensory or emotional experience; a psychedelic drug, a toxic condition or sensory deprivation; yoga, Zen, spiritual and meditative exercises may likewise interrupt our habitual associations and introduce a momentary void in awareness. In that fraction of a second when the habitual contents of awareness are knocked out there is a chance for pure awareness, "the pure light of the void" (Evans-Wentz, 1960) to shine through. This fraction of a second may be experienced as a "mystic state," satori, a peak experience or an altered state of

consciousness (Tart, 1969). It may be experienced as a moment of "fascination" or "falling in love," when the gap in one's awareness is filled by the *new* that suddenly intrudes itself.

The creative moment is thus a gap in one's habitual pattern of awareness. Bartlett (1958) has described how the genesis of original thinking can be understood as the filling in of mental gaps. *The new that appears in creative moments is thus the basic unit of original thought and insight as well as personality change.* Experiencing a creative moment may be the phenomenological correlate of a critical change in the molecular structure of proteins within the brain associated with learning (Gaito, 1972) or the creation of new cell assemblies and phase sequences (Hebb, 1963.)

The relation between psychological shock and creative moments is apparent: A "psychic shock" interrupts a person's habitual associations so that something new may appear. Ideally, psychological shock sets up the conditions for a creative moment when a new insight, attitude, or behavior change may take place in the subject. Erickson (1948) has also described hypnotic trance itself as a special psychological state which effects a similar break in the patient's conscious and habitual associations so that creative learning can take place as follows (italics are ours):

> The induction and maintenance of a trance serve to provide a *special psychological state in which the patient can reassociate and reorganize his inner psychological complexities* and utilize his own capacities in a manner in accord with his own experiential life . . . therapy results from an *inner resynthesis* of the patient's behavior achieved by the patient himself. It's true that direct suggestion can effect an alteration in the patient's behavior and result in a symptomatic cure, at least temporarily. However, such a "cure" is simply a response to suggestion and does not entail that reassociation and reorganization of ideas, understandings and memories so essential for actual cure. *It is this experience of reassociating and reorganizing his own experiential life that eventuates in a cure,* not the manifestation of responsive behavior which can, at best, satisfy only the observer.

Fine examples of this "reorganization" and "inner resynthesis" were later provided in Erickson's paper, "Pseudo-orientation in time as a hypnotherapeutic procedure" (1967b), wherein he illustrates the approach of allowing the patient's unconscious, while in a trance state, to creatively fantasize its own solutions to problems. Erickson describes this approach as follows:

Unconscious fantasies, however, belong to another category of psychological functioning. They are not accomplishments complete in themselves, nor are they apart from reality. Rather, they are psychological constructs in various degress of formulation for which the unconscious stands ready, or is actually awaiting an opportunity, to make a part of reality. They are not significant merely as wishful desire but rather of actual intention at the opportune time. . . .

In these case histories, extensive emphasis was placed upon fantasies concerning the future, and every effort was made to keep them unconscious by prohibitive and inhibitive suggestions. By so doing, each patient's unconscious was provided with a wealth of formulated ideas unknown to the conscious mind. Then, in response to the innate needs and desires of the total personality, the unconscious could utilize those ideas by translating them into realities of daily life as spontaneous responsive behavior in opportune situations. (1967b)

This approach is very different from the older more traditional hypnotherapeutic approach of simply telling the patient, while in the trance state, exactly in *what* way and frequently *how* the patient's attitudes, beliefs, and behavior are to change. This more traditional approach of directly programming the patient is in sharp contrast with Erickson's facilitation of new learning by allowing patients to *create their own solutions* in their own way and usually in their own good time.

But what, now, is the essence of Erickson's approach of allowing patients to create their own solutions? The author expected Erickson to agree that patients are actually synthesizing new psychic structures—(the phenomenological correlates of molecular change in the brain (Rossi, 1972a,b)—when they are involved with their "unconscious fantasies" during the trance state where emphasis is placed upon their future hopes. Erickson, however, tends to demur over such an interpretation. He emphasizes that in the ideal psychotherapeutic situation the therapist does not add anything new to the patient but simply helps the patient rearrange and more constructively utilize *past* learnings. He does acknowledge that this rearrangement may involve the synthesis of new associative connections, however.

This issue may be illustrated by utilizing Osgood's (1957) type of diagram of the semantic relation between complexes of meanings. In Figure 1 a circle represents a meaning-complex, while lines represent the links relating the various meaning-complexes together. In Erickson's shock approach a central neurotic complex (represented, for example, by a neurotic inhibition, behavior, or attitude) is shattered (Stage 2 in Figure 1), so its related meaning-complexes are free to rearrange themeselves in another more constructive manner (Stage 3a). A more encompassing view of hypnosynthesis (Conn, 1971) might represent the final situation as 3b, where a newly synthesized meaning-complex replaces the shattered central neurotic complex, permitting a better realignment as illustrated.

Apart from the patients cited above in his paper on pseudo-orientation in time (1967b), Erickson has recently described a unique situation in which he appears to have fostered the development of new personality structures (newly synthesized meaning-complexes) in the case of the "February Man" which is presented as the last article in this volume (see also Erickson & Rossi, 1979). In brief, this was the case of a young woman who had grown up in a materially rich but emotionally impoverished milieu such that she was afraid to have children lest they have a childhood as "miserable and lonely" as her own. In a series of interviews Erickson used hypnosis to regress her to earlier age levels (4 or 5 to 14) during which she fully experienced and enjoyed delightful conversations with Erickson playing the part of a friendly and warm-hearted "February Man." Her experiences with the February Man soon came to embody all the happy and warm feeling and associations she had missed in her actual childhood. An amnesia was maintained for all these trance experiences, so that as therapy continued, the patient in the ordinary waking state began showing less and less concern about her possible inadequacy as a mother, and repeatedly asked Erickson what he was doing with her in the trance state to give her a feeling of confidence that she would know how to share things properly with children of all ages. Although Erickson is more modest in assessing his work in this case, this author feels it to be of great significance, since it appears so clearly to illustrate psychotherapy as involving the synthesis of new psychic structures rather than a mere restructuring of old material. The author (1972a) has recently presented in great detail a number of unusually revealing examples of the spontaneous synthesis of new personality structures in series of dreams.

This, then is a basic issue which future research and practice must resolve: Is hypnotherapy (and psychotherapy, in general) to be concerned with the actual synthesis of new psychic (and behavioral) structures, or is it basically dealing with the creative reutilization of previous learnings? It is easy enough to acknowledge that both are probably involved in practical work, but the future development of both theory and practice may be greatly accelerated by clarifying just when and exactly how each are used.

Stage 1: Central Neurotic Complex
(N.C.)

Stage 2: Shattered
Neurotic Complex

Stage 3a: Newly Synthesized Connections

Stage 3b: Newly Synthesized Meaning-Complex

Figure 1. An outline of shock therapy (Stage 2) and creative moments (Stages 3a and b) involving the synthesis of new connections (Stage 3a) and/or a new meaning-complex (Stage 3b).

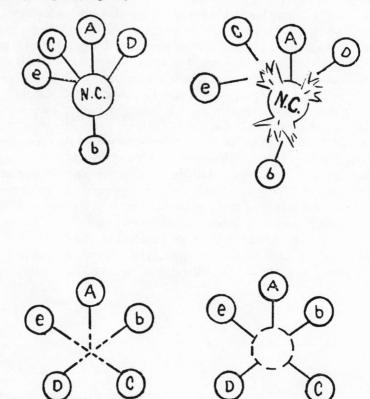

51. Facilitating a New Cosmetic Frame of Reference

Milton H. Erickson

A sophomore in college, majoring in home economics, sought therapy because of "awful inferiority feelings" that seriously restricted and hampered her daily adjustments. The essential facts of her history were few and easily understandable. She had experienced no personality difficulties until the onset of puberty. At that time, during a pleasure drive in the family automobile, an accident had caused her to be thrown out of the car. The only injury she had suffered was a "gashing of the right side of my mouth, which caused awful scarring. That's why I keep the right side of my mouth covered with my hand, or I turn my head away so that you can't see that side of my face." This mannerism had been noted as constantly present. She was unwilling to exhibit the scar to the writer, insisting that it would "disgust" him if he were to see it.

Additional inquiry disclosed that, although she was right-handed, she had learned to eat left-handedly in order to keep the scar covered while eating. Only in the family circle would she briefly discontinue her hiding behavior. She tolerated no mention of her disfigurement, however, by anyone. On the street, in social gatherings, or in the classroom she kept the right side of her mouth covered. She had escaped physical education in high school and college by means of a medical excuse from the family physician.

Because of her need to hide the scar, she was handicapped in numerous other ways. She could not drive a car because that would leave her face uncovered. Neither could she swim except in privacy. Everything she did was governed by her compulsive need to keep the right side of her mouth covered by either her left or her right hand. Even her association with men was markedly limited, despite her actual attractiveness. In fact, her social engagements with men were limited to walking on the man's right side in the dark. On such walks she would not smoke, although she enjoyed smoking, for fear that the glowing of the cigarette would light up her face. However, she would permit kissing, which she enjoyed very much, providing the darkness was deep enough.

Many efforts had been made to have her wear special cosmetics, since

Unpublished manuscript, 1927

she was "so sensitive about a little scar." This she refused to do; why, she did not know. On her own initiative she had visited a number of plastic surgeons, since her parents had "always taken a completely unreasonable attitude" about the scar. However, all three plastic surgeons had taken "the same unreasonable and unsympathetic attitude my parents took." The result was that she had intensely hostile feelings toward the medical profession.

The rest of her history was not indicative of any other problems, although it illustrated many more of her handicaps in daily behavior. Essentially, her situation was that of a young girl with one arm paralyzed and held in an awkward position covering her scar. Her object in seeking therapy was to learn how to adjust to her handicap without correcting her behavior. She was not receptive to any ideas about the possibility of altering her understandings about the "awful scar."

Not until the third interview would she permit the writer to see the scar. It was examined at great length but without comment. Finally, her extreme tension was relieved by telling her that she might again cover it with her hand and keep it covered.

CONCRETE DISPLACEMENT OF SYMPTOM

During the taking of her history it had been learned that she had considerable talent in sketching, in which she took a great deal of pride. Accordingly, she was given the assignment of going home and, in the privacy of her room, making a life-size sketch of her face, showing the exact position, shape, and size of the scar. This was to be done with every possible attention to the minutest details, and the sketch was to be "true to life and scientifically accurate."

When she succeeded in producing a sketch that she was confident was "accurate and true," she was to bring it to the writer. If she wished, she could bring it in a sealed envelope that would not be opened until she was sure that she was willing for the writer to examine it. She spent the rest of that day and a good share of the night perfecting the sketch, which she brought to the writer in a large, unsealed manila envelope. Since she expressed full willingness, a hasty glance was taken at the sketch, and it was then replaced in the envelope and filed in her case history folder. It was noted that she still kept the scar hidden but that she was much less tense and anxious. Instead, she appeared much bewildered and puzzled.

R: Her "bewildered and puzzled" state indicates that her previous attitude of fixed attention on her "ugly scar" was now depotentiated to some extent. It seems possible that the sketching of her self-portrait with the scar in detail has effected a concrete displacement of her symptom onto the picture so that she is left with a gap that leads to her puzzlement.

She is now more open and available for an inner search on an unconscious level during trance to find another frame of reference or understanding to fill that gap.*

TRANCE INDUCTION AND POSTHYPNOTIC SUGGESTION

She had previously refused to permit hypnosis, but she now readily accepted the suggestion that a trance should be induced so that she could be given a new, different, and unrelated assignment. A fairly deep trance was readily induced, during which she kept her left hand over the scar. Her next assignment, she was told, was twofold. She was to visit the college library, consult her mother, inquire of fashion experts, or consult any possible source she could discover to learn everything possible about the old-time practice of applying "beauty patches." This done, she was to make a series of sketches of women's faces showing the various shapes and locations of beauty patches. All of this was to be done in the waking state, but with no conscious awareness of why she was doing it. Nevertheless, she should know that she was doing it and wonder why. When the task was comprehensively done, she would decide to show the sketches to the writer. Each sketch would be similar to the self-portrait she had executed, and each would illustrate the use of a single beauty patch. She was then awakened with an amnesia for the trance events.

R: It was important that an amnesia be maintained for your suggestions because her negative conscious attitudes would certainly have interfered with this exploratory work wherein she is actually laying the foundation for a new frame of reference about her scar.

SHOCK AND SURPRISE: CONFLICTING FRAMES OF REFERENCE

About two weeks later she appeared with a collection of sketches amply illustrating shapes, sizes, and locations of beauty patches. She was intensely puzzled and curious about the overwhelming interest she had experienced in executing this assignment. She was asked to exhibit the sketches and to discuss them. Fortunately, all these sketches were on sheets of paper the same size as her first drawing, and all the feminine faces she had drawn were similar in outline to her self-portrait.

Advantage was taken of this to run hastily through the drawings, asking

---

*Editor's comments summarize his discussion of this case with MHE in 1978.

a simple question concerning each, and then to slip into the pile her self-portrait. She was then asked to scatter them over the table and to identify each particular type of beauty patch, whether a crescent, a star, a diamond, or whatever, and to give the reason for the site of application.

So engrossed did she become in this that she failed to recognize immediately the self-portrait. Instead, she described the scar as a six-pointed-star-shaped beauty patch applied to the corner of the mouth to attract attention to that feature as one most attractive. The fact that it was six-pointed instead of five-pointed puzzled her, and she expressed her surprise because she was certain she had only drawn five-pointed stars. As she puzzled over and examined the drawing further, she finally recognized it, with a sense of shock, as the self-portrait. For the next five minutes she faltered in her speech and stammered fragmentary utterances as she strove to integrate two conflicting frames of reference—the one centering about her "awful, disfiguring scar," and the other, her six-pointed-star-shaped beauty patch properly placed in relation to her definitely attractive mouth.

R: This is an unusually clear example of how you (1) depotentiate an old frame of reference, (2) manage to facilitate an unconscious search for a new, more adaptive one, and then (3) set them in creative conflict. As is usually the case, there is an element of shock and surprise in the process as she suddenly sees the two points of view and falls into puzzlement between them.

REINFORCING THE NEW FRAME OF REFERENCE

Finally, as she sat there, helpless in the face of her new understanding of her scar, she was told:

> Your parents, your brother, your friends were all so "unreasonable" as to think that your scar was just a beauty patch. The plastic surgeons thought so, too, and brushed you off as a silly girl who refused to recognize the scar for what it was. I, too, am sufficiently unreasonable as to see that scar as a little white star-shaped beauty patch at the corner of a very pretty mouth. *And you yourself—in fear, distress, abhorrence—drew your portrait accurately and well, and without knowing it you portrayed that scar for what it was, a beauty patch which, unguardedly, you recognized correctly.*
>
> Now, let's be scientific about this. Beauty patches are intended to draw attention to the most attractive feature. You have pretty eyes, you have a pretty dimple in your left cheek, you have a

pretty mouth. You like to be kissed, and a number of boys have kissed you. Go out with them again, one by one. Let them kiss you goodnight under the porch light. Make a mental note of where they kiss you, on the left side of your mouth, full face, or on the right side. I think they will kiss the side with the beauty patch. *You will find out.*

Now, go home, take these sketches—all of them—with you. You did them carefully and well. You learned a tremendous amount from them. You can keep the sketches, or you can give them away. *But what you learned from them you will always keep.*

R: "As she sat there helpless in the face of her new understanding of her scar," she was, in effect, in the common everyday trance wherein we are all open and receptive to the new within us as well as suggestions from the outside. You utilize this naturally receptive state to reinforce the new frame of reference.

SYMPTOM RESOLUTION AND SIX-YEAR FOLLOW-UP

Subsequently, she reported that she was invariably kissed on the right side of her mouth. (The objectivity of this report is open to serious question, however.) Moreover, she rapidly freed herself from the habit of covering her mouth and lost her feelings of inferiority. She married two years later and now has four children.

52. The Ugly Duckling: Transforming the Self-Image

Milton H. Erickson

Two young women, high school classmates but not friends, were in love with the same young man. One girl was rigid and prudish; the other girl was decidedly permissive. When the latter was about three months pregnant, she and the young man were married. Three years later the man divorced his wife for adequate reasons, and two years later he married the other girl. A baby girl was born to them two years later, much to the father's delight.

The marriage continued reasonably happy with one exception. The mother was much too puritanical with the daughter, who at the age of 25, became the writer's patient. The daughter sought psychiatric help because her marriage of four years' duration was becoming seriously unhappy. Her story was to the effect that her husband was an "intolerable, unspeakable liar," and had been since she first met him. She had excused him during their courtship and for the first year of married life because "you have to take what a man says when he is in love with lots of salt." Now, however, because her son was almost three years old and beginning to understand many things, she did not want his father "constantly telling lies."

Many times she had tried to discuss the lying with her husband but found herself unable to do so because he was "so sweet and loving" and because "I suppose I wish his lies were true. I can't help it." Nevertheless, within the past year she had become so tense and so irritable and so unable to discuss anything with her husband that she had been resorting to unprovoked temper tantrums, outbursts of screaming, threats of divorce, and ideas of suicide. At no time had she been able to discuss her husband's lying with anybody, and only his insistence that she consult a psychiatrist resulted finally in her call on the writer.

A previous visit from her husband disclosed him to be much alarmed about his wife's mental state, since he could only describe her sudden outbursts of violent temper and her bouts of weeping, which she apparently could not explain to him. He knew of no provocation whatever and considered the marriage otherwise a happy one.

Unpublished manuscript, 1933.

The patient was most unwilling to reveal what lies her husband told so repetitiously, insisting that the writer need only instruct her husband to tell the bare, simple truth. Finally, after extensive persuasion, she agreed to inform the writer. In effect, her husband, because he was in love with her as a person, out of the mistaken goodness and greatness of his love, insisted on telling her that she was pretty, that she was cute, that her hair was lovely, that he liked the tilt of her nose, "and all those silly things that men, when they fall in love, say."

She went on to state that ever since she was a tiny child her mother had "daily" told her that she was homely and unattractive, that her lack of beauty was a cross she would have to bear cheerfully and gladly. In addition, it would be only right and good for her to develop a charming personality, since that would last a lifetime, while beauty always faded away.

As a small child she had not been much concerned about her looks. In high school she had developed considerable self-consciousness, but had finally resigned herself to her fate and enjoyed "exercising her personality." She seldom accepted a second or third invitation from the high school boys because they "lied" to her about her looks. Following graduation she had obtained a secretarial job, which she continued until her marriage.

Her first social engagement with the man she married had impressed her indelibly. He had told her then that she had the most charming personality that he had ever encountered. This had been reiterated during subsequent engagements, and not until later had he told her how pretty she was. She had accepted these compliments then because he was in love with her and because they were in accord with his response to her personality. Therefore, his "lies" could be forgiven as emotional exaggerations.

With the advent of pregnancy, however, her nipples had become very deeply pigmented. Her mother had informed her that child-bearing always cost a woman whatever little beauty she had. The daughter's reaction was one of acceptance of "that fact" and strong resentment toward her mother. Thereafter, visits at the maternal home became much less frequent, and finally, they were limited to holidays and family anniversaries.

Her husband, however, had not manifested any dislike for the nipple pigmentation. In fact, he had "falsely acted pleased" about it. This, coupled with his continued expressions of his regard for her "beauty," had placed her in the unbearable situation of being constantly reminded by his compliments of her misfortune and his mendacity. She felt that a solution to her problem would be a straightforward, open, honest recognition of the fact of her unloveliness. Then the question could be dropped, and no further references need ever be made to her looks.

A careful attempt was made to get her to evaluate her features one by one, since, to the writer as well as to her husband, her features were better than averagely attractive. Her ideas were rigidly fixed, however, and she promptly accused the writer of trying to gloss over her lack of beauty to pacify her. Accordingly, the effort was abandoned. Despite her impatience about the writer's interest in "irrelevant matters," inquiry disclosed no other significant problem. Her son was described as the "spitting image" of his father. "You can tell them apart because Johnny doesn't have a moustache."

When questioned about the possibility that her husband might actually believe that she were pretty, since "people often tell lies until they actually believe them," she was rather nonplussed. After some thinking she stated that, if such were the case, therapy might help her to tolerate the situation better, so that she would not lose her temper and become so depressed by his mistaken beliefs.

THERAPEUTIC TRANCE, EXPECTANCE, AND INNER SEARCH

Since she was aware, through another patient, of the writer's use of hypnosis, it was a relatively easy task to interest her in hypnotherapy. She was a good subject, required little training, and was most cooperative. As the first measure, although extensive inquiries had been made previously of her husband, she was asked to list the various nursery tales she read to her son and to the six-year-old neighbor girl for whom she often cared on weekends. Among the tales was one she read with great frequency, "The Ugly Duckling." She was asked to recite in the trance state a number of the stories, among them "The Ugly Duckling." No special attention was apparently given the story by the writer. However, her husband stated that she had read the "Ugly Duckling" story to her son frequently since about his second birthday.

At the next session she was told in the trance state to discuss her husband's heavy, dark-brown moustache. She expressed great admiration for it, repeated how she insisted that he grow one, since it would make him look distinguished, and had refused to let him shave it off. During their courtship she had insisted that he grow one, and he had done so. Still in the trance state, she was instructed as a posthypnotic task to take a heavy, dark-brown eyebrow pencil and to paint a moustache on her son as a practical joke on her husband. Then, after they had finished laughing at it, she was to examine it and her husband's moustache and to learn to understand something of great importance to her. What this was she would not know at first, but at the right time it would become fully understood—with tremendous force.*

At the next session she was to relate her reaction to the moustache on her son. In effect, she described it as a "hideous thing" since it did not "fit" on Johnny's face, even though a moustache looked so well on his father, and despite the practically identical facial appearance of father and son. She also expressed feelings of a vague inner unrest, as if she were trying to understand something she already knew.

She was then hypnotized deeply and told that her unconscious was to remember a nursery tale and to think that tale over without letting her conscious mind know about it in any way. This nursery tale would be selected by her unconscious because it would apply to her in a most peculiar way and would fulfill her need to understand adequately certain things she had to know about herself. Furthermore, she would have to search through the nursery tales with which she was acquainted, that none of them would seem to her the right one, but that she would finally give up the task of searching and just take the handiest one, hoping that it would be the right one. Several days would have to be spent by her unconscious in its study of the tale. Also, she would probably dream about it, happy dreams, but she would not remember her dreams. Neither would her unconscious let her know what it was thinking about. Nevertheless, she would be consciously aware that something was happening within her, altering her attitudes and understandings.

At the same time, in some way, the moustache painted on her son's face, so hideous to her and so out of keeping with his face, and her husband's moustache, so attractive on him, would fit into the nursery tale in some way that would clarify all of her thinking and establish those attitudes she so greatly wanted.

Finally, just before her next session, she was to be unconsciously impelled to do something that would inform the writer, immediately as she entered the office, that her unconscious had completed its tasks adequately. Then, during the session, either in the waking or the trance state, she would begin to discuss with increasing understanding her new, altered, unconscious understandings, and thus make them a part of her total life reactions and attitudes.

She was seen five days later. She apologized as she entered the office for being late, explaining that she had been detained at the beauty shop where she had "blown the works." She added that in the past she disliked

---

*Editor's note: This is a typical approach by MHE for evoking a period of intense inner search on an unconscious level. See the five-stage paradigm of trance induction and suggestion presented as "Two-level communication and the microdynamics of trance and suggestion" in Volume One of this series.

going to beauty shops and had never had more than a permanent wave, but this time she had had everything they could offer. No comment was made except to state that she really could "follow orders." This puzzled her, but she began a casual conversation, suddenly interrupting to state that she wanted to talk about the moustache she had painted on her son and about her husband's moustache.

She was told to think over the topic carefully and to organize her thoughts. After a few minutes she began, explaining in effect that she had duplicated on her son's face a replica of her husband's moustache, in smaller size but of the same dark-brown color and shape. The effect had been grotesque and hideous because it did not "fit." The boy was too small, his appearance was too young, and hence, despite his extreme resemblance to his father, the result was a distasteful mockery. Only when he became old enough and mature enough would the dark-brown color on his upper lip be attractive.

She paused, blushed, and impulsively declared, "It's just like nipples." A further pause, "A girl's nipples should look young, but when she has matured and been pregnant, they really should look different. Why, it would be like a grownup man who had a boy's skin on his face. It wouldn't look good." After a pause she added, "Maybe I better stop trying to look at myself as if I was a little girl. My husband sees me grown up."

This observation elicited a startled silence in her. Then again she began, "I've just thought of 'The Ugly Duckling' story. All my life I've read that story over and over. I never knew why. And the last few days I've been so absentminded. I've just been keeping that story in the back of my mind. Do you know, I bet those old ducks still think that that swan is ugly. It had to join the swans to find out that it was beautiful."

Reply was made, "The old mother duck will always think the young swan is ugly, but what will the other young swans think? And what will the young swan really know about itself?" Before she could reply, she was told emphatically, "You know and you will always know.

"And now, when your husband comes home tonight, why don't you cuddle up to him at the door and ask him simply, immediately, 'Don't you want to take a pretty girl out to dinner tonight?'"

"Your next appointment will be in one week's time at the same hour." Thereupon she was summarily dismissed.

Her husband was seen before she was. He reported that she had obeyed instructions exactly and that he had been so astonished that he had forgotten a business appointment and enthusiastically agreed to her suggestion. He was most emphatic about the transformation in his wife, expressed curiosity about what had happened, but agreed to await such time as she chose to discuss the events of therapy.

At her interview the discussion was kept on a vague, casual level. About three months later she asked for an appointment. The purpose was to discuss any possible need to inform her husband of her original "silly ideas." Inquiry disclosed that he had apparently lost all curiosity. A year has passed. They were seen again because they brought to the writer a young couple, intimate friends of theirs, who were considering divorce because of marital problems, and they wished the writer to handle that problem as well as he had handled hers. Inquiry disclosed them to have been adjusting most happily.

53. A Shocking Breakout of a Mother Domination

Milton H. Erickson

Dr. X received over 300 hours of intensive psychoanalytic therapy by the past president of the American Psychoanalytic Association and of the International Psychoanalytic Association. This therapy had been without any therapeutic results. He was then taken over as a patient by another past president of the American Psychoanalytic Association and underwent another 300 hours of intensive psychoanalytic therapy with no results. He was then referred to the author.

CONSCIOUS LIMITATIONS AND HYSTERICAL DEAFNESS

About six hours were spent determining the fact that there was no approach to him to be made at the conscious level. He could narrate his obsessional fears, doubts, and compulsions, but if any comment of any sort were made to him during the hour, his eyes would glaze over, and it was entirely obvious that he would develop a hysterical deafness. This was tested by sounds that should have elicited startle reactions. Apparatus had been rigged so that a sound could be produced behind him, so there would be no possible visual awareness of what was about to happen. He made no startle or response of any kind to these unexpected sounds. It was found, however, that he would maintain sufficient visual awareness and sufficient selective hearing that he could hear and understand when the author was not speaking about him as a patient.

TRANCE INDUCTION AND TRAINING FOR POSTHYPNOTIC SUGGESTION

Having made these determinations, in the next two hours he was given the explanation that he would be hypnotized, and no effort of any sort

Previously unpublished manuscript, circa 1936.

would be made to do therapy, that every effort would be spent in training him to be a good hypnotic subject. To this he agreed readily in the same passive, accepting manner in which he had come for therapy.

He entered into a deep somnambulistic trance quite readily, and a considerable amount of time was spent in teaching him to experience the various hypnotic phenomena, particularly the execution of posthypnotic suggestion. These were of great variety, but there was a careful avoidance of anything that might be construed as therapeutic. At a later date, during a three-hour session, a deep somnambulistic trance was induced, and there was a systematic presentation to him of a long series of posthypnotic suggestions. These were explained as suggestions that he would not have to execute during the trance; that they would be without therapeutic effect in the trance; that they were posthypnotic suggestions that would be carried out at a later date in a situation far removed from the author's office and at a time when he and all others would recognize him as in the conscious state. Interwoven with these suggestions was the reassurance that he need not be afraid of listening to these posthypnotic suggestions, that he could comfort himself by knowing that, as he listened to them, they were without effect upon him as a person and as a personality; that they could have no significance until some time in what would seem to be the remote future. An example was drawn for him to the effect that he could readily accept the suggestion here and now; that two weeks from now, on a specified date, he would eat a beefsteak and that in no way need he reject that possibility. Similar parallels were drawn to ensure his full understanding that he could accept all posthypnotic suggestions and merely thoughtlessly postpone their effectiveness to what would seem to him to be the remote future.

These posthypnotic suggestions had been worked out with a great deal of care, and they were developed on the basis of the information given to the author by the patient's wife, an intelligent, cooperative, long-forebearing person who had endured her unhappy lot without complaint.

In essence the situation was that he was completely ruled by his mother. He and his wife had been married 15 years. The parents had given him and his wife a house alongside of theirs. The bride and groom had not been permitted to go on a honeymoon. His mother had insisted that he take two weeks off from his practice and honeymoon in their new home. To the bride's horror the groom's mother showed up in her kitchen the next morning to prepare breakfast. She had decided on the menu, and the bride and groom had to eat what she cooked. Mother also prepared lunch and the evening meal, besides telling them when to go to bed and when to get up. This type of behavior on the part of the husband's mother had continued for the entire 15 years of their marriage. Mother took them to church and made them sit in the pew with the young husband next to his mother and separated from his wife by his father. Mother took them out to dinner at her favorite places. Mother took them to her choice of places of entertainment. In brief, in the entire 15 years of that marriage the mother had dominated every detail of their home.

Mother belonged to the Woman's Christian Temperance Union and during medical school when he lived in the fraternity house, Sonny had imbibed alcoholic beverages. He had never dared tell his mother, and at least once a week she delivered a sermon on the evils of alcohol. Neither was he allowed to drink soft drinks, tea, or coffee. He had once ventured to request the privilege of drinking buttermilk, but his mother had expounded on the virtues of drinking only water and pasteurized milk.

Mother picked out his shirts, his ties, his shoes, and his underwear; she specified every change of clothing down to which suit he was to wear on which occasion. Mother did permit him to go to the office unescorted. But on any other trips away from home she went with him and handled him as if he were around the age of three of four years. Initially in his married life he had walked to his office; Mother said the exercise was good. But after the first year he began to leave early in the morning to avoid having people see him alone on the streets. His mother approved of long hours spent in the office, and he began working late at night in order to avoid being seen; this was not too effective, however so he began coming home by way of alleys.

In his practice of medicine he was engaged in a specialty that permitted the minimum of contact with his patients, most of whom were seen by his office help and technicians. His mother insisted that he go to medical meetings, but she always escorted him there and back. Very promptly he became too self-conscious to participate in any activities of the county medical society. In fact, he began avoiding speaking to his fellow physicians. After 12 years of this he sought therapy, and his parents begged for a special, private room at the institution where he was treated. His mother took lodgings nearby, was permitted to visit him daily and took him for walks, so that he did not participate in any of the institutional activities for patients. Since he made no improvement after over 300 hours, his mother decided to seek another therapist; she escorted him to that therapist's office and accompanied him back home. This the therapist permitted.

When Sonny was brought to the author for therapy, Mother was told in most emphatic terms that she could not accompany him to the office, that she would have to delegate that responsibility to his wife. The author finally succeeded in conveying to the mother the idea that forcing the wife to bring her husband to therapy would be an appropriate punishment for the wife, and that she in her earnest solicitude for her son's welfare should see to it that his wife undertook the punitive duty of bringing her husband for therapy.

The interview with the wife after this hoax had been perpetrated upon the mother was most delightful. She was an intelligent, capable young woman who felt herself hopelessly lost in dealing with her mother-in-law and incapable of weaning her husband away from her. It was possible to talk to her freely and frankly and to secure her promise of secrecy about the author's plans. In fact, she was most delighted with the author's intentions and most enthusiastic about cooperating. She was told to let Mother continue her domination unabated but to look forward with mirthful anticipation to what was going to happen to Mother.

The posthypnotic suggestion given to the patient in the deep trance had been worked out in extensive detail, and the patient's wife had been consulted extensively to ensure its completeness. The explanation was given to the wife that the patient could not accept therapy in the ordinary waking state and that he did not accept it in the trance state. The approach employed was to use hypnosis to impress thoroughly upon the patient's mind all the things that would lead to therapy in the trance state, but with the suggestion that they would be inoperative in that trance state. He was told that all therapeutic suggestions would become uncontrollably effective at a specified date in the future when he was in the state of full conscious awareness. In other words, the therapy was given in the trance state but remained inoperative until some later time of full conscious awareness, at which point it would become compulsively effective.

A SHOCKING BREAKOUT OF A MOTHER DOMINATION

When all of the posthypnotic suggestions had been completed, a specific date and a specific hour was set; namely, 10:00 A.M. on Sunday morning, the hour at which the mother always came to take her son, his wife, and their two children to church. That morning mother had already prepared breakfast for her son and his family and had gone home to dress for church. Her son and his wife and family had also dressed for church. The mother came in, and her son greeted her as usual; then as related by his wife, in full agreement with posthypnotic suggestion, the son said, "Mother, would you please come into the kitchen for a minute?" His mother wonderingly followed him. He walked over to one of the kitchen shelves, took down a bottle of whiskey that was only partially corked so that he could remove the cork easily, and poured out a glassful while his mother stood in shocked, silent horror; then, with a stream of profane and obscene expletives, he declared his intention to get drunker than a lord, and that she was to haul her f—— a— to church without him—whereupon he promptly drank six ounces of straight whiskey. What the patient did not remember was that immediately after breakfast he had gone to the bathroom, had inserted his finger in his throat, and had vomited up his entire breakfast. The impact of the six ounces of straight 100 proof whiskey was most startling, and it was added to by the posthypnotic suggestion. He collapsed on the floor; his wife and his mother undressed him and put him to bed, while he sang some unexpurgated songs dating back to his fraternity days; then he collapsed in a drunken stupor. His mother was so horrified that she went home and took a bath, having missed church for the first time in many many years.

She remained in bed until the next morning, when she came over to fix breakfast. As she came in, she found her son awaiting her in the breakfast room. He greeted her most profanely and obscenely, explaining, "I have been waiting for you because I am thirsty for another drink of whiskey," and thereupon he drained a glass of what appeared to be whiskey. Actually, it was tea prepared by his wife to look like whiskey. Having drained the glass, he said, "Now I had better stagger off to bed," and he began singing, "Drunk today, drunk tonight, drunker than I have ever been before." His mother left in tears and went to bed for the day and night. As soon as his mother was safely out of the house, one of the children kept watch in case the mother or father should appear. The man's wife prepared the first breakfast she ever had in 15 years of their married life. The patient notified his office that he was indisposed and he would not be in that day. At noon the patient's wife prepared lunch, and that evening, the dinner. They went to bed at the hour of their choosing. In all of this the patient's wife played a passive, submissive role in relation to her husband just as she had to her husband's mother, and in response to posthypnotic suggestion the husband began to rejoice in his wife's attitude toward him. The next morning the mother stalked into the house and said she was going to clean it out. She saw the whiskey bottle actually filled with tea and dumped it into the sink. She found another bottle of whiskey that had not been opened, and she rejoiced mightily in opening it and draining it down the sink. Then she ordered her son to march into the living room to listen to her while she "explained a few things." She also demanded that his wife and children do likewise. Very meekly the patient did as told, and as the mother began, "Now you listen to me," her son pulled out a half-pint flask of actual whiskey and drained it before his mother recovered her poise sufficiently to rush at him and take it away. The wife had immediately seized the two children aged 12 and 10 and rushed them out of the room. The patient profanely and obscenely told his mother that if she ever again came into the house without an invitation, he would promptly get drunk, and that he might even ask his wife to get drunk with him. He then ordered her with much vulgar language to get out of the house, saying that if she dared to call any physicians or any friends to come to see him, he would take extremely unpleasant measures against her.

Mother left rather frightened. For the next three months she did not appear, but her son noted that she was watching out of an upstairs window to see if he went to the office and if he was walking home. During those three months the man and his wife established a good understanding of the total situation. Also, during those three months the patient came alone to see the author to have his posthypnotic suggestions reinforced and still further elaborated. At the end of three months a new set of instructions was given the patient. He was to locate a house that he would like to live in; to make arrangements either to rent or purchase it; and then to make arrangements with the moving company to be completely moved into the new home on the other side of town during one of his parent's periodic day-long visits to an out-of-town relative.

The patient and his wife spent six weeks locating a desirable house and making appropriate arrangements with the moving company. Upon the mother's return in the evening of the day of the moving, she was utterly astonished to find a vacant house where her son had lived.

She appeared at the office the next day to find out the location of his new home. He told her coldly that he did not think she should know, and if she tried in any way to find out, he and his wife and her grandchildren would never again visit her. Greatly subdued, the mother left and made no further attempts to intrude upon her son's life.

A year later the son and his wife made a formal call on his parents, and good family relations were established. At Thanksgiving dinner the mother started to tell him what he should have on his plate and to her utter horror she saw her son, her daughter-in-law, and their two children leave the table and go home. However, they appeared for Christmas dinner, and the mother behaved herself. Thereafter good family relations were established, which the son carefully tested by offering his mother a glass of whiskey—which she politely refused—while he and his wife drank in her presence.

All together a total of not over 20 hours were spent working with this patient. (The author did not find that the previous 600 hours of psychoanalytic therapy had aided the patient's breakout in any way.) In addition to his healthy family adjustment, the patient began to participate in county medical society meetings, was elected president of the county medical society, was elected president of the state medical society, and later was elected to office in the national society of his specialty.

54. Shock and Surprise Facilitating a New Self-Image

Milton H. Erickson

The purpose of psychotherapy is to enable a patient to achieve a legitimate personal goal as advantageously as is possible. Properly, it is not a matter of advancing particular schools of thought or of attempting to substantiate interpretative psychological theories, but simply a task of appraising a patient's problem or problems in terms of the reality in which the patient lives and in the terms of the realities of the patient's continuing future as he or she may reasonably hope for it to be.

The author is well aware that this brief formulation of psychotherapy and its purposes is in marked contrast to those schools of psychotherapy which insist that, as a prerequisite for future adjustment, a painstaking, laborious one-to-three-year-or-more minute scrutiny and analysis be made of the long-dead and unchangeable past before even touching upon the patient's actual present and future needs, understandings, capabilities, and possibilities.

Yet one may consider the few troubled people who are benefitted by psychotherapy of all kinds and the countless numbers who, while also having problems, still succeed without therapy in achieving goals that they and others regard as constituting real personal and social success. Thus, after such consideration, one may well wonder at the self-reassuring dogmatism of the many self-styled "the one-and-only right" schools of interpretative, speculative psychotherapy.

After this somewhat acrimonious introduction the author wishes to present a case history in which there was employed successful psychotherapy caustically described by some colleagues as "unorthodox and not in accordance with established rules of psychotherapy." The fact that the patients had benefitted was not considered to be pertinent to the issue by those critics.

CASE 1

The first patient was a 35-year-old professionally trained woman with a

Unpublished manuscript, circa 1930s.

master's degree. She was very slightly overweight but otherwise was decidedly attractive, graceful, and possessed of a most pleasing personality. Her major defect can be summarized in the outraged statement of an unmarried man of her own age, holder of a doctoral degree in a field of work related to hers: "If that damned girl would comb her hair, wash her ears and neck, put on a dress that didn't look like an ill-fitting gunnysack, straighten her stockings, and polish her shoes, I could get seriously interested in her."

In summary, her appearance epitomized her problem, and the above outraged statement described her appearance very well. Yet Ann was a highly intelligent young woman, and in the author's six months of professional contact with her, he had been much impressed with the clarity and lucidity of her thinking and with her ability in the comprehensive appraisal of problems. The author had also developed an earnest respect for her competence as revealed in staff conferences; however, it was also noted that Ann had neither casual nor intimate friends, with the exception of one exceedingly competent, very friendly older woman who was quite obese and who suffered from arthritis.

Finally this older woman approached the author and explained that Ann was seriously depressed and definitely suicidal despite her outward facade of a comfortable, businesslike adjustment. She explained that for a long time she had attempted to coax Ann to seek therapy, and that only recently had Ann rather unwillingly agreed to see the author—but only briefly since, to quote her friend, "The darned idiot sees no hope for herself, and I want you to take her by the scruff of the neck and shove her face into a mirror and make her take a good look at herself as a real person of value. Nobody, just nobody—not even me—can talk to her; Ann just freezes and gets deaf and blind, and you lose all contact with her. But I finally have managed to make her listen long enough so that she has agreed to see you for a 'few times,' if you are willing. Please, for my sake, see her because I'm frightened by Ann's desperation."

PREPARATION FOR TRANCE INDUCTION

Ann appeared for her appointment with obvious reluctance. She was asked to take a seat beside the office door while the author sat on the opposite side of the room. She was told: "As you know, Ann, I'm very definitely crippled by anterior poliomyelitis, and anytime you want to escape from this office, you can get out of the door long before I can cross the room. Therefore you can feel safe here. And if you decide to develop hypnotic trances here, you will still have time to arouse from the trance state and get out of the office before I can cross the room. At the staff lecture on hypnosis, and at the demonstration which I gave recently and which you attended, I mentioned that several persons had unwittingly gone into and come out of hypnosis, and I refused to identify them. You, Ann, were one of those persons. Hence, I am delighted to see you here, and I hope you have come for the therapy that both Agnes and I think you need. However, therapy will not be forced on you. Agnes made this appointment for you. It will be used only to outline the situation. Your appearance here indicates that you recognize your need for therapy.

"Next, Agnes has told me that despite your salary and lack of any dependents you have so misused your income that in 12 years time you have saved only $700, and hence you are convinced that you cannot afford therapy. Let's correct your ideas on that at once. There is no charge for this interview. It is a courtesy to our friend Agnes, not a debt incurred by you.

"Subsequent interviews with you, if any, will be therapeutic, and they are to be paid for on my terms, and my terms only. These terms are absolute, full, and complete obedience in relation to every instruction I give you regardless of what I order or demand. Your one and only protection from this arbitrariness on my part is that you are free to relate everything or anything you wish to Agnes first before you act upon my instructions. If she approves, you then have no choice but to obey.

"You have told Agnes you have no time for therapy. I shall, therefore, expect the most expeditious of responses from you. No dilly-dallying, no shilly-shallying. You will be told what to do, and you will do it. That's it! If I tell you to resign your position, you will resign. If I tell you to eat fresh garlic cloves for breakfast, you will eat them. I have spoken clearly and understandably. Just as clearly do I want it understood that in psychotherapy for you, I want action and response—not words, ideas, theories, concepts. I want responses, desirable, good, informative responses of action and change, not contemplation of change, but change and action of a constructive sort. If this is understood by you, let me know and I will continue.

Ann meekly nodded her head affirmatively.

"Fine! Now listen and listen well. Think over all I have said carefully for the next three days. Understand well that for the next three long days you are to think over everything that I have said to you. If I tell you to go into a hypnotic trance, you will do so. And you and I both know, I from observation, you from your unconscious learnings and actual responses in a recent staff situation, that you can respond most adequately hypnotically. I do not care if you like that frank statement of fact or not. But you want therapy, and you have so indicated in many ways, especially to Agnes.

"After the three days you are, if you decide affirmatively for therapy, to return here for that therapy best suiting you as a potentially happy, well-adjusted person. Come at this hour prepared to stay as long as I wish, and bring your checkbook with you. Discuss this entire matter with nobody, not even Agnes, who has been told to discuss your therapeutic wishes no longer. Come prepared for and committed to therapy and to the loss of your bank account and your personality problems, but don't come back if you are not so committed. The decision must be entirely yours.

"Bear in mind that therapy is going to meet your wishes, but it will not always be comfortable and easy. You want it done rapidly, and it will be done rapidly and thoroughly. Once you come, you are committed to therapy, and your bank account belongs to me as does the registration certificate for your car, whether in my possession or not. I will tell you what to do and how to do it, and you are to be a most obedient patient, learning fully to put into action all the ideas presented by you.

"Now go home; you have a vital decision to make. Do it by yourself. If in the affirmative, return in three days at this hour, with your time my time. Goodbye.

Agnes reported that Ann went through a remarkably silent, distraught three days and that her work suffered greatly.

A SURPRISING AND RAPID TRANCE INDUCTION

Ann returned at the appointed time, entered the office hesitantly and tremulously, and stood waiting for the author to speak. She was told, "Close the door, sit down in that chair near the door, and in the process of doing those two tasks develop a deep somnambulistic trance in which you will give me your full attention mentally as well as visually and auditorily. Nod your head when you feel that you are ready for me to begin."

Moments after she seated herself, Ann began nodding her head in the typical perseverative fashion of the deep trance, her gaze fixed rigidly on the author. Her blink and swallowing reflexes were absent, and her rigid facial expression was characteristic of the somnambulistic state.

"That's fine, Ann. Continue to remain in the trance as you are now. Be receptive of everything I say. Remember you are at liberty to question Agnes on any detail that you wish, but otherwise what I say remains confidential. What I am going to say to you is not something you will expect. It will be helpful, drastically so. I will outline a course of behavior for you, and this you are to execute without fail. Do you give me your absolute promise?"

Slowly, perseveratively, Ann nodded her head.

"Are you afraid?"

Ann nodded her head affirmatively.

"You need not be afraid. I'm going to startle you greatly, and I am going to give you sharp psychological pain. Both experiences will be almost paralyzingly unpleasant, and then, as you incorporate the understandings that they signify, the pain and distress will disappear. Are you ready?"

Ann nodded her head. She was told to stand with her feet close together and her hands at her side and not to move unless there arose a good indication for moving.

As she stood waiting expectantly, the author stated, "Ann, you are 35 years old; you look at least five years or more younger than you are; you are definitely attractive in appearance; you have not had a date for at least 14 years despite your pleasing appearance, personality, and good intelligence; you are five feet three inches tall, and you weigh about 130 pounds; you have trim ankles, an excellent figure, a beautiful mouth and beautiful eyes. All this you can verify yourself."

Then in a tone of voice of utter intensity, in the manner of conveying a vitally important message, she was asked the following question: "Ann, did you know that you have a pretty patch of fur between your legs?"

For some minutes Ann stood staring at the author, blushing deeply and continuously, apparently too cataleptic to close her eyes or to move in any way.

"You really have, Ann, and it is definitely darker than the hair on your head. Now at least an hour before your bedtime, let us say at nine o'clock tonight, after you take your shower, stand in the nude before the full-length mirror in your bedroom. Carefully, systematically, thoroughly examine your body from the waist down. Be pleased with your belly button, curious about that pad of fat between your belly button and your pretty pubic hair.

"Try to realize how much you would like to have the right man caress your pretty pubic hair and your softly rounded belly. Think of how you would like to have him caress your thighs and hips. Stand there in front of the mirror and keep standing there until you have realized all of this. Then, as you become pleasingly tired physically, go to bed happy, blushingly happy, knowing that you do have a pretty piece of fur between your legs, and fall restfully into physiological sleep, and sleep restfully the whole night. You do not need to remember your dreams, nor will they disturb your sleep; but the next day, outwardly calm and composed but inwardly warm and happy, work well and comfortably.

"Do you understand all of this instruction, and are you prepared to do it as I have outlined it? Nod your head affirmative if you understand fully."

Slowly Ann nodded her head, continuing to blush constantly and to breathe irregularly.

"Now listen carefully, Ann. Shortly you are to awaken from your trance. You are to have a complete amnesia for all that has happened here, has been said here, has been experienced by you here. Go home, take your tub bath or shower early, dry yourself, then suddenly find yourself standing in front of your full-length mirror, staring at yourself from the waist down, and then remember in full detail everything that was said to you here, every comment, every instruction; and, Ann, execute them fully. This you will do to the full satisfaction of my instructions and to the full satisfaction of your needful understandings of the therapeutic advances you need to make.

"Then tomorrow, at this same hour, come for your second appointment. Come dressed as you are today, in the same dress, outwardly appearing exactly as you do today. Now arouse from your trance with the total amnesia I have asked for and go about your duties, unconsciously awaiting the right time tonight. And in the process of arousing gently, sit down comfortably in the chair there and then become fully alert but not curious because I dismiss you."

Ann sat down, obviously aroused from her trance state, and looked expectantly at the author. She was told not to be curious about the passage of time (she had looked at her watch and had showed marked astonishment), that all was well and that she would, without further instruction, keep her next appointment. With a most puzzled look she departed.

She appeared a half-hour early for her next appointment, but spent that extra time pacing back and forth in front of the office as if attempting to make up her mind whether or not to keep her appointment. Exactly on time she entered the office, her face bursting red with blushes. Precipitously she declared, "I remember everything. I don't know what to say."

"Just close the door and sit down in that chair."

She did so, immediately developed a profound trance, and sat looking wide-eyed at the author, still blushing.

"I see that you want therapy and that you did as you were instructed."

Blushing more deeply she nodded her head perseveratively.

"Now stand up in the same way as you did yesterday. Thank you! Now listen to me well, carefully, thoughtfully. Yesterday, quite drastically, in a fashion which you could not avoid understanding and which precluded any possibility of suppression or repression, I asked you to become fully aware of the badge of femininity which you wear, a badge of femininity which you should rightly treasure in all ways.

"But that is not all of which you are to become aware. Tonight, even as last night, in the same sequence of events as I described yesterday, find yourself unexpectedly in the nude in front of the mirror, then suddenly recall all the instructions I have already given you here in the office and which I will give you today.

"Tonight, as you stand in the nude in front of the mirror, look at your badge of femininity, be pleased with it, even blush, and then suddenly, as if it were for the first time that you saw them, look well at the two emblems of womanhood you wear on your chest.

"Examine them carefully, both visually and tactually, thinking over carefully all the things that you know I could tell you to think—all of the things I could tell you to think over. Is it necessary for me to elaborate?" She slowly shook her head.

"Will you do it even more elaborately than you think I would order you to do the task?"

Ann began blushing in waves as she tried to turn her head aside, and then, yielding, she nodded her head affirmatively.

She was then instructed to return the next day and to appear in the same dress and outwardly unchanged. Next, she was told to sit down, to arouse from hypnosis with a complete amnesia for everything until the crucial moment before the mirror that night.

As she aroused from the trance, she was told, "That's all for today." Her face expressed bewilderment, she looked at her watch in a most puzzled fashion, but she departed without saying anything.

She appeared on time the next day, blushing deeply as she entered the office. Without any hesitation she promptly closed the door, sat down in the chair, and immediately developed a profound somnambulistic trance; her blushes disappeared.

She was immediately asked, "Do you want to say something?" She nodded her head.

"All right, say it now to your full satisfaction."

Promptly she stated, "I did all you said, I did it better, I think, than you could have asked." Then with many blushes she asked, "Do I have to tell you?"

"No, Ann, the fact that you have obeyed instructions fully, even better than I could expect, and since your question implies your willingness to cooperate in therapy by relating things you reasonably can expect me not to know, your progress is entirely satisfactory."

Ann ceased blushing and waited expectantly.

"Did you remember everything both times upon awakening, yet handle your awarenesses well throughout the following day?"

Ann nodded affirmatively.

"Now stand up as before, beside your chair. Today's task is much harder, much, much harder, much more troublesome, much more painful. Upon leaving here you will notify your office that you will not be there the rest of the day. You will leave here with an amnesia for what I am about to say to you, but still fully consciously aware of the learnings you have acquired the past two nights.

"Listen well! You have heard how many a mother gets her small child neat and clean and declares that it seems to her that in only a few moments' time he becomes unbelievably untidy. Now listen, Ann! This is the third day you have been in the office. It is not the first time you have worn a dress three days in succession. I merely ensured no accidental change of dress. Now listen carefully, storing every word in your unconscious mind for sudden, full conscious memory when you find yourself in front of your mirror promptly upon returning to your apartment after leaving this office. Do you understand?"

Ann nodded her head slowly, apparently bewildered by the author's rather sharp tone of voice.

"Ann, our dress looks horrible. It's saggy and baggy and it fits you like any old potato sack, and it is wrinkled and perspiration-stained, and you don't have a decent-fitting, decent-looking dress in your entire wardrobe. Every one is an insult to the eye. No taste, wrong colors, wrong everything, and yet you wear them to the office, on the street. When you find yourself in front of the mirror today, with full conscious memory of all that I have said and will say in this office today, examine each and every dress you have, model it, note the ill fit, the sweat stains, spots, rips, loose buttons on blouses—see how competently you dress to be an eyesore.

"And worse, Ann. Look at your hair. Never have I seen it properly combed in the six months I have known you. Always at least a couple of snarls, and that parting of your hair, how do you make it so outrageously crooked? Take a hand mirror and use it to help you to see in the large mirror. A woman's hair is 'her crowning glory' or, in your case, Ann, your crowning disgrace.

"More yet! Have you a personal prejudice about washing your ears and behind them? Don't answer, but look in the mirror and get an answer then! And your neck! You take a shower or a tub bath, but how do you forget to wash your neck? It must be an art, an undesirable art. Who would want to neck with a dirty-necked girl, a dirty-necked girl like you? Shudder about that a bit as you look in the mirror. If you want feminine corroboration of all I'm saying, get Agnes to let loose some of her suppressed feelings. You will like them less that what I am saying to you.

"How often do your fingernails go into mourning with that line of black dirt under your poorly trimmed fingernails? Do you think it is pleasing to hold hands with a girl whose fingernails are in mourning? Don't answer. The questions are rhetorical. For six months I have known you with mussy hair, dirty ears and neck, displeasing, disgusting fingernails, and ill-fitting, untidy dresses, wrinkled stockings—take a look at those, too, tonight. What a slob you are outwardly!"

"You have $700 in the bank. You can borrow money. Go downtown to Department Store X. Seek out Miss Y. I know her; Agnes knows her; I've spoken to her sufficiently about your needs. Tell her that you want her to teach you that vast amount of learning you lack but which every woman should have as second nature. Miss Y will be reasonable; accept instruction fully, buy everything you need, get some pretty dresses that fit you, some deodorants and antiperspirants, learn to comb your hair—say a happy goodbye to your $700 and what more you borrow. Arrange for time off work—this I know is possible. There is more I could say, but it really isn't necessary to elaborate.

There is just one question that intrigues me, but do not answer. It is, where did you get the good sense to go to the dentist to keep your teeth in such good shape, or do you just naturally have such beautiful teeth? Well, use them to sink into the task before you.

"Now you are to leave here with a total amnesia for all that has occurred today in this office. For any reason that comes to mind, notify the office of your absence for the rest of the day. Go to your apartment. Look around happily. It is neat and tidy. Agnes has told me so. Feel pleased with it. Then step to the mirror and let the 'horror show' begin, and stay to the bitter end and then realize what happiness can be yours.

"A closing remark to you is this: awaken and leave promptly upon grasping the meaning of what next I say. Let me see no more of you until you keep your next appointment as a 'vision of delight.' Now get out of here and close the door from the other side."

She left hurriedly in puzzled bewilderment.

A month passed, and late one afternoon Ann entered the office blushing furiously, smiling happily but embarrassedly, most beautifully gowned. She explained that she was going to a very "special" dinner and dance with a very "special boy friend" and that she would tell the author all about it later, as indeed she did, and she added with much self-consciousness that she hoped she was a "vision of delight."

Within a year Ann was engaged to a physician; she married him shortly thereafter and moved to another part of the country. Occasional news was received about her. At the age of 45 Ann was encountered unexpectedly while she and her family were on a vacation trip. She was the mother of four children; she appeared to be not over 40 years of age, and she was exceedingly happy. Her husband had achieved marked recognition in his specialty, and the entire family was obviously happy and well-adjusted. One careful comment was made by Ann to the effect that, bit by bit, as her daughter grew old enough to understand each item, she intended to teach the child progressively "how to be a vision of delight."

55. Correcting an Inferiority Complex

Milton H. Erickson

A 29-year-old man, employed as a clerk, sought therapy in an ambivalent manner. He explained that, while he wanted therapy, he did not amount to enough to warrant anybody wasting time on him. He had sought therapy from other psychiatrists but had always discontinued because the amount of time that seemed indicated for results was so greatly out of proportion to his worth as a person. He always felt the time spent on him could be better spent on less inferior patients. He had come to the writer in the hope that hypnosis would be used and that his therapy could be expedited without depriving more deserving patients of needed time with the writer.

The suggestion was offered that he probably wished limited therapy that would meet his minimal needs. He agreed with as much enthusiasm as he could muster. He also agreed reluctantly to the idea that preliminary interviews would be spent in securing a necessary factual history, but was somewhat reassured by the statement that he could abbreviate the time by giving freely whatever information the writer wished.

His history can be summarized by first giving the recurrent theme of it and listing illustrative items. "I have never done anything very good, no matter what. I'm completely inferior in everything." He was the only child of shiftless, ne'er-do-well parents. He had failed to attend the eighth grade graduation ceremonies and felt that he had not really graduated. High school required four and a half years because of time spent in changing schools. Even so, he failed to graduate because he lacked one credit. He was always a hanger-on at social activities in school, and his diffidence and lack of self-confidence precluded any active participation. In high school, despite his excellent physique, he succeeded only in being waterboy for a brief time. He was, in his own words, "a wash-out as a waterboy." In essence, he was one of those "nice fellows" for whom the general tendency of people is to feel contemptuous pity.

His parents died when he was nearly 18. His first employment had been scattered odd jobs at manual labor. Finally, he secured employment washing cars in a large garage and graduated to the position of handyman and errand boy for everything. This led to his placement in the automobile parts department, where he actually manifested good ability. However,

---

Unpublished manuscript, 1937–1938.

his willingness to work hard for a minimal salary earned him only job security and general disrespect.

On inquiring into minute details of what he could do, numerous, consistent items were discovered. A few of these may be listed:

1. He could not knot his tie neatly, nor could he tie his shoestrings neatly.
2. He was invariably five minutes late coming to work and about 20 minutes late in quitting.
3. Time after time he ruined social engagements arranged on a joint basis for him by associates by making some inept remark, such as telling his girl companion, "He [the other man] always gets the prettiest girl."
4. A final item, which he had mentioned repeatedly in giving his history, was his handwriting. It was practically illegible, and his records at work were a constant source of embarrassment, even though they constituted an insurance against his discharge.
5. One other and highly important theme in his story, reiterated again and again, was "If I could only do one thing good, just one thing, I'd have some pride in myself. Can't you learn me just one thing good?"

TRANCE INDUCTION UTILIZING THE PATIENT'S INFERIORITY COMPLEX

When he had completed his story, he was told that hypnotherapy would be employed. To accomplish this, it was explained that he would be used as a demonstration subject for the writer's medical students and that the therapy would be an incidental part of the instruction of the medical students. This type of cavalier offer to help him utilized his need for inferiority even in the therapeutic situation and actually pleased him. His general pattern of submissiveness aided greatly in inducing a deep trance without difficulty. He learned to manifest readily all the general hypnotic phenomena.

Extensive use was made of posthypnotic suggestions to create situations in which his general inept behavior was brought into sharp contrast with the competent behavior of the medical students. In this way an attitude of dependence upon and security in relation to the writer as a completely tolerant, forgiving protector was established to satisfy his neurotic needs.

HYPNOTIC ROLE-PLAYING FACILITATING
OBJECTIVE SELF-PERCEPTION

After about 12 hours of this sort of activity, intermingled with instructional work with the medical students, he was deeply hypnotized and depersonalized. He was then induced to assume the identity of that medical student with whom the writer felt he could most easily identify. This accomplished, the selected medical student, who was an amateur actor, was hypnotized deeply and instructed to assume the patient's identity.

There followed a repetition of various of the procedures previously employed to create special situations with the pseudo-patient duplicating the patient's previous inept behavior. During this the patient, in his identity as a student, participated in the discussion of the induced behavior portraying himself. Thus he was enabled to see himself in an objective, detached fashion and, from unrecognized inner knowledge, to appreciate exactly what was occurring.*

When it seemed that there had been sufficient demonstration of his ineptness, one final item not previously employed was utilized. This was a systematic calling upon various but not all of the medical students, one by one, to write and sign the statement, "This is a beautiful day in June." In each case the students were urged to write clearly and legibly. Each written production was then critically examined by the entire group, except the pseudo-patient. Among those not called upon to write was the actual patient.

Next the pseudo-patient was asked to write the same sentence. A horribly illegible scrawl with an indecipherable name was produced. (This student had previously been shown the patient's handwriting and had been asked to study it.) The pseudo-patient was urged again and again to write more legibly, but each production remained illegible.

After discussion of this with the group, the writer explained at length that the "patient" could be taught to write easily and legibly by the utilization of a special technique. Thereupon the medical student, in his role as the patient, was regressed to an earlier childhood level and asked to write simple statements. He did this in a typical childish handwriting, but legibly so. After securing samples of his handwriting at various age

*Editor's note. This is another approach to facilitating objective self-perception. See also "Hypnotic Psychotherapy" reprinted in this volume as Article 4. Compare the hypnotic role-playing in this case with that in "Latent homosexuality: Identity exploration in hypnosis," which is Article 43.

levels, he was reoriented to the original trance state. Again he produced illegible scrawls.

SERIAL POSTHYPNOTIC SUGGESTIONS AND AUTOMATIC WRITING

He was then given a series of posthypnotic instructions to awaken and, at a specified cue, to write clearly and legibly, "It is not raining tonight" and to sign it with the names of several classmates. This writing, it was explained, would be done automatically, and he would not know who wrote it since it would be written with such legibility. Also, at a second cue he would write the same sentence again with great care and still not know that he had written it. In fact, he would vigorously deny having written either production, insisting that he could not write that legibly.

The pseudo-patient obeyed instructions in full, and his illegible and legible productions were passed around the group for criticism and discussion, while he vigorously claimed that he had not written them, a claim rendered recognizably valid by his posthypnotic amnesia.

Following this, the patient, still in a trance, was reoriented hypnotically and his identity restored. He was immediately regressed to various childhood levels at each of which he was asked to write clearly and legibly the sentence, "This is a beautiful day in June," signing his name each time and recording his age and the date. At the 14-year level a prolonged series of suggestions was given him to the effect that when he was a grown man, he would be called upon to do the same thing, and a promise was elicited that he would. He was then reoriented to the current situation with an amnesia for trance events, though still in a deep trance.

With great emphasis and care he was given a long series of posthypnotic suggestions to the effect that upon certain specified cues he would, after awakening, write automatically the sentence, "It is a beautiful day in June," and sign it with his name. He would not know he was doing this, and he would vigorously deny having written it. Furthermore, while writing it, he would be engaged in discussing with the medical students some topic that would be raised. (The medical students were posted to have in readiness such topics as the city's population 10 years ago, the street location of some building, etc.)

Additionally, the posthypnotic cue would be repeated a number of times, and each time the writer would raise some question as, "I wonder if the same writing will appear on the next sheet," or, "I expect the next signature will have the full middle name, instead of the initial." Each such question was to be responded to by the execution of the implied suggestion.

When it seemed reasonably certain that he understood, he was awakened. After a few casual remarks, at a glance from the writer, one of the students began discussing a topic. The writer drummed briefly on his desk with his fingers. The patient abstractedly picked up a pencil and, while attending to the discussion directed at him, wrote the sentence and signed it with his first and last names and middle initial, all in legible fashion.

This sheet was quietly removed, a new topic raised, the cue given, and the question voiced by wondering if the sentence would be written. The patient responded exactly as he had been instructed. This time his attention was called to the completed writing, and he was asked if he had done it.

There followed his denials and the animated assertions of the students that he had written it. The patient "proved" his contention by copying the same sentence in his usual illegible script underneath his automatic writing. His "proof" was accepted with a show of much reluctance, and the writer took advantage of this development by asking him to scrutinize that page most carefully, to memorize its appearance thoroughly, and to be prepared to recognize it when shown it again. The sheet was then quietly put out of sight along with the first.

He was asked to count the sheets of paper on the desk and to examine them carefully, one by one, to determine if there were any writing on them. When he affirmed that there was none, he was engaged in a new topic of conversation, the cue was given as the writer "wondered" if his name would appear on the uppermost sheet. Automatically his hand wrote legibly without his knowledge.

Again the procedure was repeated, this time the writer wondering if the top sheet would be placed underneath the other sheets and if his full name would be written on the next. Absentmindedly he straightened out the sheets, slipping the top one underneath and writing his full name on the exposed sheet.

The procedure continued with the items listed below written, one by one, clearly and legibly. Repeatedly his attention was called to the fact that everybody was fully 10 feet away from him. The repetition of this puzzled him greatly.

Sheet 3: "My birthday is November 9th. I was born in Lodi."
      4: "Natalie Williams."
      5: "2 3 8 1 9 2 9"
      6: "Look on the next sheet for the name of the person writing this sentence."
      7: "John Robert Doe."
      8: "You don't believe it, do you?"
      9: "You will—you really will."
     10: "Didn't know you could write well, did you, John R. Doe?"

11:    "You are about to find out that you can write well, and you will
really know it. You will watch yourself writing and you will see
it with your own eyes."

This last sheet was placed at the bottom of the pile. He was then
interrupted and asked if any further writing had appeared on the paper
since that sentence. He shook his head, remarked that the group was too
far away, glanced at the stack of paper, and added that it was ready for
writing if anybody wished to do any. He was asked if he still remembered
the sheet he had been asked to memorize. He nodded his head, and the
writer stepped over and handed it to him. He pointed at the "strange
writing" and his own and showed it to each one in the group.

He was asked to be most certain about his statements concerning the
writing and to hand it to the writer. While the patient's attitude was
distracted for a moment, the first sheet was substituted and he was again
asked if he were certain about the writing. As he asserted he was, the first
sheet was extended to him for apparently a reinspection. He was
tremendously startled to find that "his writing" had disappeared and that
the "strange writing" had moved to a different position on the sheet.
Further manipulation of the sheets bewildered him still more, until he
declared that he did not know what to think since he knew the author was
not a magician. He was assured at once that he would soon know what to
think, and he would then be right.

Next he was asked to examine the stack of paper in front of him and to
see if there was writing on the various sheets. He asserted that he knew
there was none, but upon request he started examining them one by one.

The first few sheets were of course blank. When he came to Sheet No.
3, he commented in astonishment, "That's the same as my birthday, and I
was born in Lodi. That's funny." At Sheet No. 4 he was even more
startled, commenting in amazement that that was his mother's maiden
name.

Sheet No. 5 bewildered him completely, and he disclaimed any
understanding. However, when asked for his present street address and
any other past addresses he remembered, he complied and then suddenly
recognized the house number where he had lived in 1929. Immediately he
looked at the next sheet, hastily read it, and then uncovered Sheet 7. He
read his name aloud to himself, declaring that it was his name, that
nobody else there knew his middle name, that it was not his writing, that it
could not be. He reexamined the other sheets, including the first two. This
discovery of the first sheet and the second as two different written
productions confused him still further.

Upon reading Sheet 8 he was too dumbfounded to speak, except to say,
"I can't; I didn't." Then, after looking hesitantly around, almost furtively,
he looked at Sheet 9, shook his head uncertainly, and slowly lifted the

sheet to see No. 10. This he read aloud to himself in a puzzled, bewildered fashion and finally asked, "What is going on? What is happening?"

The reply was offered, "You are learning something most important. Why not look at the next sheet?" Obediently he uncovered the next sheet, read it carefully, and turned to the writer as if waiting.

Immediately, a posthypnotic cue previously employed to induce a trance was given. He developed a deep trance at once and was instructed, "You know unconsciously the whole truth about the writing unconsciously, and you are now ready to know it consciously. You can write well, you can take pride in doing something well, and more than that, you know, really know, that you can do many things well. Only one thing remains to be done before you can use all this understanding to change your ways of doing many things. That one thing that needs to be done will be done shortly.

VISUAL HALLUCINATIONS TO FACILITATE OBJECTIVE SELF-PERCEPTION

"I want you to look in that crystal ball right there and see yourself writing in the unhappy, miserable fashion you have for so long. See yourself plainly. Now that that is done, see a second crystal ball alongside that one. In it you now see yourself writing legibly, and as you watch, a tremendous flood of joy and happiness and confidence and pride will well up in you, ready to become shown as soon as you awaken and watch your handwriting, 'This is a beautiful day in June. Signed: John R. Doe.' You will watch your hand write this and then write it a second time. Then you will put the sheet away and turn to me and tell me from the bottom of your heart that you can write well and you will show me by writing whatever you wish. And then all the happiness in the world will well up in you, just like in a happy little boy, a growing boy, just like in a teenager who has won first place, like a young man that has succeeded in his first big job. This joy you will really share with everybody, and we will enjoy your happiness because it means everything in so many ways to you. Now awaken and watch first how your hand writes."

Instructions were followed fully, and the writing he did of his own determining was, "I can really write—I can really do a lot of things I am going to do. John R. Doe."

Upon reading it through, he leaped to his feet and, at first childishly, then boyishly, then youthfully, demanded over and over that each of the medical students, as well as the writer, read his writing, comment on it favorably, and watch him do further writing. About 15 minutes was spent in this emotional display. Then suddenly he gathered up his papers, handed them to the writer, and said "Thank you." Turning to the students he said, "Excuse me a moment, gentlemen," sat down, undid his knotted shoestrings, and tied them in neat bows.

Straightening up, he addressed them, "I want to thank you gentlemen, too. If you ever need any automobile parts, I'll give you the best service in the world." After shaking hands all around, he took his departure, but he was observed entering the men's room. When he came out, his tie was neatly knotted.

He was seen two weeks later. He reported that he had been working overtime, extensively recopying for his employer all the past records of parts received and sold, so that his employer would have decent records. A month later he had received a promotion and a marked increase in salary. He had developed his social life and had joined an amateur theatrical group and was at the present rehearsing regularly for one of the leading roles. He had also been having social engagements with a young woman of his age.

A year later he was decidedly happy in a minor executive position in a large automobile-accessory firm and was considering marriage. Several years later word was received indirectly that he was happily married and still employed by the same firm.

56. The Hypnotherapy of Two Psychosomatic Dental Problems

Milton H. Erickson

In the practice of psychiatry one frequently encounters patients whose problems center around some physical attribute with which they are dissatisfied. Too often they seek help from those trained to deal with such physical aspects of the body, but who have not had the training or the experience necessary to recognize that the primary consideration is the patient's personality reaction, not the patient's physical condition.

Consequently, efforts to alter the physical state, regardless of the technical skill employed and the excellence of the results obtained, are not appreciated, since the patient's hopeful expectations are not limited to the actual possibilities of the physical realities. Particularly is this true in the fields of dentistry and plastic surgery, where sometimes the most skillful work may fail to meet the emotional demands of the patient.

To illustrate this general type of psychosomatic problem in the field of dentistry, two case histories are to be cited below. In each instance the patient seized upon a dental anomaly as the explanation of a definite personality maladjustment. For each, the problem of therapy was not a correction of the dental problem but a recognition of emotional needs.

Several examples of the first type of patient have been seen. Among them was one who underwent an extraction and a fitting with a denture. Her maladjustment continued, increased by her permanent dissatisfaction with the dental work. Another had centered all her life around her neurotic reactions, scorning any type of treatment. A third had been comfortingly told, when she sought dental intervention, that she should take pride in being unique, and so well had the dentist done this that she had adjusted satisfactorily.

Two examples of the second type have been seen. Both of those bitterly resented the dental correction that had been made, since they had been left with their primary personality problem unsolved.

Neither of the writer's patients reported here had sought correction of their dental anomalies nor had their dentists suggested any need for correction.

Reprinted with permission from the *Journal of the American Society of Psychosomatic Dentistry and Medicine*, 1955, *1*, 6–10.

While the cases to be cited represent primarily problems best handled by a psychiatrist, there is a need for those in allied fields to be aware of the nature and possible seriousness of seemingly minor psychosomatic reactions and of the opportunities of dealing more adequately with them.

PATIENT A

A high school girl sought psychiatric help because she was failing her second-year work and because she had barely succeeded in meeting the first year's requirements. Her reason for coming to the writer was that she knew he was a hypnotist and because she had been much impressed by an extracurricular lecture he had given at the high school. As she entered the office, she remarked that she would probably be hypnotized by a single glance from the writer and that she probably would not even know she was in a trance. No effort was made to disillusion her.

She had come without her parents' knowledge because she felt that they would not understand her problem. Nor could she go to anybody else she knew because they would only minimize her problem and reassure her "falsely."

Her complaint was that she was an "absolute freak" in appearance because she had only one double-sized upper incisor tooth. This had not troubled her until the development of physiological maturity and a concurrent change in residence, making necessary admission to a high school where she knew nobody.

Her reaction to her personal and school situation had been one of withdrawal, seclusiveness, and the development of much wishful thinking in which her teeth were "normal." She found herself extremely self-conscious, was unwilling to eat in the school cafeteria, and avoided smiling or laughing at every cost: her enunciation of words was faulty because of her voluntary rigidity of her upper lip. However, her attitude in the office was one of ease, which she explained was because she was probably hypnotized.

During the interview it was noted that she relied almost exclusively on slang and "jive talk." Even in making serious remarks, she couched them in extravagances of slang.

For the next two interviews she was encouraged to display her actually extensive knowledge of, and fluency in, past and current slang, and she was delighted to display her ability. Additionally, she was an excellent mimic and had a remarkable command of accents, which she was most ready to display. Accordingly she was asked to demonstrate at length the "choppy" speech of the British and the "bitten off" enunciation of the Scotch. Also, she had an extensive knowledge of popular songs, past and present, comic strips, nursery tales, and light literature of all sorts.

The next interview was devoted to an extensive discussion of the picturesqueness of slang. This conversation unnoticeably and deviously led into a discussion of expressions, such as L'il Abner's "chompin' gum," "what big teeth you have, Grandmother," "Ol' Dan Tucker, who died with a toothache in his heel," "putting the bite on Daddy for more pocket money," "sinking a fang in a banana split," and various other expressions or phrases containing references to teeth or dental activity.

She was interested and pleased but also amused by the writer's effort to talk in "hep" style. She contributed gladly and readily to the discussion by calling upon her extensive knowledge of references to teeth in popular songs, nursery tales, comics, and slang, without seeming to note the personal implications.

For the next interview she promised to "rattle the ivory" with every reference she could "dig up, from China Choppers to the Elks' Club."

The next session was fascinating. In response to a request, in rapid-fire fashion, alternating from the British to the Scottish pattern of speech, utilizing slang to do so, she proceeded to give, from song, stories, ditties, doggerel, comics, fables, and slang old and new, innumerable references to teeth.

When she finally began to slow down, the remark was made, "When you put the bite on a job, you really sink your fang into it, but then, you've got the really hep accessory for that. Use your choppers now to chop off a bit more of the British and your fang to bite off a bit more Scotch."

She paused abruptly, apparently suddenly realizing both the personal implications and the fact that teeth could be an interesting, amusing, and pleasingly fascinating subject. Immediately, since she also liked puns immensely, she was reminded of the comic, "That's my Pop," and told to go home, look into the mirror, smile broadly, and then say, "That's my maw." If she did not understand, she was then to consult a dictionary.

At the next interview she was full of smiles and laughter, greeting the writer with a wide grin and saying, "Yes sir, that's my maw."

Asked what she had been doing since the last interview, she replied that she had been having a good time "chewing international fat" (talking with various accents), thereby bewildering her teachers and entertaining her schoolmates. Asked if she felt that she were a freak, she stated that she did not but that her instructors surely did when she "chewed the frog, the sauerkraut, or the cornpone" (French, German, and Southern accents).

Subsequently, one of her high school teachers, in discussing pedagogical problems with the author, commented on a remarkable transformation of one of his students. He had first noted her as a shy, withdrawn, and inept student, one whose speech was faulty and whose recitations were unsatisfactory. Then one day she had given a faultless recitation with a strong British accent, repeating the performance on another day with a Scottish accent. Subsequently, he had heard her chattering to a group in the corridor with a Norwegian accent. He regarded her as a decidedly brilliant student, though rather inexplicable in her adolescent behavior.

Still later another instructor, in discussing his Ph.D. thesis on aspects of high school behavior, cited the instance of this same girl's remarkable transformation and her amazing linguistic abilities, which had rendered her a popular and well-adjusted, competent student.

PATIENT B

A 21-year-old girl, employed as a secretary for a construction firm, sought therapy because "I'm too inferior to live, I think. I've got no friends, I stay by myself. I'm too homely to get married. I want a husband, a home, and children, but I haven't a chance. There's nothing for me but work and being an old maid, but I thought I'd see a psychiatrist before I committed suicide. I'm going to try you for three months' time and then, if things aren't straightened out, that's the end."

She was utterly final in this attitude, and consented to only two therapeutic hours a week for three months. She paid in advance and stipulated that she be discharged at the close of the thirteenth interview. (She checked the calendar and counted the number of possible interviews.)

She was not communicative about her past history. Her parents, neither of whom had wanted her, had been unhappy as long as she could remember. They were killed in an automobile accident shortly after her graduation from high school. Since then she had lived in rooming-houses and had worked at various stenographic and secretarial jobs. She changed jobs frequently because of self-dissatisfaction.

Concerning herself and her feelings of inferiority, she listed them bitterly as follows:

1. There is an unsightly wide space between my two upper front teeth. It's horrible and I don't dare to smile. (With difficulty she was persuaded to show this. The spacing was about an eighth of an inch.)
2. I can't talk plain. (From holding her upper lip stiff.)
3. My hair is black, coarse, straight, and too long.
4. My breasts are too small, and my hips are too small.
5. My ankles are too thick.
6. My nose is hooked. (Actually very slightly.)

7. I'm Jewish.

8. I'm an unwanted child, always have been, always will be.

In explaining this list of defects, all emphasis was placed upon the spacing of her upper incisors. To her that was the causation of all her difficulties. She felt that she could adjust to the "other things," but this "horrible spacing" rendered impossible for her any hope of adjustment.

After her unhappy description of herself, she sobbed and then endeavored to leave, declaring, "Keep the money, I won't need it where I'm going." However, she was persuaded to keep to her original plan of three months' therapy.

Contrary to her description of herself, she was definitely a pretty girl, well-proportioned, and decidedly attractive. She was graceful in her movements and had good posture, except for her downcast head.

Her general appearance, however, was most unattractive. Her hair was straggly, snarled, and uneven in length. (She cut it herself.) The part was crooked and careless. Her blouse lacked a button, there was a small rip in the skirt, the color combination of the blouse and the skirt was wrong, her slip showed on one side, her shoes were scuffed, and her shoestrings were tied in unsightly knots. She wore no makeup, and while her fingernails were well-shaped, remnants of fingernail polish were on only one hand. (She had started to apply fingernail polish a few days previously but was too discouraged to complete the task or to remove the evidence of her attempt.)

During the next four sessions she was sullen and uncooperative, insisting that the writer earn his fee by doing all the talking.

However, it was learned that she was intensely attracted to a young man two years older than she who also worked at her place of employment. She usually arranged to observe him when he went to the drinking fountain down the corridor, but she ignored him and never spoke to him, although he had made overtures. Inquiry disclosed that the fountain trips were rather numerous. She made it a point to go whenever he did, and apparently he behaved similarly. This had been taking place for the last two months.

She proved to be a rather poor hypnotic subject and only a light trance could be induced. Hence, all these and subsequent interviews were conducted in the light trance.

The next four sessions were primarily devoted to building up the general idea that, by a certain date, she was to acquire a completely new, but quiet and modest outfit of clothes and to have her hair dressed at the beauty shop. Then, at a date set by the writer, she was to go to work in her new clothes. (During this period of time she continued to wear the same clothes she had worn at the first interview). The rationalization was offered her that since she was not optimistic about the future, she might as well have "one last fling."

The next two sessions were spent on the subject of her "parted teeth." She was given the assignment of filling her mouth with water and squirting it out between her teeth until she acquired a practiced aim and distance. She regarded this assignment as silly and ridiculous, but conscientiously practiced each evening because "it doesn't really matter what I do."

The two following sessions were devoted, first indirectly and then more and more directly, to the idea that she would make use of her newly acquired skill of squirting water as a practical joke at the expense of the desirable young man.

At first she rejected the idea, then accepted it as a somewhat amusing but crude fantasy, and finally she accepted it as a possibility to be definitely executed.

The final plan evolved was that the next Monday, dressed in her new outfit, her nails polished and her hair having been dressed the previous Saturday at the beauty shop, she would await a favorable opportunity to precede the young man to the drinking fountain. There she would await his approach, fill her mouth full of water, and spray him. Then she was to giggle, start to run toward him, turn suddenly and "run like hell down the corridor."

As was learned later, she carried out the suggestions fully. Late in the afternoon she had seized an opportunity to execute the plan. His look of consternation and his startled exclamation of, "You damn little bitch," evoked her laughter at him. When she ran, he, quite naturally, pursued her and caught her at the end of the corridor. Upon seizing her he declared, "For that kind of a trick, you're going to get a good kissing" and suited his action to his words.

The next day, rather timid and embarrassed, she warily went to the fountain for a drink. As she bent over the fountain, she found herself being sprayed with a water pistol by the young man concealed behind a telephone booth. She immediately filled her mouth with water and charged him, only to turn and run wildly as he met her charge head on. Again she was caught and kissed.

The patient failed to keep her next two appointments, and then came in at the next regular time, thoroughly well groomed in appearance.

She gave the foregoing account, and stated that the second episode had resulted in a dinner invitation. This had been repeated two days later. Now she was considering the acceptance of another invitation for dinner and the theater.

She explained further that the outcome of the silly prank suggested to her by the writer had caused her to spend many thoughtful hours "taking inventory of myself." As a result she had one request to make of the writer—namely, would he coldly, judiciously, and honestly appraise her in detail? When this was done, she would terminate therapy. The smile with which she made this statement was most reassuring.

Accordingly, her request was met by discussing:

1. Her original woebegone, desperate emotional attitude.
2. Her unkempt, frumpish appearance.
3. Her unwarranted derogation of her physical self.
4. Her misconception of a dental asset as a liability.
5. Her sincerity and cooperation in therapy, however bizarre had seemed the ideas presented.
6. The readiness with which she had assumed self-responsibility in reacting to pleasurable life situations.
7. The obvious fact that she now recognized her own personal values.
8. Her need to review her objectives in life as stated in the original interviews.
9. Her personal attractiveness, not as seen only by herself but as appreciated from the masculine point of view.

She listened attentively and, at the close of the interview, thanked the writer graciously and took her departure.

Several months later a marked copy of the local newspaper was received in the mail containing an announcement of her engagement. About six months later an announcement of her marriage to the young man was received. Then, 15 months later, a letter was received containing a snapshot of her home, the announcement of her son's birth, and a newspaper clipping announcing her husband's promotion to junior member of the construction firm. Since then no direct word has been received, but she has referred to the writer several patients who speak glowingly of her.

DISCUSSION

Although both of these patients emphasized their dental complaint as the fundamental consideration in their maladjustment, the case histories have been reported without distortion. Instead, an effort has been made to present the general situation of which the dental aspect constituted merely the one item which had been seized upon to represent completely a total problem.

Therapy for both was predicated upon the assumption that there is a strong normal tendency for the personality to adjust if given an opportunity. The simple fact that both patients had centralized their complaints upon one single item of a psychosomatic character, which was alterable if necessary, suggested that prolonged, extensive probing into the experiential life of the patients and elaborate reeducation were not necessarily indicated.

The therapeutic results obtained indicate that an uncomplicated psychotherapeutic approach may be most effective in a circumscribed psychosomatic reaction. Had this method failed with these two patients, there would still have remained the possibility of a more elaborate psychotherapeutic procedure.

57. The Identification of a Secure Reality

Milton H. Erickson

Reality, security, and the definition of boundaries and limitations constitute important considerations in the growth of understanding in childhood. To an eight-year-old child the question of what constitutes power and strength and reality and security can be a serious matter. When one is small, weak, and intelligent, living in an undefined world of intellectual and emotional fluctuations, one seeks to learn what is really strong, secure, and safe.

A 27-year-old mother began to encounter serious difficulty with her eight-year-old son, who was becoming progressively defiant and seemed to find a new way to defy her each day. The mother had divorced her husband two years previously for adequate reasons recognized by all concerned. In addition to her son she had two daughters, aged nine and six. After some months of occasional dating with men in the hope of marriage, she found her son had become rebellious and an unexpected problem. The older daughter had joined him briefly in this rebelliousness. The mother was able to correct the daughter by her customary measures of discipline through anger, shouting, scolding, threatening, and then an angry spanking followed by an intelligent, reasonable, objective discussion with the child. In the past this had always been effective with the children. However, her son Joe refused to respond to her usual measures, even when she added repeated spankings, deprivations, tears, and the enlistment of her family's assistance. Joe merely stated, quite happily and cheerfully, that he planned to do whatever he pleased and nothing, just nothing, could stop him.

The son's misbehavior spread to the school and to the neighborhood, and literally nothing was safe from his depredations. School property was destroyed, teachers defied, schoolmates assaulted; neighbor's windows were broken and their flower beds destroyed. The neighbors and teachers, endeavoring to take a hand in the matter, succeeded in intimidating the child, but nothing more. Finally the boy began destroying things of value in the home, especially after the mother was asleep at night, and then he would infuriate her by boldfacedly denying guilt the next morning.

This final mischief led the mother to bring the boy in for treatment. As the mother told her story, Joe listened with a broad, triumphant smile.

Reprinted with permission from *Family Process*, September, 1962, *1*, 294–303.

When she had finished, he boastfully declared that the author could not do anything to stop him and he was going to go right on doing as he pleased. The author assured him, gravely and earnestly, that it was unnecessary for him to do anything to change the boy's behavior because he was a good, big, strong boy and very smart, and he would have to change his behavior all by himself. The boy was assured that his mother would do just enough to give him a chance to change his behavior "all by himself." Joe received this statement in an incredulous sneering manner. Then he was sent out of the office with the statement that his mother would be told some simple little things that she could do so that he himself could change his behavior. He was also earnestly challenged in a most kindly fashion to try to figure out what those simple little things might be. This served to puzzle him into quiet reflective behavior while he awaited his mother.

Alone with the mother, the author discussed a child's demand for a world in which he could be certain that there was someone stronger and more powerful than he. To date her son had demonstrated with increasing desperation that the world was so insecure that the only strong person in it was himself, a little eight-year-old boy. Then the mother was given painstakingly clear instructions for her activities over the next two days.

As they left the office, the boy challengingly asked if the author had recommended spankings. He was assured that no measure would be taken except to give him full opportunity to change his own behavior; no one else would change it. This reply perplexed him, and on the way home his mother administered severe corporal punishment to compel him to let her drive the automobile safely. This misconduct had been anticipated; the mother had been advised to deal with it summarily and without argument. The evening was spent in the usual fashion by letting the boy watch television as he wished.

The following morning the grandparents arrived and picked up the two daughters. Joe, who had plans to go swimming, demanded his breakfast. He was most puzzled when he observed his mother carry into the living room some wrapped sandwiches, fruit, one Thermos bottle of fruit juice and one of coffee, and some towels. She put all these items securely on a heavy couch with the telephone and some books. Joe demanded that she prepare his breakfast without delay, threatening physical destruction of the first thing he could lay his hands on if she did not hurry. His mother merely smiled at him, seized him, threw him quickly to the floor on his stomach, and sat her full weight upon him. When he yelled at her to get off, she replied mildly that she had already eaten breakfast and she had nothing to do except to try to think about ways to change his behavior. However, she pointed out that she was certain she did not know any way; therefore it would all be up to him.

The boy struggled furiously against the odds of his mother's weight, strength, and watchful dexterity. He yelled, screamed, shouted profanity and obscenities, sobbed, and finally promised piteously always to be a good boy. His mother answered that the promise did not mean anything because she had not yet figured out how to change his behavior. This evoked another fit of rage from him, which finally ceased, followed by his urgent plea to go to the bathroom. His mother explained gently that she had not finished her thinking; she offered him a towel to mop up so he would not get too wet. This elicited another wild bit of struggling, which soon exhausted him. His mother took advantage of the quiet to make a telephone call to her mother. While Joe listened, she explained casually that she had not yet reached any conclusion in her thinking and she really believed that any change in behavior would have to come from Joe. Her son greeted this remark with as loud a scream as he could muster. His mother commented into the telephone that Joe was too busy screaming to think about changing his behavior, and she put the mouthpiece down to Joe's mouth so that he could scream into it.

Joe lapsed into sullen silence, broken by sudden surges of violent effort, screams, demands, and sobbing interrupted by piteous pleas. To all of this his mother gave the same mild, pat answers. As time passed, the mother poured herself coffee, fruit juice, ate sandwiches, and read a book. Shortly before noon the boy politely told her he really did need to go to the bathroom. She confessed a similar need. She explained that it would be possible if he would agree to return, resume his position on the floor, and let her sit down comfortably upon him. After some tears, he consented. He fulfilled his promise, but almost immediately launched into renewed violent activity to dislodge her. Each near success led to further effort, which exhausted him still more. While he rested, she ate fruit and drank coffee, made a casual telephone call, and read a book.

After over five hours Joe surrendered by stating simply and abjectly that he would do anything and everything she told him to do. His mother replied just as simply and earnestly that her thinking had been in vain; she just did not know what to tell him to do. He burst into tears at this, but shortly, sobbing, he told her he knew what to do. She replied mildly that she was very glad of this but she did not think he had had enough time to think long enough about it. Perhaps another hour or so of thinking might help.

Joe silently awaited the passing of an hour while his mother sat reading quietly. When over an hour had passed, she commented on the time but expressed her wish to finish the chapter. Joe sighed shudderingly and sobbed softly to himself while his mother finished her reading.

With the chapter finally finished, the mother got up and so did Joe. He timidly asked for something to eat. His mother explained in laborious detail that it was too late for lunch, that breakfast was always eaten before lunch, and that it was too late to serve breakfast. She suggested instead that he have a drink of ice water and a comfortable rest in bed for the remainder of the afternoon.

Joe fell asleep quickly but awakened to the odors of well-liked foods. His sisters had returned, and he tried to join them at the table for the evening meal. His mother explained—gravely, simply, and in lucid detail—that it was customary first to eat breakfast and then lunch and then dinner. Unfortunately, he had missed his breakfast, therefore he had to miss his lunch. Now he would have to miss his dinner, but fortunately he could begin a new day the next morning. Joe returned to his bedroom and cried himself to sleep. The mother slept lightly that night, but Joe did not arise until she was well along with breakfast preparations.

Joe entered the kitchen with his sisters for breakfast and sat down happily while his mother served his sisters with pancakes and sausages. At Joe's place was a large bowl. His mother explained that she had cooked him an extra-special breakfast of oatmeal, a food not too well liked by him. Tears came to his eyes, but he thanked her for the serving, as was the family custom, and ate voraciously. His mother explained that she had cooked an extra supply so that he could have a second helping. She also cheerfully expressed the hope that enough would be left over to meet his needs for lunch. Joe ate manfully to prevent that possibility, but his mother had cooked a remarkably large supply.

After breakfast Joe set about cleaning up his room without any instruction. This done, he worked hard picking up the stones he had thrown on the lawn. When he asked his mother if he could call upon the neighbors, she had no idea what this portended but gave permission. From behind the window curtains she watched him while he went next door and rang the bell. When the door opened, he apparently spoke to the neighbor briefly and then went on up the street. As she later learned, just as systematically as he had terrorized the neighborhood, he canvassed it to offer his apologies and to promise that he would come back to make amends as fast as he could. He explained that it would take a considerable period of time for him to undo all the mischief he had done.

Joe returned for lunch, ate buttered, cold, thick sliced oatmeal, helped voluntarily to dry the dishes, and spent the afternoon and evening with his schoolbooks while his sisters watched television. The evening meal was ample but consisted of leftovers, which Joe ate quietly without comment. At bedtime Joe went to bed voluntarily while his sisters awaited their mother's usual insistence.

The next day Joe went to school, where he made his apologies and promises. These were accepted warily. That evening he became involved in a typical childish quarrel with his older sister, who shrieked for her mother. As the mother entered the room, Joe began to tremble visibly. Both children were told to sit down, and the sister was asked to state her case first. When it became his turn to speak, Joe said he agreed with his sister. His mother then explained to Joe that she expected him to be a normal eight-year-old boy and to get into ordinary trouble like all regular eight-year-old boys. Then she pointed out to both of them that their quarrel was lacking in merit and was properly to be abandoned. Both children acquiesced.

GAINING MOTHER'S COOPERATION

The education of Joe's mother to enable her to deal with her son's problem by following out the instructions was a rather difficult task. She was a college graduate, a highly intelligent woman with a background of social and community interests and responsibilities. In the interview she was asked to describe, in as full a way as possible, the damage Joe had done in the school and the community. With this description the damage became painfully enlarged in her mind. (Plants do grow back, broken windowpanes and torn dresses can be replaced, but this comfort was not allowed to be a part of her review.)

Next she was asked to describe Joe "as he used to be"—a reasonably happy, well-behaved, and actually a decidedly brilliant child. She was repeatedly asked to draw these comparisons between his past and present behavior, more briefly each time, but with a greater highlighting of the essential points. Then she was asked to speculate upon the probable future of Joe both "as he used to be" and as was "quite possible" now in the light of his present behavior. Helpful suggestions were given to aid the mother in drawing sharply contrasting "probable pictures of the future."

After this discussion she was asked to consider in full the possibilities of what she could do over the weekend and the kind of role she ought to assume with Joe. Since she did not know, this placed her completely in a passive position, so the author could offer plans. Her repressed and guilty resentments and hostilities toward her son and his misbehavior were utilized. Every effort was made to redirect them into an anticipation of a satisfying, calculated, deliberate watchfulness in the frustrating of her son's attempts to confirm his sense of insecurity and to prove her ineffectual.

The mother's apparently justified statement that her weight of 150 pounds was much too great to permit putting it fully on the body of an eight-year-old child was a major factor in winning the mother's full cooperation. At first this argument was carefully evaded. The mother was helped systematically to marshal all of her objections to the author's proposed plans behind this apparently indisputable argument that her weight was too great to be endured by a child. As she became more entrenched in this defense, a carefully worded discussion allowed her to wish with increasing desire that she could do the various things the author outlined as he detailed possibilities for the entire weekend.

When the mother seemed to have reached the right degree of emotional readiness, the question of her weight was raised for disposal. She was simply assured that she need not take medical opinion at all but would learn from her son on the morrow that her weight would be inconsequential to him. In fact it would take all of her strength, dexterity, and alertness in addition to her weight to master the situation. She might even lose the contest because of the insufficiency of her weight. (The mother could not analyze the binding significance of this argument so simply presented to her. She was placed in the position of trying to prove that her weight was really too much. To prove this, she would need her son's cooperation, and the author was certain that the boy's aggressive patterns would preclude any passive yielding to his mother's weight. In this way the mother would be taught by the son to disregard her defenses against the author's suggestions, and she would be reinforced in her acceptance of those suggestions by the very violence of his behavior.) As the mother later explained, "The way that bucking bronco threw me around, I knew I would have to settle down to serious business to keep my seat. It just became a question of who was smarter, and I knew I had a real job to do. Then I began to take pleasure in anticipating and meeting his moves. It was almost like a chess game. I certainly learned to admire and respect his determination, and I got an immense satisfaction out of frustrating him as thoroughly as he had frustrated me.

"I had one awfully bad time though. When we came back from the bathroom, and he started to lie down on the floor, he looked at me so pitifully that I wanted to take him in my arms. But I remembered what you said about not accepting surrender because of pity but only when the issue was settled. That's when I knew I had won, so I was awfully careful then to be sure not to let any pity come in. That made the rest of it easy, and I could really understand what I was doing and why."

A LATER REINFORCEMENT

For the next few months, until midsummer, all went well. Then for no apparent reason except an ordinary quarrel with his sister settled unfairly to her advantage, Joe declared quietly but firmly that he did not have "to take that kind of stuff." He said he could "stomp" anybody, particularly the author, and he dared his mother to take him to see the author that very evening. At a loss what to do, his mother brought him to the office immediately. As they entered, she declared somewhat inaccurately that Joe had threatened to "stomp" the author's office. Joe was immediately told, disparagingly, that he probably could not stomp the floor hard enough to make it worthwhile. Irately, Joe raised his foot and brought his cowboy boot down hard upon the carpeted floor. He was told, condescendingly, that his effort was really remarkably good for a little eight-year-old boy and that he probably could repeat it a number of times, but not very many. Joe angrily shouted that he could stomp that hard 50, 100, 1,000 times if he wished. Reply was made that he was only eight years old, and no matter how angry he was he couldn't stomp 1,000 times. In fact he couldn't even stomp hard half that number of times, which would only be 500. If he tried, he would soon get tired, his stomp would get littler and weaker, and he would have to change off to the other leg and rest. Even worse, he was told he couldn't even stand still while he rested without wiggling around and wanting to sit down. If he didn't believe this, he could just go right ahead and stomp. When he got all tired out like a little boy, he could rest by standing still until he discovered that he could not even stand still without wiggling and wanting to sit down. With outraged and furious dignity Joe declared his solemn intention of stomping a hole in the floor even if it took a hundred million stomps.

His mother was dismissed with instructions that she was to return in the "square root of four," which she translated to mean "in two hours." In this way Joe was not informed of the time when she would return, although he recognized that one adult was telling another a specific time. As the office door closed upon his mother, Joe balanced on his right foot and crashed his left foot to the floor. The author assumed a look of astonishment, commenting that the stomp was far better than he had expected of Joe, but he doubted if Joe could keep it up. Certainty was expressed that Joe would soon weaken, and then he would discover he couldn't even stand still. Joe contemptuously stomped a few more times before it became possible to disparage his stomp as becoming weaker.

After intensifying his efforts, Joe reached a count of 30 before he realized that he had greatly overestimated his stomping ability. As this realization became evident in Joe's facial expression, he was patronizingly offered the privilege of just patting the floor 1,000 times with his foot, since he really couldn't stand still and rest without wiggling around and wanting to sit down. With desperate dignity, he rejected the floor-patting and declared his intention of standing still. Promptly he assumed a stiff upright position, with his hands at his sides, facing the author. He was immediately shown the desk clock, and comment was offered about the slowness of the minute hand and the even greater slowness of the hour hand, despite the seeming rapidity of the ticking of the clock. The author turned to his desk, began to make notes in Joe's case record, and from that he turned to other desk tasks.

Within 15 minutes Joe was shifting his weight back and forth from one foot to the other, twisting his neck, wiggling his shoulders. When a half-hour had passed, he was reaching out with his hand, resting some of his weight on the arm of the chair beside which he was standing. However, he quickly withdrew his hand whenever the author seemed about to look up to glance reflectively about the room. After about an hour the author excused himself temporarily from the office. Joe took full advantage of this, and of several repetitions, never quite getting back into his previous position beside the chair.

When his mother knocked at the office door, Joe was told, "When your mother comes in, do exactly as I tell you." She was admitted and seated, looking wonderingly at Joe as he stood rigidly facing the desk. Signaling silence to the mother, the author turned to Joe and peremptorily commanded, "Joe, show your mother how hard you can still stomp on the floor." Joe was startled, but he responded nobly. "Now, Joe, show her how stiff and straight you can stand still." A minute later two more orders were issued, "Mother, this interview between Joe and me is a secret between Joe and me. Joe, don't tell your mother a single thing about what happened in this office. You and I both know, and that's enough. O.K.?"

Both Joe and his mother nodded their heads. She looked a bit mystified; Joe looked thoughtfully pleased. On the trip home Joe was quiet, sitting quite close beside his mother. About halfway home Joe broke the silence by commenting that the author was a "nice doctor." As the mother later stated, this statement had relieved her puzzled mind in some inexplicable way. She neither asked nor was given any explanation of the office events. She knew only that Joe liked, respected, and trusted the author and was glad to see him occasionally in a social or semisocial fashion. Joe's behavior continued to be that of a normal, highly intelligent boy who now and then misbehaved in an expected and warrantable fashion.

Two years passed, and Joe's mother became engaged. Joe liked the prospective stepfather but asked his mother one demanding question—did the author approve of the man? Assured the author did approve, there was then unquestioning acceptance.

COMMENT

In the process of living the price of survival is eternal vigilance and the willingness to learn. The sooner one becomes aware of realities and the sooner one adjusts to them, the quicker is the process of adjustment and the happier the experience of living. When one knows the boundaries, restrictions, and limitations that govern, then one is free to utilize satisfactorily whatever is available. But in an undefined world, where intellectual and emotional fluctuations create an enveloping state of uncertainty that varies from one mood and one moment to the next, there can be no certainty or security. Joe sought to learn what was really strong, secure, and safe, and he learned it in the effective way one learns not to kick a stone with the bare foot or to slap a cactus with the bare hands. There are relative values of effort and purposes and rewards, and Joe was given an opportunity to strive, think, assess, compare, appraise, contrast, and to choose. Thereby he could learn and hence could adjust.

Joe is not the only patient on whom this type of therapy has been employed. Over the years there have been a number of comparable instances, some almost identical. In some of these cases the author's practice of keeping in contact with patients over the years has yielded information repeatedly affirming the value of reality confrontation as a successful measure for defining a secure reality.

58. The Hypnotic Corrective Emotional Experience

Milton H. Erickson

An unintentional, completely hypnotic, Corrective Emotional Experience occurred under unusual circumstances at a medical meeting where the author had been asked to present a general lecture on hypnosis without a demonstration. In attendance there was a group of seven physicians, among them psychoanalytically trained psychiatrists, who sat together in the rear to one side of the auditorium. They had previously spoken most adversely about hypnosis and had opposed inviting the author to address the group. Scattered in the audience were a number of other physicians who were also unreceptive of hypnosis, a fact of which the official host for the meeting had informed the author. During the question-and-answer period numerous requests were made that a demonstration of hypnosis be given. Since it was obvious that the vast majority of those present were decidedly in favor of a demonstration, volunteers were called for—but there were none. The author asked if the audience would be agreeable to his choosing at random someone in the audience, and a most favorable response was received. Thereupon a physician was singled out and invited to the speaker's platform. After a moment's hesitation he rose and strode up briskly. As he was doing this, the author's host frowningly shook his head negatively and held up his hand in the "thumbs down" position to indicate that a bad choice had been made. But the author saw no immediate solution to the problem.

(Two explanatory paragraphs will be inserted here so that the reader may better understand the unexpected course of events. After the meeting the author was apprised that his subject was a rather unusual and even somewhat eccentric character. He had never married, and had two interests—his medical practice and his studies. He was a man of high intelligence and integrity, and he was well-respected. He had intensely strong, even extreme likes and dislikes, and he was not hesitant about making them freely and bluntly known. For years he had been bitterly resentful toward psychiatry, and the author's random choice of him as a subject caused considerable apprehensiveness in the audience.

Reprinted with permission from *The American Journal of Clinical Hypnosis,* January, 1965, 7, 242–248.

As for his "studies," he was always engaged upon some new course of intensive study which was invariably detailed, comprehensive, and systematic, and which he always completed. Usually with the advent of any new or striking development in medicine, he embarked upon an intensive course of study for months at a time, yet devoted himself untiringly to his extensive general practice in a large rural community. Because he was extremely well informed, he was frequently consulted by physicians in other fields—except psychiatry, toward which he manifested a well-verbalized, violent dislike. Also he often freely exhibited unreasonable antagonism toward psychiatrists in general. Even his presence at the lecture had distressed a number of people, who anticipated a disagreeable outburst from him. The author's chance selection of him as a subject caused those in charge of the meeting serious alarm, but they could think of nothing to do to avert the expected catastrophe.)

As the man approached the author at the podium, he was asked for his name. His reply was simply the rather brusque question, "Is it really necessary for you to know my name to demonstrate hypnosis?"

He was answered with the statement, "Not at all; just seat yourself comfortably in that armchair while I make a few remarks to the audience." After a momentary pause he moved the chair so that he would face the author and present his profile to the audience; then he sat down.

Addressing the audience, the author reminded them of his comments earlier on ideomotor responses, their involuntary character, and the frequent development of a sense of physical dissociation. Peripheral vision disclosed the subject to be listening with utter intensity. The author continued with an explanation that a voluntary motor response, once initiated, could be converted easily into an involuntary continued response. "For example," it was stated, "if I take this physician's wrist and extend it at shoulder level in front of him [suiting action to the words], and then gently, with my right hand, place his hand in a position of dorsiflexion [again suiting action to the words], and ask him to fixate his gaze intently on his thumbnail, and begin the action of moving his hand slowly toward his face [doing so], his elbow will bend gently more and more, and the movement soon becomes involuntary [releasing the hold upon the wrist with a wavering, uncertain, altering, and constantly decreasing pressure of first one finger and then another until, unnoticeably, contact with his wrist ceased, a technique described in a previous article (Erickson, 1964)], and there results an unexpected catalepsy and the rather rapid development of a deep trance state."

It was at once apparent that exactly what the author had just described was occurring, since this procedure is an indirect, unchallengeable technique seemingly addressed to others, but which puts the subject in the position of listening and trying to understand and thus becoming responsive by virtue of the very effort of trying to understand, thereby to be enabled to challenge the operator. But most astonishingly, as the subject's hand slowly approached his face, he slowly twisted his body and tilted it forward until he seemed to be in a position to look directly at the group of hostile physicians in the far corner of the room. As his hand came close to his face, there was a slow spreading of the digits, the development of a slightly amused, sardonic expression on his face, and his hand came to rest in the nose-thumbing position. At a total loss to understand this behavior, the author simply watched him for at least three minutes. The man was obviously cataleptic, his blink and swallowing reflexes were absent and no startle response was manifested when the author surreptitiously pushed a heavy pointer off the table to fall noisily on the floor. The audience, however, showed an overreactive startle response to this disturbance, but the author merely attributed this to the unusualness and rigidity of the subject's behavior they were witnessing.

At a loss to understand the situation, the author addressed the subject and instructed him to lean comfortably back in his chair, to let his hand slowly lower until it rested comfortably in his lap, to understand fully that henceforth, whenever he wished, he could go into a profound somnambulistic trance, and to take three deep breaths slowly and then to awaken with an amnesia for having been in a trance.

The subject responded as instructed, but immediately upon awakening, he said most earnestly, "Dr. Erickson, I owe you an apology. I came up here for only one reason, to prove that hypnosis is a fraud, a miserable hoax. That's why I didn't tell you my name. It's W——, but all my friends call me Jim, so just call me Jim. Then, when you asked me to sit down on the chair, I began to do some fast thinking, I went into high speed and I realized that all the things you said here tonight made complete sense. The trouble is, I've been too busy listening to a bunch of blowhards [nodding his head toward the far corner of the room] that I didn't like anyway and actually believing what they said about hypnosis, when all the time they were just showing off their ignorance. I'm a very intolerant man when it comes to somebody shooting off his mouth about something he doesn't know a thing about, and should keep his mouth shut and his mind open. And when I sat down in this chair, I realized that I was doing the same thing toward them [again nodding his head toward the far corner of the room] that they were doing toward you, and I was joining them. But I didn't come up here to tell you this, I just want you to know I'm sorry for being rude. And now I'm ready to learn everything you can teach me. What stuns me is how fast what you said tonight has sunk in. And next I'm going to apologize to those fellows [nodding his head indicatively a third time] for being so close-minded and learn from them everything they can teach me. And Mister, I sure mean that—you don't know what I'm talking about but everybody else here probably does. Now with that off my chest, I'm pleased to be your subject, you can be sure I'll try to cooperate."

The author made no effort to understand this explanation but simply asked him if there were any special technique he would like used. He answered, "Mister, I don't know a thing about techniques, so use some technique where I can sort of look in and see what's happening."

"In what field of medicine do you practice?"

"Well, I do a lot of general medicine, but I do a lot of anesthesia for my colleagues, so that would be interesting."

"Local or general?"

"Oh, you mean me—that is, what kind of anesthesia? Well, it would have to be local if I get to look in on it in me."

During those questions and answers the author's study of the patient disclosed him to be in a somnambulistic trance. Turning to the audiience, the author stated that the situation they had just witnessed was marked by an actual continuation of the somnambulistic state, despite the subject's appparent state of waking awareness; that the subject's interest in hypnosis was obviously so great that his desires would literally become self-suggestions, and that the author would play only a minor part in the subject's development of hypnotic phenomena. In fact, the specific request for anesthesia would become manifest in accord with previously observed behavior, and suggestions would not be necessary. As this was said, the author took advantage of his standing position, which shielded his right arm, and as he said the words, "It will be here," the author drew attention to his right arm by moving it. Neither the audience nor the subject grasped the meaning implied, and the subject said, "I don't follow you at all." He was told, "It's all right, you will."

The subject answered, "I still don't get it, but something is happening to me. Look, Mister, I mean Dr. Erickson, that's just a speech habit of mine, especially when I'm excited, but look Mister, there I go again, but my whole right arm is numb. In fact, I can't even feel it being there. I can see it hanging there, but I can't move it, and look, I can't even feel this [pinching the back of his right arm vigorously]. Now you haven't hypnotized me, how come I've got an anesthesia of the arm? I don't understand this." The author gave the following explanation, apparently addressed to him but which was actually intended to inform the audience. "A few minutes ago the audience watched right arm behavior. You wished to have a local anesthesia. The previous arm behavior [the ideomotor activity] set up a pattern or focus for further hypnotic behavior. There was really no awakening from that trance by you, only the continuance of a profound somnambulistic trance, which often occurs in highly intelligent, vitally interested subjects. As can be noted, your blink reflex has been continuously absent as has been the swallowing reflex. Additionally, despite the fact I am addressing the audience, your behavior is entirely in response to me without a single glance in the direction of the audience, since you [a nod of the head similar to that the subject made previously] are out of rapport with them. Hence, there isn't any turning toward or attention directed to the audience as I speak, which would be so natural in the waking state. You are looking to me only for a resolution of the obvious confusion expressed by your face."

The subject spoke, "Mister, I just don't get you at all. I just don't know what you are talking about. What I'm interested in is this arm anesthesia. I've got an old lady with cancer, and this anesthesia I've got in my arm is the thing she needs for her pain. Oh, Ruth, Ruth." Previous comparable experience allowed the author to recognize immediately what had happened; the subject was promptly asked for the benefit of the audience, "By the way, where are we?" The reply startled the audience, "Oh, didn't I tell you? This is my office, and the girl will bring in the record on the old lady with the cancer."

A few questions clarified for the audience that in the subject's intense interest in hypnosis and in his earnest desire to seek information, he had spontaneously reoriented himself to his office, his favorite place to study.

By intruding upon the subject's wishes, the author was enabled to have him demonstrate all of the various phenomena of deep somnambulism to the satisfaction of the severest critic in the audience. Nobody questioned the validity of the hypnotic responses.

At the conclusion of the demonstration the subject was dismissed with the statement that he could now awaken from the trance, that he could remember any and all of his trance experiences if he so wished, that he could develop a trance state whenever he wished, and that he could now return to his seat in the audience. He aroused, started to leave the stage, paused, turned excitedly, and declared, "Listen! You've had me hypnotized. I'm remembering a lot of things. I didn't know you did that! That anesthesia was certainly real. And I am interested! I do have an old lady with cancer. Maybe I can do something for her besides narcotizing her."

As a final demonstration the author asked, with special intonation, "And you can develop a complete amnesia for everything, can you not?" His response was an immediate development of a trance, whereupon the author in a casual tone of voice said, "Fine, thank you very much, that's all except that Louis [the author's host] might want to ask you if you can go into a trance."

The subject aroused immediately, whereupon Louis asked him, "Jim, do you really think you could go into a trance?"

The answer was, "Well, this afternoon I was completely certain that hypnosis was a lot of hocus pocus, but after the lecture tonight and the thinking I've done, I'm completely certain it's psychosomatic interrelationships that are definitely applicable in various medical conditions, and I can promise you that I'm going to make a sufficiently intensive study so that I can convince those fellows back there"—nodding his head toward the hostile group. "But first I want Dr. Erickson to induce a trance in me and let me experience some hypnosis, and then, Mister, I'm going to get every book on hypnosis that Dr. Erickson recommends, some good books on psychology that Joe [indicating a member of the audience] can recommend. And [smiling broadly] I'll have those fellows back there recommend some books on psychiatry and psychosomatics and I'll get out my anatomy and neurology texts, and Mister, I'm going to have me a time, and when I finish, I'll know something about hypnosis, and then I'm going to see how hypnosis fits into medicine the way it should be practiced."

Upon leaving the stage, Jim strode to the back of the room and shook hands cordially with each of the special group. In the general discussion that followed Jim discovered that he could recall all of the events of the trance and forget them practically at will. This intrigued him as greatly as it did the audience.

In the time that has elapsed since then, well over a year, Jim has followed his plan of study, and now uses hypnosis extensively in his general practice. Of remarkable note was the fact that Jim's long-continued resentment toward psychiatrists and psychiatry, so much in evidence for years, vanished that evening in the hypnotic state. Warm professional friendships and a new view of a medical specialty resulted from that apparently unintentionally developed Corrective Emotional Experience in the hypnotic state.

DISCUSSION

The foregoing account is an excellent example of a Corrective Emotional Experience hypnotically induced. The situation in its setting and nature made it easy to describe and explain. It demonstrates additionally the unimportance of the therapist's complete awareness of everything without being necessarily handicapped in directing or aiding the patient's progress. It clearly illustrates the need and the value of actual behavior in enabling a patient to make therapeutic progress. Also of importance was the author's unconcerned acceptance of the patient's behavior and his utilization of the total setting and the patient's behavior as measures of indirectly suggesting an interweaving and an integration of the forces governing the patient. Addressing remarks to the audience and to the patient—actually separately, though simultaneously, by having the choice of words convey one meaning to the patient and another to the audience—is always a most effective means of promoting therapy. In his many lectures before the professional public the author has many times deliberately undertaken therapy for patients not seen previously, but who "volunteered" as "demonstration subjects." In the guise of suggestions leading to the demonstration of hypnotic phenomena, therapeutic suggestions can be indirectly given without the audience becoming aware of the pertinences to the subject. Subsequent inquiries have disclosed that many corrective emotional experiences on the lecture platform have been of sustained value. Often, too, the author has found out that the "volunteering" as a "demonstration subject" is a trial by the patient, to test for himself his readiness to accept therapy with subsequent good results.

For example, a woman who was a lifetime enuretic "volunteered" as a demonstration subject. Just previous to the demonstration she had been asked in the waking state if there were anything she wished the author to do. She stated that a physician friend of hers in the audience was particularly interested in enuresis in small children, and as the author turned to the audience, a physician nodded his head affirmatively. Nevertheless, the author, being a psychiatrist, wondered if there might be a more personal application to the requester. With subtle but strong emphasis, he asked the woman, "Do *you* mind if *I discuss* this matter *helpfully with you here* on the platform?" She answered agreeably, but a slow flush covered her face, not deeply enough to be apparent to the audience.

Juvenile enuresis was discussed at length with various careful emphases while the woman went into a trance, and she was then used as a demonstration subject immediately after the discussion of enuresis.

Two years later, while lecturing there again, the same woman was noted to be present. She was sought out and taken aside and asked if she wished to volunteer again. She replied simply, "No, not really. I don't need to now." The implication of this last statement suddenly became apparent to her. She flushed deeply and hesitantly said, "You knew, didn't you?"

"Yes, but tell me, please, what happened."

"As you discussed it, I knew that you were talking to me as well as the audience, and I sat in frozen horror because I knew one little slip of your tongue would expose me to the audience. It was horrible. I guess I went into a trance to escape. Then when you finished discussing it, you explained a posthypnotic suggestion in which you told a patient that it was over with and done with, and belonged to the past, and to go on to other and pleasing things. I knew you were saying that to me; and my horror and terror disappeared, and I felt so happy and relieved and comfortable. Then you began demonstrating things, but I just felt like I was in heaven. And that was the end of it—that horrible terror, that sudden feeling of peace and comfort, and the end of my problem. I don't understand, I don't want to understand. I'm just happy. Many, many thanks to you."

Many other instances of a Corrective Emotional Experience could be cited, since the author utilizes it in psychotherapy extensively. Why and how it serves the individual's needs is usualy difficult to understand. Sometimes it is used without employing hypnosis, but this is more difficult. Hypnosis allows freedom and ease in structuring the therapeutic situation and renders the patient much more accessible. Also, hypnosis allows ready retreat if the patient is not yet ready, without there being any loss of therapeutic gains already made. One can easily and safely reinterpret a structured Corrective Emotional Experience for which the patient is not yet ready, and thus leave the way open for a future approach. The Corrective Emotional Experiences vary in relation to the individual and in relation to his problem. The essential task is to structure the therapeutic situation in such fashion that emotions are greatly intensified, all behavior inhibited, and the need for behavior intensified. Then, and not until then, an opportunity for directed behavior with a special significance is given.

In the case of the physician reported above, the author was aware of a difficult situation from the "thumbs-down" signal, and was then made more acutely aware of it by the challenge in the refusal by the volunteer to give his name.

If the readers will review the handling of this situation, they will note an immediate inhibition of the physician by instrumentalizing him as a display object for the audience, the initiation of passive directed behavior, the careful shifting of the intense emotional state that the man already had into an intense emotional interest in his own subjective experience, which he himself augmented by his intense emotional interest in his cancer patient. This was followed by a redirection of his interests toward his colleague Louis, which, perhaps unnecessarily, intensified his behavior in relation to his other colleagues. Thus, a very marked reorientation of this physician in his life situation and his total life adjustment was effected by simple little items of behavior which he progressively enlarged into a revision of his emotional and intellectual attitudes.

As for the enuretic woman, she became hopelessly trapped by the author's clinical attentiveness, and rapidly led in a terrifying, bewildering, threatening sea of emotions, inhibited in all of her behavior and helpless until suddenly she was propelled into doing *the things the author wanted her to do,* and doing these things well and competently. This created a feeling and an attitude which she carried over into the field of her enuresis problem, where, without explicitly so declaring, she wanted the author's aid to tell her to do well and competently the things that she knew the author would tell her to do. Thus, a long-continuing pattern of behavior was set into action, tremendously reinforced by the woman's own emotional history.

In brief, the Hypnotic Corrective Emotional Experience, however simple it may appear, is a highly complex restructuring of subjective understandings of one's subjective experiences that can be initiated very simply and then gently guided toward a therapeutic goal. Essential is good clinical attentiveness to the patient's behavior, a confident awareness that one can delay, even halt, and nullify hypnotically whatever is taking place, and postpone, modify, or reinforce the structured situation leading to a therapeutic goal. More than once this author has found himself in the need of arresting the patient's behavior hypnotically in some distracting, harmless manner while he carefully revised his own understandings, thus to meet better the patient's needs.

What happens if a hoped-for Corrective Emotional Experience gets out of hand and becomes uncontrolled? Merely a disagreeable experience for the patient and properly increased awareness by the therapist of the problem at hand, with a need to repair rapport lest the patient seek help elsewhere. Even at the worst, the patient may be benefitted by the debacle which serves to render the patient more aware of his needs. More than once this author has deliberately structured a Corrective Emotional Experience wrongly and watched the patient react unfavorably; and then, with carefully mended rapport, he began again, aided by the patient's unexpected unconscious wisdom in restructuring the Corrective Emotional Experience. As for actual harm this can be best summarized by comments from patients, of which the following is an excellent example: "Things really went all wrong there for a while, and that shook me awfully. I didn't think I could ever get straightened out, but then things would begin to slide together so smoothly, and I would begin to think that being so badly shook just kind of speeded things up."

In conclusion, the Hypnotic Corrective Emotional Experience is a relatively easy and effective psychotherapeutic measure in the hands of an attentive clinician. It is, as is illustrated in the instances cited, best "played by ear" with no elaborate plans formulated, but with a multitude of possibilities floating freely in one's mind ready for adaptation to each new development presented by the patient. It is easily arrested and nullified if not properly structured, and at the worst can only lead the patient to seek a more competent therapist. Used with care and discrimination, the Hypnotic Corrective Emotional Experience is of great value in shortening psychotherapy and in bringing about a therapeutic reordering of the patient's adjustments to his life situation.

59. The February Man: Facilitating New Identity in Hypnotherapy

Milton H. Erickson and
Ernest L. Rossi

Up to this point we have emphasized that hypnotherapy involves the utilization of the patient's own life experiences and that the indirect forms of suggestion are the means of evoking those experiences for therapeutic change. What happens, however, when the patient has been severely deprived in some basic life experiences? Can the therapist supply them vicariously in some way? Sensitive therapists have long recognized their role as surrogate parents who do, in fact, help their patients experience life patterns and relationships that have been missed.

In this final chapter we will present some of the senior author's approaches to supplying a patient with a personal relationship in a manner that anchors her within a more secure inner reality around which she can create a new identity for herself. This is the case of a young woman who so lacked the experience of being mothered that she gravely doubted her own ability to be one. Through a series of age regressions the senior author visited her in the guise of the February Man: A kindly granduncle type who became a secure friend and confidant. A series of such experiences enabled her to develop a new sense of confidence and identity about herself that led her eventually to a rewarding experience of motherhood with her own children.

The senior author has actually played the role of the February Man with a number of patients throughout his career. So complex are some of the details of his work in these situations, however, that he never quite completed any of his manuscripts about them. The following case is thus a synthesis of several of the senior author's original manuscripts together with commentaries on them by the junior author.

The reader is invited to explore with us some of the approaches and issues involved in the work of the February Man. There is much about this work that is beyond our own understanding. The use of indirect suggestions to integrate hypnotic and real-life memories to create a

---

This case material is reproduced from Erickson & Rossi, *Hypnotherapy: An Exploratory Casebook* (Irvington, Chapter 10, 1979).

self-consistent internal reality is an art that does not entirely lend itself to rational analysis. We do try, however, fully realizing we have fallen short and are in need of the reader's creativity to fill some of the gaps and to carry the work further.

Initial Interview: A Lonely Childhood

At midterm of her first pregnancy the wife of a young doctor on our hospital staff approached the senior author for psychiatric help. Her problem was that although happily married and pleased with her pregnancy, she was fearful that her own unhappy childhood experiences would reflect themselves in her handling of her child. She stated that she had "studied too much psychology" since it made her aware of the possible inadvertant unfortunate handling of a child, with resulting psychological traumatization.

She explained that she had been a most unwanted child. Her mother never had any time for her. Her care rested in the hands of her mother's unhappy spinster older sister who, in return for a home, acted as nursemaid, housekeeper, and general factotum. Her preschool days had been spent almost exclusively in her nursery, and she was left to devise her own games and entertainment. Occasionally, when her mother gave a social tea, she would be trotted out briefly for exhibition and told what a sweet, pretty little girl she was and then dismissed. Otherwise, her mother, between social engagements, looked in upon her in the nursery briefly and casually. She had been sent to a special nursery school and later to various private schools for her grade school and high school education. During the summers she was sent to special camps to "further" her education. During these years her "mother took time out from her round of pressing social engagements and trips abroad" to see her daughter as often as was "humanly possible." Essentially she and her mother had remained strangers.

As for the father, he, too, was a busy man, greatly absorbed in his business enterprises and traveling much of the time. He did have a genuine affection for his daughter, however, and had frequently found time to take her, even as a small child, out to dinner, to the circus, to amusement parks, and to other memorably delightful places. He also had bought her toys and presents befitting her needs, in contrast to the "horribly expensive" dolls with which her mother showered her, but with which her aunt would not let her play because they were "beautiful" and "valuable." She had received only "the best of everything" from her mother, but her father had always given her "many little things that were really nice." At the age of eighteen she had rebelled against "finishing" school and, to her mother's intense distress and resentment, had insisted on attending a state university. Her mother's chief argument was the debt the daughter owed her for "practically ruining" her figure in order to give birth to her. The father, greatly dominated by his wife but much in love with her, had secretly abetted his daughter in her decision and had encouraged and aided in every possible way, but without trying to overindulge her.

Her university adjustments had been good scholastically, but she felt that she had made insufficient use of her social opportunities. Early in her senior year she had met an intern, five years older than she, with whom she fell in love. She had married him a year later. This had distressed her mother, since the intern lacked "social position," but the father had privately expressed his approval.

Because of this history she now wondered what kind of mother she would be. Her psychological reading had convinced her that her rejection by her mother and her emotional starvation as a child would in some way adversely affect the handling of her own baby. She wanted to know if, through hypnosis, her unconscious could be explored and either her anxieties relieved or she could be made aware of her deficiencies and thus make corrections. She asked the senior author to consider her problem at length and to give her another appointment when he felt he might be able to meet her needs.

She was told that before this could be done, it would be necessary for her to relate at length all her anxieties, fears, and forebodings. In so doing she was to give as comprehensive a picture of their nature, variety, and development as possible. It was explained that the primary purpose of this report was to make certain that the senior author appreciated as fully as possible her feelings and thoughts before any attempts were made to ascertain causes and remedies. From this additional material, of course, he privately hoped to learn more details of her life history that he could use to facilitate the hypnotherapeutic work.

Second Interview: A Spontaneous Catharsis

At the next interview the patient was exceedingly fearful, anxious, and tearful. She expressed disconnected fears of hurting, neglecting, and resenting her child. She feared feeling tied down by it, of being overly anxious, of giving overcompensatory attention to it, of making it a hideous burden in her life instead of a pleasure, of losing her husband's love, of never loving the child, and so on.

She elaborated upon these ideas poorly but in relationship to every possible stage of the child's eventual development.

She wept throughout the interview, and while intellectually she regarded her fears as groundless, she declared that their "strong obsessional character" was causing insomnia, anorexia, and severe depressive reactions that terrified her.

If she tried to read or to listen to the radio, the printed page or the program would be obscured by vivid, compelling memories of her own childhood unhappiness. She recognized that all her fears were abnormally exaggerated, but she felt helpless to do anything about them.

Except for innumerable anxieties little actual history was obtained. She asked tearfully if the writer thought he could help her, since she felt she was breaking down more rapidly than ever. She was assured that before her next appointment a therapeutic plan would be worked out for her.

Third Interview: The Interpolated Trance, Age Regression and Amnesia

At the next interview she was assured that an elaborate program had been worked out and that the results would undoubtedly be most satisfying to her. What the plan was could not be disclosed to her yet, but through hypnosis her unconscious would acquire adequate understanding. All that she needed to know consciously was that hypnosis would be employed and that the task could be begun immediately if she wished. She acquiesced eagerly. In this session approximately five hours were spent training her adequately as a hypnotic subject. Particular emphasis was placed upon age regression. Her intelligence and excellence as a subject made possible the elaborate training considered necessary for the planned procedure.

During the training slowly and cautiously she was regressed in time repeatedly to some safe past situation into which, in some fashion, the writer could enter directly or indirectly, without distorting the regression situation. Thus the first regression was to the first interview with her. In having her relive that interview, it became easily possible to introduce a new element not actually belonging to the situation but that could easily fit into it. In accord with her revivification of that interview the writer merely remarked, "Do you mind if I interrupt and introduce a thought that just came to my mind? It just occured to me that you could easily be a good hypnotic subject, and I wonder if you would mind closing your eyes and sleeping hypnotically for a few moments, and then arousing and continuing from where I interrupted?" Thus an interpolated trance was introduced into that reliving of the first interview, in which no hypnosis had occurred.

> R: The first trance has the effect of dissociating the patient away from the surrounding reality into her internal environment. When you then interpolate a second trance into the first, it effects an even deeper regression into herself. The basic purpose of the interpolated trance is to get the patient further removed from outer consensual reality. It's particularly useful for age regression.

> E: Yes, I don't have to help her withdraw from the outer

environment with the interpolated trance. When she gets back to reality, it will be much more difficult for her to recover that interpolated trance for which she has an amnesia even in the trance state.

R: So an interpolated trance is another way of effecting a deeper hypnotic amnesia.

E: In future trances she's going to have an amnesia for the interpolated trance, but she would have to go through it to get a complete memory of the first trance in which it took place. I gave her many positive supportive suggestions during the interpolated trance. This served to reinforce all the positive values of that initial interview.

R: It's like a feedback loop, where what comes later reinforces the positive values of what occurred earlier.

E: Yes, and it's reinforcing what happens now by virtue of the "past" that I've transplanted into the initial interview. I work in all directions. In everyday life when strangers meet they may speak casually in a general way until they discover something common in their past: They might have vacationed in the same place or come from the same state or town or gone to the same school. Sometimes they discover to their delight that they have a few acquaintances in common and can now share more intimate details of their lives. They have now created a strong rapport in the present based entirely on experiences from the past.

R: They have created a shared "phenomenal world in common" (Rossi, 1972a). They have built associative bridges that now bind them together in friendship. This is a common everyday process of social relating that you are now utilizing to enhance your rapport with this patient. The interpolated trance is a way of rapidly creating a positive "history" that enhances current relations.

Rapport Protection: Indirect Suggestion and Contingent Possibilities

She was then regressed to an intern's party at which there was a number of the senior author's former medical students. In the process of regression the suggestion was implanted that she might meet him at that party or that someone would mention his name, and undoubtedly this would happen when someone approached her and attracted her attention by gently squeezing her wrist. Then, when this unexpected thing happened, she could make a full response to the wrist pressure and react in accord with whatever situational need developed. Primarily, this was to introduce a physical cue to permit ready induction of a trance state at any time, even during the reliving of past events that had occurred long before meeting the senior author. Various such regressions were induced, aided by special information that had been privately supplied by the husband. These were utilized to condition her for trance induction in any set of psychological circumstances.

> E: I was building rapport protection with this procedure. I once regressed a subject at Clark University to ten years of age. While regressed, he explained that he was on an errand to buy a loaf of bread for his mother. We could all see the abject terror on his face because he did not know anyone in that room (where as an adult he was being hypnotized). I spent a wretched four and a half hours trying to get back into rapport with him because he was afraid of me and afraid of everyone else. That taught me that thereafter I'd have a secondary way of establishing rapport with the subject such as touching a wrist. It's an attention-attracting but otherwise meaningless cue. The subject cannot easily incorporate it into the age-regressed pattern of behavior.

> R: You did not directly tell her that pressure on her wrist was a cue to enter trance or to pay close attention to what you were suggesting.

> E: If I had said it that directly, she could reject it. Therefore I put it in an indirect framework of *contingent possibilities:* She *might* meet me. Someone would approach her; she *could* make a full response to the wrist pressure and react in accord with *whatever situational need developed.* These (the italicized words) are all undefined. There is no demand or threat in all this, and therefore no need for resistance or rejection.

> R: We usually don't reject undefined possibilities in everyday life. Rather, possibilities and contingencies usually evoke our sense of wonder, speculation, and expectation. Possibilities actually initiate pressures of *unconscious search* within us that may trip off useful unconscious processes. "Whatever situational need" also covers all possibilities, including whatever suggestions you give her. You give her the most general form of an indirect suggestion here.

> E: A most general form that can be filled in by the patient's specific understannding.

Interpolating New Life Experiences: The February Man

She was trained to develop in good fashion extensive regressions that were made to serve merely as a general background and situation for new, interpolated behavioral responses. She was regressed to past situations, and that frame of reference was employed merely as a background into which new hypnotic behavior could be interpolated. When sufficient training had been completed to ensure good responses, she was regressed to childhood at the age of four. The month of February was selected because it was her birthday. She was oriented to the living room of her childhood in the act of merely walking through it. She had often walked through her living room. Since the state of regression was limited to that act, it would constitute only a frame of reference. The walking through could be arrested and new behavior introduced into that setting without altering or falsifying the situation. Thus the new behavior intruded into that situation could be related temporally to the events of that age-regression period.

As she roused somnambulistically in this regressed state, she was greeted by the senior author: "Hello, little girl. Are you your Daddy's girl? I'm a friend of your Daddy's, and I'm waiting for him to come in to talk to me. He told me yesterday that he brought you a present one day and that you liked it very much. I like your Daddy, too. He told me it would soon be your birthday, and I'll bet he brings you an awful nice present." This was followed by silence, and the senior author apparently absentmindedly snapped open and closed his hunting case watch, with no further effort to engage her in conversation or to attract her attention. She first eyed him, then became interested in the watch, whereupon he held it to his ear and stated that it went "tick, tick" very nicely.

E: "Hello, little girl" assigns her a hypnotic role.

R: In that first second when she opens her eyes in somnambulistic trance you immediately reinforce the age regression so there could be no doubt about it. Is she going to see you as Dr. Erickson or as someone she does not know in her past? Your opening remark orients her into the past.

E: And there have been people in her past who have said just such a thing.

R: You then attract her attention appropriately by playing with your watch. This is just about right for a four-year-old; you do not introdue yourself in a direct or demanding way. You behave very much as a visitor to her house might when she was a child.

Wrist Cue as a Nonverbal Signal for Metasuggestions Orienting the Somnambulistic State

After a few moments the suggestion was offered that she might like to snap the case open or to listen to the watch. She nodded her head shyly and extended her hand. Taking hold of her wrist as if to help her, the senior author handed her the watch. She looked at it and played with it. The suggestion was offered that if she listend to it for a little while, it would make her very sleepy. This was followed by the comment that soon the senior author would have to go home, but that some time he would come back, and, if she wished, he would bring his watch so she could open and close it and listen to it.

She nodded her head, and her hand holding the watch was guided to her ear. Her wrist was slowly squeezed, and trance suggestions were given accompanied by suggestions that maybe next summer the senior author would come again, and maybe she would recognize him.

> E: I had to get out of her house. I ended that interpolated life experience with the wrist cue in an appropriate way (guiding her hand with the watch to her ear) and suggesting she would get sleepy as she listened to it.

> R: Having her go to sleep is fairly appropriate behavior for a four-year-old listening to a watch, and her sleep allowed you to leave. It also enabled you to give her the posthypnotic suggestion about seeing her again next summer *maybe,* and *maybe* she would recognize you. These possibilities are appropriate for her age because a four- to five-year old child might not recognize a friend after a year. But why did you give her the rapport cue by squeezing her wrist as you added these suggestions?

> E: Although she was in a somnambulistic trance, further hypnosis would be needed to effect an alteration of that state to induce other phenomena.

> R: I see. Even during a somnambulistic state special rapport is needed to effect important suggestions. The wrist cue is an orienting signal for the metasuggestions you will use to guide the somnambulistic state; it tells her important suggestions are coming. I have had the difficulty of working with some subjects who were so obstinate during the somnambulistic state that I could hardly get a word in edgewise. Like self-centered children, such subjects would soon take over the situation and simply live out an inner experience without my being able to relate to them. This may be valuable for cathartic purposes, but it does not permit the therapist to interpolate new experience as you are doing here.

> E: You need another hypnotic frame of reference to orient her to important suggestions without verbally defining it as such and without altering my role as a stranger, Daddy's friend.

R: Classical age regression has typically been a simple reliving of a past life experience. A catharsis or process of desensitization is relied upon as the therapeutic means of resolving pent-up emotions of life traumas.

E: That does not add anything. Here I'm adding to the past.

R: That's the object of the entire procedure. You regress her to establish a frame of reference into which you can interpolate therapeutic life experiences. You are adding new experiences to her memory bank; you're adding new elements of human relating that she missed in reality.

E: You can add belief to something that does not exist if you repeat it often enough. That's why I had to give her many experiences with me as the February Man. I'm adding reality to a nonexistent thing.

R: It becomes "real" in terms of internal reality. With this approach you can alter a patient's belief system; you cannot really change her past, but you can change her beliefs about her past.

E: You can change beliefs and values. It's not really that we can believe lies; rather, we discover more things. Patients believe their limited reality until they discover more reality.

R: I wonder if we can equate "discover more reality" with creating new consciousness? There is still a basic question here, however. Are you (1) really adding something new to the personality, or are you (2) simply helping her discover and experience a natural, inherent pattern of human relating (the archetypal child-parent relationship) that she very much needed and wanted? Utilization theory would emphasize the second alternative; you are structuring circumstances that allow her to evoke and utilize inherent (species-specific) behavior patterns that must be expressed for normal development. But you are certainly adding a new content within the framework of this inherent pattern.

Continuing Experiences with the February Man: Ratifying the Historical Reality of Age-Regressed Experience

She was then permitted to experience about fifteen minutes of profound hypnotic sleep. This sleep was a passage of time during which my departure and eventual return (as had already been suggested) could take place. Her wrist was then again gently squeezed, and suggestions were offered that she better be in the yard because the flowers were blooming for the first time since her birthday last winter, and perhaps her Daddy's friend might come again. At all events she could really open her eyes very, very wide to see the flowers. She opened her eyes and was apparently enjoying her visual hallucinations when the writer, from behind, addressed her, "Hello, little girl. Do you remember me?" She turned, eyed him carefully, smiled, and said, "You're Daddy's friend." The reply was made, "And I remember your name. It is R." In this way the senior author became established as an actual figure in her past life without impinging upon realities or distorting them, but merely by adding to them by a simple process of temporal association. Thereupon a casual conversation was initiated at a childish level about the red and pink and yellow flowers (she said they were tulips), whereupon she reminded the writer about his watch, and essentially the same course of events ensued as had previously. Many more comparable instances were developed to ensure the possibility of the writer's intrusion into her past without invalidating the regression state. She was given extensive experience with the February Man, a figure that became more and more established in her life history.

E: I had learned from the initial interviews that her childhood home did have extensive flower gardens with red, pink, and yellow flowers. I would further ratify the historical aspects of the experience by pretending to have an unclear memory of my previous visits with her. How clear does anyone remember an experience of a year ago? Two years ago? Four years ago? I also introduced changing views. As she gets older, she gets a different perspective on things. I'd say, "That first doll you had was really very nice." "Remember your enthusiasm for that first circus?" I might make such remarks to the ten- or twelve-year-old girl about the six-year-old girl.

R: You built associative bridges between the trance experiences at different age levels that established the historical reality of your visits with her.

Indirect Posthypnotic Suggestion

Finally she was placed in a profound trance and given extensive posthypnotic suggestions to ensure a comprehensive amnesia for all trance events and to ensure continued cooperation. I'd gently squeeze her wrist and say "You have now completed that task. I want you to go into a profound trance at this time. I want you to enjoy resting. I want you to feel fresh after you've awakened, comfortably enjoying the feeling of being wide awake, prepared for a new day's activities."

E: That latter suggestion, "prepared for a new day's activities," implies that she will be ready for more work; we are just beginning.

R: That's how you also imply a posthypnotic amnesia without directly telling her she would not remember. You could then put her back into trance for another experience with the February Man.

Time for Hypnotic Work

In subsequent sessions, usually of several hours' duration, essentially the same procedure was followed.

E: I had to have several hours in order to let her have an experience with the February Man at one age level, rest, and then another experience at another age level. Time is expandable and compressible, but a certain amount of real clock time is still needed for careful work. Initially you really don't know what the patient's capacities are. Time is needed to explore them.

Integrating Hypnotic and Real-Life Memories: Creating a Self-Consistent Internal Reality

A number of hypnotherapeutic sessions now took place following this same pattern. She was regressed to many different periods of her life, usually in a chronologically progressive fashion, taking care not to let the created situation impinge contradictorily upon the actual realities of the past. For example, on one occasion, regressed to a nine-year-old level, she manifested intense astonishment upon opening her eyes and seeing the senior author. Cautious inquiry disclosed that she was visiting a distant relative for the first time and had just arrived the previous night. A few questions elicited enough information to orient the senior author so that he could claim a business friendship with her relative. This laid a foundation very necessary for the subsequent ubiquity of him in her life experience. Aiding in the acceptance of his ubiquity was the fact that both of her parents traveled extensively and often unexpectedly, and that they had innumerable acquaintances and friends. Hence it was easily assumed that the same was true of the senior author as "Daddy's friend." Also of importance was the February Man's knowledge of various cities she had visited and the fact that he, as well as she, had studied psychology, all of which provided a wide background permitting her to accept him unquestioningly. As the procedure continued, the technicalities of securing responsive behavior became minimal, and a dozen regressed states could be developed in an hour's time. These were all utilized to secure a report by her of things and attitudes current to the regression period, as well as an account of expected or anticipated events. Anticipated events served admirably in enabling the senior author to direct regression states to "safe" periods. However, care had to be exercised, since anticipations were not always fulfilled. Frequently, however, the "visit" was devoted to an account of what had happened since the last "visit" that is, the preceding regressed state. She learned to look upon the senior author as a recurrent visitor and as a trusted confidant to whom she could tell all her secrets, woes, and joys and with whom she could share her hopes, fears, doubts, wishes, and plans.

From time to time it became necessary to induce comprehensive amnesias, obliterating various of the senior author's "visits," and to regress her to an earlier age and to go over an already partially covered period of her life more adequately. Thus, some sudden change in her life, not anticipated at an earlier age regression, might have become established before the period of the next age regression, thereby creating a situation at variance with established understandings. On such occasions the last age regression would be abolished by amnesia suggestions, and a new regression to an earlier time would be induced to permit the securing of pertinent data.

R: You made a very careful and extensive effort to integrate hypnotic and real memories so they were molded into a self-consistent inner reality. This would ensure the permanence of the new attitudes you were facilitating in her. If there were contradictions and a lack of consistency between the hypnotic and real memories, self-corrective processes within the unconscious would have tended to gradually eliminate the hypnotic suggestions as foreign intrusions. This may be why so much hypnotic work in the past has had only temporary or partial effect. Direct suggestions made even while a patient is in a deep somnambulistic state are not programmed within the mind forever in a rigid way. The human mind is a dynamic process that is continually correcting, modifying, and reformulating itself. Inconsistencies are either worked out in a satisfactory manner or are expressed as "problems" (complexes, neuroses, psychosomatic symptoms, etc.). There is thus nothing magical or mysterious about the effectiveness of your approach: It is based on very careful, thorough work integrating real memories with hypnotic experience.

Facilitating Therapeutic Attitudes: A Therapy of Life Perspectives: Dreams and Hypnosis

The consistent and continual rejection she experienced from her mother presented many opportunities to reorganize her emotions and understanding. By this procedure the senior author's role became one of friendship, sympathy, interest, and objectivity, thereby giving him the opportunity to raise questions concerning how she might later evaluate a given experience. Thus, in expressing her grief over breaking a cheap little china doll her father had given her and which she treasured, she could declare that, when she grew up and became a mother and had a little girl who broke her doll, she would know that it wasn't something "awful bad" but that she would know just how her little girl would feel. Similarly, a fall on the dance floor in her teens was regarded by her as an utterly and completely devastating experience. Yet she manifested a readiness to understand the senior author's comment that she should rightly appreciate it as such in the present but that at the same time she could also understand how, in the future, it could really be regarded as a minor and completely unimportant event, perhaps even amusing. Her first adolescent infatuation, her jilting by the boy, and her tremendous need to understand herself in relation to that event were dealt with. Her resolution to leave the finishing school, to enter the university, her choice of studies, her scholastic struggles, and her limited social life were all covered. The meeting with the man who became her husband, her doubts and uncertainties about him, the eventual engagement, and the mother's attitude toward him, toward the marriage, and toward the subsequent pregnancy were all detailed to the senior author in "current" accounts of what was happening to her. Numerous other instances of rejection, neglect, and disappointment by her mother and father were relived and discussed with the February Man. Real happy memories were also relived and integrated with the hypnotic memories to ensure a comprehensive integration of them.

R: Whenever she had a traumatic life situation, she could now discuss them with her father's friend, the February Man. In effect you became a therapist at such times. This is a curious state of affairs, you as her current therapist became a therapist in her past, helping her deal with her difficult life situations as they occurred. I've noticed something similar in dreams. Some patients seem to relive their past in dreams but correct the traumatic aspects of their past with their current adult perspectives (Rossi, 1972a; 1973c). This again points out the self-corrective aspect of the psyche; it is in a continual process of reformulating or resynthesizing itself to achieve a more integrated pattern of functioning. You utilize and facilitate this resynthesizing aspect of psychic functioning with your role as the February Man. You are doing hypnotically what frequently happens naturally during dreams.

E: Yes. [The senior author now recalls such a dream of his

own, when the adult Dr. Erickson observed himself as a child (Erickson, 1965a).] Dreams give us the opportunity to relive past events and appraise them critically from an adult perspective.

R: Dreams are autotherapeutic processes that help the mind correct and integrate itself. I also believe we are synthesizing new phenomenological realities in our dreams that become the basis of new patterns of identity and behavior (Rossi, 1971; 1972 a, b; 1973 a, b, c.).

A Reversal of Realities: Deepening the Therapeutic Frame of Reference

Toward the end of this extensive reorganization of her attitudes about her past, a new memory was recalled: Her secret resolve years ago to have hypnotic anesthesia should she ever marry and become pregnant. As she now again considered this possibility, she received a letter of foreboding from her mother requesting that the term "grandmother" never be used—in essence, rejecting the unborn baby. This letter intensified the patient's anxieties and fears anew.

To deal with these renewed anxieties a variation in our hypnotic procedure was developed. In this variation a blanket amnesia was first induced for all her previous hypnotic work, and she was asked to again relate all her fears and anxieties. In this state, as expected, her account was comparable to her original expression of her problems before hypnotherapy.

A new trance state was then induced in which the blanket amnesia was removed. She was then regressed to a week *before* the arrival of her mother's letter. In this state of hypnosis she was asked to recall fully all the many visits, talks, and discussions over the years she had had with the senior author as Daddy's friend. As she recalled his many visits and their conversations on so many subjects, the suggestion was offered that she ought to consider the present minor worries against that total background. As she began this correlation of her unhappy ideas in the past as she conceived it at the moment, she began to develop amazing insights, understandings, and emotional comfort.

Having reestablished the new attitudes developed in the hypnotic work, the senior author next led her into an age-regression state covering the period just *after* the receipt of the mother's letter. After expressing some sensible views about her mother's problem, she was asked to give the reactions she could develop if she did not include in her thinking "all she knew about her past." She was told that she ought to speculate aloud on how she could really enlarge her reactions into exaggerated fears and anxieties by just "not being comprehensive in her thinking." She was urged to offer "speculative statements" expressing such anxieties. She then proceeded to verbalize them as she thought would be possible if she "did not think intelligently." This speculative account was identical with that which she had originally given just before therapy began and the previous account with the blanket amnesia for all the hypnotherapeutic work. But it was given as a "speculative" account which was decidedly different from the new reality of her emotional life that now included the new frames of reference she had developed with the February Man.

Subsequent regression states were similarly utilized. Her "speculations" about how she could exaggerate her fears always gave accounts similar to the one she gave originally before hypnotherapy. These speculations were always in sharp contrast to her "real attitudes" developed with the help of Daddy's friend, the February Man. She now drew extensively upon her "actual" past history, with all its interpolated experiences with Daddy's friend. During this period a tremendous amount of her past history came out in clear relevance to her entire current problem. As this type of activity continued, she developed insights that were remarkably corrective.

R: This is an ingenious twist: what was originally a painful reality now becomes the "speculative account," while the new attitudes introduced by hypnosis become the abiding reality. That is, she is now accepting her expanded frame of understanding developed with the February Man as her "real" views, while her previous behavior is now seen merely as a speculative account of how badly things could be if she "did not think intelligently." This procedure may be helping her integrate the February Man frame of reference at an even deeper level. This is particularly the case because she is already in a deep hypnotic state as she experiences this reversal of realities.

Termination: A Final Conscious Integration of All Trance Work

Finally, as she progressed in this regard, the topic of hypnotic anesthesia for the delivery of her child was mentioned increasingly by her while she was in trance. She was reassuringly told that as the months of pregnancy passed, it was absolutely certain that all of her anxieties would be comprehensively and comfortably understood and thus become a resolved experience of the past. In their place would be a realization that in some way she would meet someone who would teach her to understand herself happily. Since she was in an age-regressed state, this was naturally a reference by implication to the senior author as someone she would meet in the future. In so doing she would be trained to become an excellent hypnotic subject and thereby her college resolve for a hypnotic delivery would be fulfilled.

The termination of therapy was accomplished rather simply. She was regressed to the time of preparation for her first visit to the senior author's office. She was assured by him—still in the role of Daddy's friend—that her trip would be fully successful in many more ways than she really expected. The scene was then shifted to the office, and she was much astonished to see the February Man. The senior author was also astonished! She was puzzled at his presence, explained that she had come to see Dr. Erickson. She was assured that she would see Dr. Erickson and that he would meet her wishes fully, but that, for a few minutes, she should sleep most profoundly. During this trance approximately one half-hour was spent instructing her so that after she awakened she would recall from the beginning, in chronological order, every trance experience she had had, together with all insights and understandings that she had developed up to the date shown by the day's newspaper on the desk. At the close of the interview she was told to spend a few delightful days reviewing her memories, making certain that she understood, remembered, and accepted all her past in an adjusted fashion. As for the hypnotic anesthesia, she would be certain of it, but the minor details would be arranged in the next interview.

R: This was a final summation for a final conscious integration of all her therapy. She now finally learns how you played the role of the February Man, how you reversed her realities, and so on. Yet this does not undo the effectiveness of the new attitudes and frames of reference you helped her develop. Why doesn't it? After all your incredibly complex efforts to develop a new frame of reference, integrate it, and deepen it, why do you end the therapy with this complete denouement?

E: Because I may have made some errors. She may have made some errors. Let's make sure we get the whole set of errors corrected.

R: You are not afraid of undoing your therapeutic work because you actually have helped her develop new frames of reference and understandings that have therapeutically altered her emotional life. This case contrasts sharply with those cases in which you like to maintain an amnesia for all hypnotherapeutic work. What is the difference?

E: Some personalities need amnesia, some do not. It's a matter of clinical experience to distinguish them.

R: Those patients whom you judge to have destructive conscious attitudes toward the therapy might do better with an amnesia.

E: This patient was actually left with some amnesia for the negative emotions she experienced in relation to her mother. My final posthypnotic suggestion to her was to "spend a few delightful days reviewing her memories, making certain that she understood, remembered, and accepted all her past in an *adjusted* fashion." This precluded any regression into the catastrophically negative affects and anxieties she was experiencing before therapy.

Traing the Obstetrical Analgesia: A Two-Year Follow-up

At the next session some days later she stated that she had been interested primarily in thinking about her hypnotic delivery. After much discussion with her husband, during which he was primarily the listener, she had decided on an analgesia if it were possible. She explained that she wished to experience childbirth in the same fashion as she had, as a child, sensed the swallowing of a whole cherry or a lump of ice, feeling it pass comfortably and interestingly down the esophagus. In a similar manner she would like to feel labor contractions, to sense the passage of the baby down the birth canal, and to experience a sense of distension of the birth canal. All this she wished to experience without any sense of pain. When questioned about the possibility of an episiotomy, she explained that she wanted the sensation of the cutting without pain and that she wanted to feel in addition the suturing that would be done. When asked if she wished at any time to experience any feeling of pain merely as a measure of sampling it, she explained: "Pain shouldn't have any part in having a baby. It's a wonderful thing, but everybody is taught to believe in pain. I want to have my baby the way I should. I don't want my attention distracted even a single minute by thoughts of pain." Accordingly, as a measure of meeting her wishes, she was taught to develop complete hypnotic anesthesia. (Usually the procedure is to proceed from numbness to analgesia to anesthesia.) Since in this instance an analgesia was the primary goal, anesthesia was induced extensively and then systematically transformed into an analgesia. (That a complete transformation of anesthesia to analgesia could be effected is doubtful, but the patient's wishes could be met in this manner, and whatever anesthesia remained would only supplement the effectiveness of the analgesia.)

When she had been trained sufficiently to meet various clinical tests for analgesia, extensive training was given to her to effect the development of a profound somnambulistic posthypnotic trance with "that degree and type of analgesia you have just learned," so that she could enter into labor without any further contact with the senior author.

Additional instructions were that she would awaken at the completion of labor with a full and immediate memory of the entire experience. Then, when she returned to her room, she would fall into a restful, comfortable sleep of about two hours' duration, and thereafter she would have a most pleasant hospital stay, planning happily for the future.

About seven weeks after the delivery she and her husband and baby daughter visited the senior author. They reported that, as she entered the hospital, she had developed a somnambulistic trance. During the labor and delivery her husband was present. She had talked freely with her husband and the obstetrician and had described to them her labor contractions with interest. She had recognized the performance of the episiotomy, the emergence of the head from the birth canal, the complete delivery of the baby, and the suturing of her episiotomy—all without pain. The expulsion of the placenta caused her to ask if there was a twin because she felt "another one moving down." She was able to laugh at her error when informed it was the placenta. She counted the stitches in the repair of her episiotomy and inquired if the doctor had "cheated" by giving her a local anesthetic because, while she could feel the needle, it was in a numb, painless way that she associated with the numb feeling of her cheek after a local dental anesthetic. She was relieved when informed that there had been no local anesthetic.

She was shown the baby, looked over it carefully, and asked permission to awaken. She had been instructed to be in full rapport with her husband and the obstetrician and to do things as needed to meet the situation. Hence, inexperienced in the situation, she carefully met the need of abiding by the situation by making sure it was in order to awaken. She again looked the baby over. Then, upon telling her husband that she had full memory of the entire experience and that everything had occurred exactly as she desired, she suddenly declared that she was sleepy. Before she left the delivery room, she was sound asleep, and slept for one and a half hours. Her stay in the hospital was most happy.

Two years later she announced to the senior author she was having another baby, and asked that she be given a "refresher course, just to make certain." One session of about three hours in the deep trance sufficed to meet her needs. Much of this time was used to secure an adequate account of her adjustments. They were found to be excellent in all regards.

REFERENCES

Barron, F. *Creative person and creative process*. New York: Holt, Rinehart & Winston, 1969.

Bartlett, F. *Thinking: An experimental and social study*. New York: Basic Books, 1958.

Bass, M. Differentiation of the hypnotic trance from normal sleep. *Journal of Experimental Psychology*, 1931, *14*, 382–399.

Beck, F. Hypnotic identification of an amnesia victim. *British Journal of Medical Psychology*, 1936, *16*, 36–42.

Brennan, M. Dreams in hypnosis. *Psychoanalytic Quarterly*, 1949, *18*, 455.

Brickner, R., & Kubie, L. A miniature psychotic storm produced by a superego conflict over simple posthypnotic suggestion. *Psychoanalytic Quarterly*, 1936, *5*, 467–487.

Carkhuff, R., & Berenson, B. *Beyond counseling and therapy*. New York: Holt, Rinehart & Winston, 1967.

Chapel, J., Brown, N., & Jenkins, R. Tourette's disease: symptomatic relief with haloperidol. *American Journal of Psychiatry*, 1964, *121*, 608–610.

Conn, J. Hypnosynthesis. *American Journal of Clinical Hypnosis*, 1971, *13*, 208–221.

Cooper, L., & Erickson, M. *Time distortion in hypnosis*. Baltimore: Williams & Wilkins, 1954.

Cushing, M. The psychoanalytic treatment of a man suffering with ulcerative colitis. *Journal of the American Psychoanalytic Association*, 1953, *1*, 510.

Eisenberg, L., Ascher, E., & Kanner, L. A clinical study of Gilles de la Tourette's disease (maladie des tics) in children. *American Journal of Psychiatry*, 1959, *115*, 715–723.

Erickson, M. Possible detrimental effects of experimental hypnosis. *Journal of Abnormal Psychology*, 1932, *27*, 321.

Erickson, M. The investigation of a specific amnesia. *British Journal of Medical Psychology*, 1933, *13*, 143–150.

Erickson, M. A brief survey of hypnotism. *Medical Record*, 1934, *140*, 609–613.

Erickson, M. A study of an experimental neurosis hypnotically induced in a case of ejaculatio praecox. *British Journal of Medical Psychology*, 1935, *15*, 34–50.

Erickson, M. The development of apparent unconsciousness during hypnotic reliving of a traumatic experience. *Archives of Neurology and Psychiatry.* 1937, *38,* 1282–1288. (a)

Erickson, M. The experimental demonstration of unconscious mentation by automatic writing. *Psychoanalytic Quarterly,* 1937, *6,* 513–529. (b)

Erickson, M. A study of clinical and experimental findings on hypnotic deafness: I. Clinical experimentation and findings. *Journal of General Psychology,* 1938, *19,* 127–150. (a)

Erickson, M. A study of clinical and experimental findings on hypnotic deafness: II. Experimental findings with a conditioned response technique. *Journal of General Psychology,* 1938, *19,* 151–167. (b)

Erickson, M. An experimental investigation of the possible anti-social use of hypnosis. *Psychiatry,* 1939, *2,* 391–414. (a)

Erickson, M. An experimental study of age regression. Address delivered before The American Psychiatric Association in Chicago, 1939. (b)

Erickson, M. Experimental demonstrations of the psychopathology of everyday life. *Psychoanalytic Quarterly,* 1939, *8,* 338–353. (c)

Erickson, M. The induction of color blindness by hypnotic suggestion. *Journal of General Psychology,* 1939, *20,* 61–89. (d)

Erickson, M. Experimentally elicited salivary and related responses to hypnotic visual hallucinations confirmed by personality reactions. *Psychosomatic Medicine,* 1943, *5,* 185–187. (a)

Erickson, M. Hypnotic investigation of psychosomatic phenomena: A controlled experimental use of hypnotic regression in the therapy of an acquired food intolerance. *Psychosomatic Medicine,* 1943, *5,* 67–70. (b)

Erickson, M. Hypnotic investigation of psychosomatic phenomena: Psychosomatic interrelationships studied by experimental hypnosis. *Psychosomatic Medicine,* 1943, *5,* 51–58. (c)

Erickson, M. Hypnotic investigation of psychosomatic phenomena: The development of aphasia-like reactions from hypnotically induced amnesias. *Psychosomatic Medicine,* 1943, *5,* 59–66. (d)

Erickson, M. Hypnotic psychotherapy. *The Medical Clinics of North America.* May, 1948, New York number, 571–583.

Erickson, M. Special techniques of brief hypnotherapy. *Journal of Clinical and Experimental Hypnosis,* 1954, *2,* 109–129.

Erickson, M. An application of implications of Lashley's researches in a circumscribed arteriosclerotic brain condition. *Perceptual and Motor Skills,* 1963, *16,* 779–780.

Erickson, M. Pantomime techniques in hypnosis and the implications. *American Journal of Clinical Hypnosis,* 1964, *7,* 64–70.

Erickson, M. A special inquiry with Aldous Huxley into the nature and character of various states of consciousness. *American Journal of Clinical Hypnosis,* 1965, *8,* 14-33.

Erickson, M. Deep hypnosis and its induction. In J. Haley (Ed.),

Advanced techiques of hypnosis and therapy: Selected papers of Milton H. Erickson, M.D. New York: Grune & Stratton, 1967. (a)

Erickson, M. Pseudo-orientation in time as a hypnotherapeutic procedure. In J. Haley (Ed.), *Advanced techniques of hypnosis and therapy: Selected papers of Milton H. Erickson, M.D.* New York: Grune & Stratton, 1967. (b)

Erickson, M., & Brickner, R. Hypnotic investigation of psychosomatic phenomena: The development of aphasia-like reactions from hypnotically induced amnesias. *Psychosomatic Medicine*, 1943, *5*, 59–66.

Erickson, M., & Erickson, E. The hypnotic induction of hallucinatory color vision. *Journal of Experimental Psychology*, 1938, *22*, 581–588.

Erickson, M., & Erickson, E. Concerning the nature and character of posthypnotic behavior. *Journal of General Psychology*, 1941, *24*, 95–133.

Erickson, M., & Hill, L. Unconscious mental activity in hypnosis—psychoanalytic implications. *Psychoanalytic Quarterly*, 1944, *13*(1), 60–78.

Erickson, M., & Kubie, L. The use of automatic drawing in the interpretation and relief of a state of acute obsessional depression. *Psychoanalytic Quarterly*, 1938, *7*(4), 443–466.

Erickson, M., & Kubie, L. The permanent relief of an obsessional phobia by means of communications with an unsuspected dual personality. *Psychoanalytic Quarterly*, 1939, *8*(4), 471–509.

Erickson, M., & Kubie, L. The translation of the cryptic automatic writing of one hypnotic subject by another in a trance-like dissociated state. *Psychoanalytic Quarterly*, 1940, *10*(1), 51–63.

Erickson, M., & Kubie, L. The successful treatment of a case of acute hysterical depression by a return under hypnosis to a critical phase of childhood. *Psychoanalytic Quarterly*, 1941, *10*, 583–609.

Erickson, M., & Rossi, E. *Hypnotherapy: An exploratory casebook.* New York: Irvington Publishers, 1979.

Erickson, M., Rossi, E., & Rossi, S. *Hypnotic realities.* New York: Irvington Publishers, 1976.

Evans-Wentz, W. *The Tibetian book of the dead.* New York: Oxford University Press, 1960.

Farber, L., & Fisher, C. An experimental approach to dream psychology through the use of hypnosis. *Psychoanalytic Quarterly*, 1943, *2*, 202–216.

Ferenczi, S. Psychoanalytic observations on tic. In S. Ferenczi, *Further contributions to the theory and technique of psychoanalysis.* London: Hogarth Press, 1950.

Fisher, C. Hypnosis in treatment of neuroses due to war and to other causes. *War Medicine*, 1943, *4*, 565–576.

Fisher, C. Studies on the nature of suggestion: Experimental induction of dreams by direct suggestion. *Journal of the American Psychoanalytic Association*, 1953, *1*, 222.

From-Reichmann, F. *Principles of intensive psychotherapy.* Chicago: University of Chicago Press, 1950.

Gaito, J. (Ed.) *Macromolecules and behavior.* (2nd ed.) New York: Appleton-Century Crofts, 1972.

Garnett, R., Jr. & Elberlik, K. Torticollis: Its dymanics and therapy. *Southern Medical Journal*, 1954, *47*.

Gerard, M. The psychogenic tic in eye development. In A. Freud et al. (Eds.), *Psychoanalytic study of the child.* Vol. 2. New York: International University Press, 1946.

Gill, M. Psychotherapy and hypnosis. Unpublished article.

Gill, M., & Brenman, M. Treatment of a case of anxiety hysteria by a hypnotic technique employing psychoanalytic principles. *Bulletin of the Menninger Clinic*, 1943, *7*, 163–171.

Haley, J. *Uncommon therapy: The psychiatric techniques of Milton H. Erickson, M.D.* New York: Norton, 1973.

Harriman, P. A note on "An experimental investigation of the possible anti-social use of hypnosis." *Psychiatry*, 1941, *4*, 187–188.

Harriman, P. Hypnotic induction of color vision anomalies: I. The use of the Ishihara and the Jensen tests to verify the acceptance of color blindness. *Journal of General Psychology*, 1942, *26*, 289–298. (a)

Harriman, P. Hypnotic induction of color vision anomalies: II. Results on two other tests of color blindness. *Journal of General Psychology*, 1942b, *27*, 81–92.

Hebb, D. The semi-autonomous process, its nature and nurture. *American Psychologist*, 1963, *18*, 16–27.

Huston, P., Shakow, D., & Erickson, M. A study of hypnotically induced complexes by means of the Luria technique. *Journal of General Psychology*, 1934, *11*, 65–97.

Jung, C. *Psychology and alchemy.* Princeton: Princeton University Press, 1953.

Jung, C. On the discourses of the Buddha. In *The symbolic life: Miscellaneous writings.* Vol. 18. *The Collected Works of C. G. Jung.* Bollingen Series XX, Princeton: Princeton University Press, 1976.

Klein, M. A contribution to the psychogenesis of tics. In *Contribution to psychoanalysis,* International Psychology Library, No. 34. London: Hogarth Press, 1948.

Kuhn, T. *The structure of scientific revolutions.* (2nd ed.) Chicago: University of Chicago Press, 1970.

Liebman, M. Traumatic amnesia during hypnosis. *Journal of Abnormal and Social Psychology*, 1941, *36*, 103–105.

Luria, A. *The nature of human conflicts*. Trans. W. H. Gantt. New York: Liveright, 1932.

MacAlpine, I. The development of the transference. *Psychoanalytic Quarterly*, 1950, *19*, 501.

Nunberg, H. Transference and reality. *International Journal of Psychoanalysis*, 1951, *32*, 1.

Osgood, C., Suci, J., & Tannenbaum, P. *The measurement of meaning*. Urbana, see: University of Illinois Press, 1957.

Platonow, K. Experimental age regression. *Journal of Experimental Psychology*, 1933, *9*, 190–210.

Raeder, O. Hypnosis and allied forms of suggestion in practical psychotherapy. *American Journal of Psychiatry*, 1933, *13*, 69–76.

Rosen, H. Discussion of Seitz' article "Symbolism and organic choice in conversion reactions: II. Further hypnotic experiments in symptom substitution." *Psychosomatic Medicine*, 1953, *15*, 422. (a)

Rosen, H. *Hypnotherapy in clinical psychiatry*. New York: Julian Press, 1953. (b)

Rosen, H. The dangerous effects of hypnosis (when utilized by unskilled, inept, untrained or emotionally sick hypnotists). Paper read at the Fourth Annual Meeting of the Society for Clinical and Experimental Hypnosis, September 26, 1953. (c)

Rosen, J. *Direct analysis*. New York: Grune & Stratton, 1953.

Rossi, E. Growth, change and transformation in dreams. *Journal of Humanistic Psychology*, 1971, *11*, 147-169.

Rossi, E. *Dreams and the growth of personality*. New York: Pergamon Press, 1972. (a)

Rossi, E. Self reflection in dreams. *Psychotherapy*, 1972, *9*, 290–298. (b)

Rossi, E. Dreams in the creation of personality. *Psychological perspectives*, 1972, *3*, 122–134. (c)

Rossi, E. The dream-protein hypothesis. *American Journal in Psychiatry*, 1973, *130*, 1094-1097. (a)

Rossi, E. Psychological shocks and creative moments in psychotherapy. *American Journal of Clinical Hypnosis*, 1973, *16*, 9-22. (b)

Rossi, E. Psychosynthesis and the new biology of dreams and psychotherapy. *American Journal of Psychotherapy*, 1973, *27*, 34-41. (c)

Sears, R. An experimental study of hypnotic anesthesia. *Journal of Experimental Psychology*, 1932, *15*, 1–22.

Seitz, P. Symbolism and organic choice in conversion reactions: II. Further hypnotic experiments in symptom substitution. *Psychosomatic Medicine*, 1953, *15*, 422.

Tart, C. (Ed.) *Altered states of consciousness*. New York: Wiley, 1969.

Vogel, V. Treatment of stuttering by suggestion under hypnotism. *The Hospital News*, U.S. Public Health Service, Vol. 1, No. 6, 1934.

Watzlawick, P. *The language of change: Elements of therapeutic communication*. New York: Basic Books, 1978.

Weisman, A. Nature and treatment of tics in adults. *Archives of Neurology and Psychiatry*, 1952, *68*, 444.

White, R. A preface to the theory of hypnotism. *Journal of Abnormal and Social Psychology*, 1941, *36*, 477–505.

Whitehorn, J., & Zilboorg, G. Present trends in American psychiatric research. *American Journal of Psychiatry*, 1933, *13*, 303–312.

Williams, G. Comparative study of voluntary and hypnotic catalepsy. *American Journal of Psychology*, 1930, *42*, 83–95.

Wolberg, L. *Hypnoanalysis*. New York: Grune & Stratton, 1945.

Wolberg, L. Discussion of Rosen, H., "The hypnotic and hypnotherapeutic control of severe pain." *American Journal of Psychiatry*, 1951, *107*, 917–925.

SUBJECT INDEX

[Page numbers in **bold face** type are major references.]

NAME INDEX